Introduction to the Pharmaceutical Sciences

An Integrated Approach

SECOND EDITION

Nita K. Pandit, B.S. Pharm, PhD

Professor of Pharmaceutics
College of Pharmacy and Health Sciences
Drake University
Des Moines, Iowa

Robert Soltis, B.S. Pharm, PhD

Professor of Pharmacology
College of Pharmacy and Health Sciences
Drake University
Des Moines, Iowa

 Wolters Kluwer | Lippincott Williams & Wilkins
Health

Philadelphia · Baltimore · New York · London
Buenos Aires · Hong Kong · Sydney · Tokyo

Acquisitions Editor: David B. Troy
Product Manager: Sofia De Jesus/Meredith Brittain
Senior Marketing Manager: Joy Fisher-Williams
Designer: Teresa Mallon
Compositor: Aptara, Inc.

Second Edition

351 West Camden Street   Two Commerce Square
Baltimore, MD 21201   2001 Market Street
                                Philadelphia, PA 19103

Printed in China

Library of Congress Cataloging-in-Publication Data

Pandit, Nita K.
  Introduction to the pharmaceutical sciences : an integrated approach /
Nita K. Pandit, Robert Soltis. – 2nd ed.
    p. ; cm.
  Includes bibliographical references and index.
  ISBN 978-1-60913-001-5
  1. Pharmacology. 2. Pharmacokinetics. I. Soltis, Robert P., 1964-
II. Title.
  [DNLM: 1. Pharmacokinetics. 2. Pharmacology. QV 38]
  RM300.P26 2011
  615.7–dc23

                                        2011025428

DISCLAIMER

Care has been taken to confirm the accuracy of the information present and to describe generally accepted practices. However, the authors, editors, and publisher are not responsible for errors or omissions or for any consequences from application of the information in this book and make no warranty, expressed or implied, with respect to the currency, completeness, or accuracy of the contents of the publication. Application of this information in a particular situation remains the professional responsibility of the practitioner; the clinical treatments described and recommended may not be considered absolute and universal recommendations.

The authors, editors, and publisher have exerted every effort to ensure that drug selection and dosage set forth in this text are in accordance with the current recommendations and practice at the time of publication. However, in view of ongoing research, changes in government regulations, and the constant flow of information relating to drug therapy and drug reactions, the reader is urged to check the package insert for each drug for any change in indications and dosage and for added warnings and precautions. This is particularly important when the recommended agent is a new or infrequently employed drug.

Some drugs and medical devices presented in this publication have Food and Drug Administration (FDA) clearance for limited use in restricted research settings. It is the responsibility of the health care provider to ascertain the FDA status of each drug or device planned for use in their clinical practice.

To purchase additional copies of this book, call our customer service department at (800) 638-3030 or fax orders to (301) 223-2320. International customers should call (301) 223-2300.

Visit Lippincott Williams & Wilkins on the Internet: http://www.lww.com. Lippincott Williams & Wilkins customer service representatives are available from 8:30 am to 6:00 pm, EST.

9 8 7 6 5 4 3 2 1

Think simple as my old master used to say, meaning reduce the whole of its parts to the simplest terms, getting back to first principles.　　　　　　　　　　*—Frank Lloyd Wright*

This is the second edition of *Introduction to the Pharmaceutical Sciences;* the first edition was published in 2007. Many improvements have been made in the second edition, the most important being the addition of a distinguished coauthor, Dr. Robert Soltis, a Drake colleague who team-teaches the *Introduction to the Pharmaceutical Sciences* course with me. His expertise in pharmacology has greatly improved many chapters in the book.

The philosophy of the second edition remains unchanged. It is an introductory book that provides a simple, integrated, and coherent overview of pharmaceutical science concepts for the beginner or nonspecialist. We introduce and explain fundamental principles that underlie all pharmaceutical science disciplines, reveal the connections between them, and point to their pharmaceutical and therapeutic applications.

The integration of various disciplines is particularly important to us and is reflected in the new subtitle "An Integrated Approach." Pharmacists must be able to integrate their knowledge of the pharmaceutical and clinical sciences to solve drug therapy problems. Pharmaceutical scientists in drug discovery and development must have a broad understanding of the field as they participate in interdisciplinary project teams.

The target audiences are first-year pharmacy students, junior-level science undergraduates, and other scientists new to the pharmaceutical field. We assume that readers have at least 2 years of college-level science and mathematics, with a basic background in general chemistry, organic chemistry, biology, and algebra. Some knowledge of introductory biochemistry and calculus is helpful but not required. Physiological concepts are introduced as needed.

In our experience, students who understand the language of the pharmaceutical sciences, the key concepts, and links between these concepts are better able to appreciate more advanced material in specialized courses that come later. They are less likely to treat each discipline as a silo and often find connections that faculty miss!

The text could be used for a one-semester or a full-year course, depending on the desired depth of coverage. All topics may not be necessary for a one-semester course; selection of material could depend on the course objectives and subsequent curriculum. A full-year course may use the entire book with detailed discussion and additional readings as desired. For a pharmacy student, an understanding of the basic concepts in this book will be followed by courses in pharmacology, pharmaceutics, pharmacokinetics, and medicinal chemistry. For graduate students, this book will provide a broad context in which to study and investigate problems in their chosen pharmaceutical specialty. Although this book is written as a text, it will be valuable to scientists new to the pharmaceutical industry who need a simple overview of the pharmaceutical sciences.

It is important to state what this book is not intended to be. It is not meant to be an encyclopedia of the pharmaceutical sciences, a "how-to" book for laboratory researchers, or a book for the specialist in one of the pharmaceutical science disciplines. Because we wish to emphasize common concepts underlying this field, discussion of special topics and details of any one discipline are generally limited. There are several other courses and excellent books that fill these needs, and suggestions are provided at the end of each chapter.

We continue to aim for simplicity, clarity, and brevity so that students will actually read the book. Historical development of theories and hypotheses has been omitted. To provide coherence and readability, material is not referenced to primary literature; however, every attempt has been made to ensure that statements reflect generally accepted scientific views. Need-to-know concepts are emphasized; nice-to-know content and material that will be taught later in pharmacy curricula or that is not directly relevant have been minimized.

Features

Every chapter has received critical attention and has been updated. A couple of chapters were eliminated, while others were combined to improve the flow. Like the first edition, each chapter builds on previous material, so we recommend that the sequence in the book be followed for best outcomes.

Practice Problems

Practice problems have been added to more chapters, if appropriate. These elements help students to work with material discussed and to develop their quantitative and problem-solving skills. Solutions are provided only to the instructor to retain control over how to use the problems (homework, in-class discussion) and when and how to reveal solutions

to students. We hope that this feature enhances student learning and problem-solving abilities.

Cases

Cases at the end of many chapters are an important new addition to the second edition. Cases are multifaceted and realistic scenarios that teach students to apply their knowledge to solve problems. Some background information is provided, and students are led through a series of increasingly complex questions. Clinical application of basic pharmaceutical science concepts is introduced wherever appropriate. Cases in early chapters are fairly short and increase in complexity through the book, requiring students to integrate knowledge from preceding chapters. Instructors will be provided with detailed answers and suggestions on ways to expand the case discussions.

Key Concepts and Review Questions

Key Concepts are summarized at the end of each chapter so that readers know what they should have learned from a particular chapter. A list of Review Questions is provided at the end of each chapter. These broad questions test understanding of the concepts rather than the details.

Additional Reading

All chapters include a list of Additional Reading at the end to which a reader can turn for further information on a topic.

We hope that this text will make it easier for faculty to develop and teach a truly integrated course in the pharmaceutical sciences. We would also like to see this book used in other degree programs so that students in chemistry, biology, or premedical programs can appreciate the applications of pharmaceutical sciences and see this field as a career opportunity. Lastly, we want to emphasize that this book continues to be a "work in progress"; feedback from readers is always welcome.

Resources for Instructors

Approved adopting instructors will be given access to the following additional resources:

- Answers to practice problems
- Answers to case study questions in the text
- Additional integrated case studies not included in the text

In addition, purchasers of the text can access the searchable Full Text Online by going to the *Introduction to Pharmaceutical Sciences,* second edition Web site at https://thepoint.lww.com/Pandit2e. See the inside front cover of this text for more details, including the passcode you will need to gain access to the site.

Nita K. Pandit, PhD
Robert Soltis, PhD

ACKNOWLEDGMENTS

As with any book, this text has benefited from contributions of many people. Students at Drake have been our primary audience, and we thank them for their suggestions in shaping the second edition. We are also grateful to our colleagues at the Drake University College of Pharmacy for their support and encouragement in this endeavor.

The second edition has also improved as a result of feedback from our audiences outside Drake. Their input has been valuable in making the book suitable not just to the needs of Drake students but to students, teachers, and readers elsewhere.

We particularly thank the wonderful people at Lippincott Williams & Wilkins, whose enthusiasm, commitment, professionalism, and patience made this a rewarding undertaking.

CONTENTS

Preface iii
Acknowledgments vi

  1. Introduction 1

Part I: Drug Chemistry   7

  2. Drugs and Their Targets. 8
  3. Ionization of Drugs 26
  4. Solubility and Lipophilicity 42

Part II: Drug Delivery   58

  5. Transport Across Biological Barriers 59
  6. Drug Absorption 89
  7. Drug Delivery Systems 105

Part III: Drug Disposition   119

  8. Drug Distribution. 120
  9. Drug Excretion 138
  10. Drug Metabolism 155
  11. Pharmacokinetic Concepts 183

Part IV: Drug Action   200

  12. Ligands and Receptors. 201
  13. Mechanisms of Drug Action 226
  14. Dose–Response Relationships 246

Part V: Drug Therapy   262

  15. Therapeutic Variability. 263
  16. Drug Interactions. 278
  17. Pharmacogenomics. 294

Part VI: Special Topics   313

  18. Biopharmaceutical Drugs. 314
  19. Drug Discovery and Approval 340

Index 355

CHAPTER 1

Introduction

The pharmaceutical sciences are a group of interdisciplinary areas of study that deal with the design, action, delivery, disposition, and use of drugs. This field draws on many areas of the basic and applied sciences, such as chemistry (organic, physical, and analytical), biology (anatomy and physiology, biochemistry, molecular and cell biology), mathematics, physics, and chemical engineering, and applies their principles to the study of drugs.

The pharmaceutical sciences may be further subdivided into several specialties, for example:

- Pharmacology: study of the biochemical and physiological effects of drugs on organisms.
- Pharmacodynamics: study of the cellular and molecular interactions of drugs with their targets.
- Pharmaceutical toxicology: study of the harmful or toxic effects of drugs.
- Pharmacokinetics: study of factors that control the concentration–time relationship of drug at various sites in the body.
- Medicinal chemistry: study of drug design to optimize pharmacokinetics and pharmacodynamics, and synthesis of new drugs.

- Pharmaceutics: study and design of drug formulation for optimum delivery, stability, pharmacokinetics, and patient acceptance.
- Pharmacogenomics: study of the influence of genetic variation on drug response in patients.

As new discoveries advance and extend the pharmaceutical sciences, subspecialties continue to be added to this list. At the same time, boundaries between these specialty areas of pharmaceutical sciences are beginning to blur. Many fundamental concepts are common to all pharmaceutical sciences. In this book, we will focus on these shared concepts to understand their applicability to all aspects of pharmaceutical research and drug therapy.

What Is a Drug?

Broadly, a drug is any substance used in the diagnosis, treatment, or prevention of a disease. It may be a synthetic, semi-synthetic, or naturally occurring compound or mixture of compounds. Most drugs interact with a part of the body to alter an existing physiological or biochemical process. A drug can either decrease or increase an existing function of an organ, tissue, or

1

cell, but cannot impart a new function to them. For example, drugs are available to decrease blood pressure, decrease acid formation in the stomach, increase urine production, and increase bone density. Some therapies, such as vaccines and gene therapy, are not drugs in the traditional sense but are also used in management of diseases.

An ideal drug is one that:

- Has a desirable pharmacological action
- Has no side effects
- Reaches its intended location in the right concentration at the right time
- Remains at the site of action for the necessary period of time
- Is rapidly and completely removed from the body when no longer needed.

All these goals cannot be achieved fully when developing a new drug, but need to be considered and optimized during the research and development process. The success of a new drug depends on how close it comes to meeting these objectives.

How Do Drugs Work?

The site of action of a drug is the location in the body where the drug performs its desired function. For example, a drug may act in the brain, heart, eye, or kidney. Within the organ, the drug may act on a particular component of the organ, such as a certain type of cell. Drug action may be extracellular, where the drug performs its function outside the cell, or intracellular, in which case the drug has to enter the cell to work. Alternatively, the action may be on the cell surface, at the cell membrane.

Drugs work by interacting with target molecules found at the site of action, and altering their activity in a way that is beneficial to health. Drug targets are usually biomolecules such as proteins, protein complexes, or nucleic acids that play a role in a particular disease process. In most cases, the drug must temporarily attach

(*bind*) to the target to exert its action. The drug–target binding can either stimulate the target or block the normal activity of the target, resulting in a physiological effect. A common type of drug target is a receptor, generally a protein on the cell membrane, that can bind with a specific molecule (such as an endogenous compound or a drug) to alter the cell's behavior. The interactions between a drug and its receptor and succeeding events that lead to pharmacological action of the drug are broadly considered the field of pharmacodynamics.

A simple analogy often used to describe drug–target interactions is that of a *lock and key*—the target is a lock on a door that only a certain drug (the key) can bind to and open, this is illustrated in Figure 1.1. Ideally, the key should not fit any other lock, and different keys should not open this lock. Some keys may fit in the lock, but not perfectly. Consequently, these imperfect keys cannot open the door. Yet, by fitting into the lock, imperfect keys prevent the original key from fitting into the lock; they therefore block the door from opening.

Using this analogy, the target is a molecular lock that contains a "keyhole" with a very specific and consistent size and shape. This molecular keyhole is termed the active site of the target and can interact with only molecular keys of a complementary size,

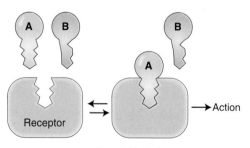

Drug **A** binds to receptor
Drug **B** cannot bind to receptor

Figure 1.1. A simplified diagram illustrating drug–receptor binding. Drug A has a structure that is complementary to the receptor and therefore can bind to it. The structure of Drug B is not compatible with the receptor, and thus no binding occurs.

shape, and charge. The three-dimensional shape of the drug molecule must fit exactly into the structure of the target to activate it. Therefore, just like locks and their keys, the interactions between drugs and their targets are highly specific.

In reality, most targets are not as rigid as locks and the active site can somewhat change its shape and size depending on the environment. Most drugs, also, are not as specific as a key. Thus target–drug interactions are much more complex than the simple lock-and-key analogy leads us to believe. Few drugs interact exclusively with their intended target. Many drugs bind to more than one type of target and influence physiological or biochemical processes that were not targeted. This leads to undesirable side effects of drugs, or toxicity.

How Are Drugs Designed?

Drug design is the process of finding new drugs based on the understanding of the disease and the structure and function of a biological target molecule involved in the disease. Once these are known, chemical compounds are synthesized with structures that allow them to bind to and alter the behavior of the target. The structures of these compounds are progressively refined, often using computer-modeling, to fit even better with the target. In addition to being able to bind to the target, a drug must be able to pass through barriers our body puts in its path. It must be able to adequately withstand the body's protective mechanisms that reject or decompose it. Ultimately, the body should be able to eliminate and remove the drug. This systematic approach to new drug discovery is called rational drug design.

In the past, most drugs were discovered through a search of natural sources such as plants and microorganisms, or by the synthesis of an extensive number of compounds of varying structures. These synthetic or natural compounds were then tested for various kinds of biological activities in the laboratory. This type of trial-and-error approach, called random screening, resulted in the discovery and development of many important drugs. It still has a place in drug discovery and is often used by pharmaceutical companies to identify *lead compounds*. These lead compounds are then synthetically modified to give new compounds with improved properties.

Most drugs are small organic molecules produced through chemical synthesis, but biopharmaceutical drugs (also known as *biologics*) produced through biological processes are becoming increasingly more common.

How Are Drugs Administered?

A drug can exert its intended action only after reaching its intended target at the site of action. This means a drug that acts on the heart must reach appropriate target biomolecules in the heart, and a drug that acts on the brain must reach its targets in the brain. It is often inconvenient or impossible to apply a drug directly at its site of action; instead, drugs must be given at an administration site far removed from the site of action. For accuracy and convenience of dosing, the drug is almost always incorporated into a dosage form or drug delivery system (such as tablets, patches, inhalers). Delivery systems can also be designed to provide *controlled* or *sustained* release of the drug.

The method and form of administration must consider the body's protective barriers, the drug's physical and chemical properties, clinical need, and patient acceptance. Most drugs are given orally because patients prefer this administration method. After oral dosing, the drug must be released from the delivery system and enter the bloodstream (a process called absorption) so that it can reach the site of action. Another common but less convenient administration route is by injection, which is usually reserved for drugs that cannot be absorbed orally, or in

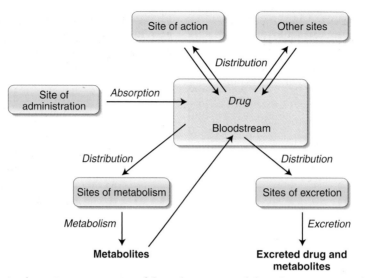

Figure 1.2. A schematic representation of drug absorption and drug disposition processes that follow drug administration.

situations where a patient cannot take an oral medication.

How Are Drugs Transported in the Body?

The term drug disposition refers to distribution, metabolism, and elimination of drugs after entering the bloodstream. After absorption, circulating blood carries the drug throughout the body in a process called distribution. How much drug reaches each tissue, and how long it remains in the tissue, depends on the properties of each drug and of the tissue.

After the drug has carried out its intended action, the body must be able to inactivate and eliminate the drug by normal physiological processes. Enzymes in the body break down drugs (by a process called metabolism or biotransformation) and convert them into inactive products. Drugs and their breakdown products are removed from the body in waste fluids such as urine (by a process termed excretion). The acronym ADME (using the first letters from the words absorption, distribution, metabolism, and excretion)

describes the absorption and disposition behavior of a drug in the body. Figure 1.2 shows a simple representation of these processes.

How Are Drugs Used Clinically in Patients?

The study of the therapeutic uses and effects of drugs in patients is called pharmacotherapeutics. The focus of pharmacotherapy is the patient, not the drug or the disease. Drugs do not behave in the same way in all individuals, and patient-to-patient variability in drug response is very common. Therapeutic variability may be caused by differences in patient body size and composition, age, disease, environmental factors, and genetic influences. It may also be attributable to drug interactions that result from two drugs competing for the same mechanisms during a pharmacodynamic or an ADME process. A thorough understanding of pharmaceutical sciences is essential in providing appropriate pharmacotherapy, and in anticipating and avoiding drug interactions.

How Do Genetic Factors Affect Drug Therapy?

An important challenge for pharmaceutical and clinical sciences is to understand why individuals respond differently to drug therapy, and then to design drugs considering this variability. The field of pharmacogenomics promises to illuminate many difficult questions about the nature of disease and drug therapy that have been unanswerable so far. It is the study of how genetic inheritance affects an individual's response to drugs. Greater knowledge of genes and their proteins will help pharmaceutical scientists to understand the cause of disease and design better drugs. Many pharmaceutical companies are now taking a pharmacogenomic approach in drug research to come up with drugs that have consistent and predictable behavior in defined patient populations. Knowledge of genes and proteins and of their functions will also allow scientists to "fix" a genetic defect and cure diseases as an alternative to drug treatment.

How Are New Drugs Developed and Approved for Marketing?

The U.S. Food and Drug Administration (FDA) is the government agency that regulates marketed drug products and approves marketing of new drug products. The FDA defines a drug product as a finished dosage form (e.g., tablet, capsule, or solution) that contains the drug (called the drug substance or active ingredient) in a particular strength, generally in association with one or more other ingredients. The FDA considers the different strengths and dosage forms of a drug as separate and distinct drug products.

The process of new drug development and discovery is long, complex, and risky. Typically, it takes an average of 10 years for a drug to make it to pharmacy shelves after its first discovery. The major steps in this discovery, development, and approval process are summarized in Figure 1.3.

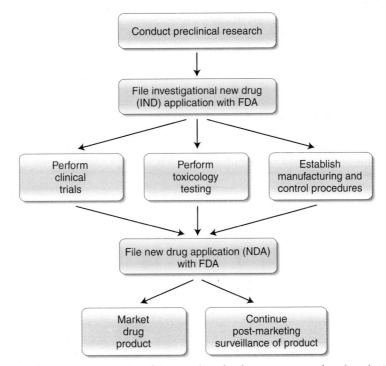

Figure 1.3. A schematic representation of the new drug development, approval, and marketing process.

Concluding Remarks

The pharmaceutical sciences comprise a broad range of interconnected disciplines whose main goal is to design safe and effective drug products for patients based on an understanding of drug action and disposition.

In this book, we will gain an understanding of the fundamental concepts of the pharmaceutical sciences. Early chapters will lay out the first principles, derived from the basic sciences, on which the pharmaceutical sciences are founded. A thorough knowledge of these principles will set the groundwork for the remainder of the book. Subsequent chapters will examine the application of these principles to drug delivery, drug disposition, and drug action, and finally to pharmacotherapy and new drug development, using an interdisciplinary and integrated approach.

Drug Chemistry

If you want to understand function, study structure
—Francis Crick

Chapter 2   Drugs and Their Targets

Chapter 3   Ionization of Drugs

Chapter 4   Solubility and Lipophilicity

Drugs and Their Targets

In the overview presented in Chapter 1, a drug was broadly defined as any substance used in the diagnosis, treatment, or prevention of a disease. In this chapter, we will consider the actions of drugs from the perspective of the drug as a chemical or molecule. In order for a drug to produce its beneficial effects, it must accomplish two major tasks: (1) travel to its site of action and (2) interact with its target which is often another molecule found in the body. The chemistry of these molecules dictates how well the drug achieves these steps and subsequently how effective it will be. At times, the characteristics of the molecule needed to accomplish both actions are in opposition to one another.

When a drug is administered, it will encounter many biological systems that represent barriers and potential targets.

- Anatomical barriers—membranes that prevent passage of the drug from its site of administration to its intended site of action.
- Chemical barriers—bodily fluids whose pH and aqueous content vary and may affect the solubility and ionization of the drug.
- Biochemical barriers and targets—transporters, enzymes, and receptors that bind the drug resulting in movement of

the drug into or out of a cell, destruction of the drug or production of a target response or unintended response.

In order to get a drug to work optimally, that is, get to its site of action and interact with its target without unintended effects, the structure of the drug molecule may need to be altered so that it can get past barriers or act appropriately at the target. The structural and chemical properties and how they may influence drug action include the following:

- Physicochemical properties such as solubility, partition coefficient, and ionization can influence how well the drug is absorbed from the gastrointestinal tract and where it travels in the body.
- Chemical properties such as resonance structure and inductive effects may play a role in the drug's ability to bind to targets and other proteins.
- Stereochemistry takes into account the shape and size of the molecule and can influence how the drug interacts with targets and whether it can produce the appropriate target response.

In the drug discovery process, a balance will often times need to be struck between those characteristics of the molecule that allow the drug to get to its site of action and those characteristics that allow it to produce the desired effect. As a result, most drugs on the market were not initially discovered in their final form but went through a process of experimentation and modification to make the best possible therapeutic agent. The starting point is identification of a substance that possesses the desired target response and then the molecule is altered to address any unfavorable properties such as toxicity, problems with one or more absorption, distribution, metabolism, and excretion (ADME) processes, or an unusually complex or expensive manufacturing process. Therefore, the initial compound may be modified to enhance the desired activity and to eliminate or minimize unwanted properties. The following sections of this chapter will discuss the basics of how a drug produces a desired target response and then examine ways in which the drug can be altered to address potential problems but still retain the desired actions. Chapters 12 and 13 will examine in greater detail the actions of drugs at their targets.

Targets and Biological Activity

Recall the simple analogy of the lock and key presented in Chapter 1; a drug must fit with or into its target in order to produce a target response. This concept is known as complementarity. The drug and the target must have three-dimensional shapes that allow them to fit together in a complementary fashion. The target response then occurs as a result of this binding or interaction between the drug and its target.

The vast majority of drug targets are proteins made by the body. Exceptions include antibiotics and antiviral medications that bind to proteins made by microorganisms. Drugs will bind to a specific site or pocket within the protein to alter the activity of the protein. The function that the protein normally carries

out determines what ultimately happens when the drug binds to it. One of the most important concepts regarding drug action is that a drug cannot create or confer a new biological function. That is, a drug can only increase or decrease the normal function of its target. For example, the pain and inflammation associated with an injury is caused by the synthesis and release of several substances. Ibuprofen (Motrin®), a nonsteroidal anti-inflammatory agent, inhibits the enzyme associated with the synthesis of those substances. The drug is not conferring a new function; it is preventing something from occurring by inhibiting the actions of a target protein. Therefore, to understand the action of drugs, you will first need to understand the actions and functions of proteins.

Proteins—What Are They?

Proteins play a multitude of roles including regulating the activation of genes, relaying signals within and between cells, and driving metabolic processes. Proteins are required for the structure, function, and regulation of the body's cells, tissues, and organs. For cells and tissues to remain healthy they must be able to make proteins, and the proteins they make must be able to function correctly. Changes in the composition or the amount of critical proteins can lead to disease.

Drug–protein interactions play a vital role in almost all aspects of a drug's behavior and function. Many of today's drugs work by fitting into pockets, channels, or pores in proteins. Furthermore, drugs are transported, metabolized, and excreted with the help of proteins. Thus, proteins can be the intended targets for drug actions and drugs can be the targets for certain protein actions.

The structure of a protein can be divided into four levels of complexity: primary, secondary, tertiary, and quaternary (Fig. 2.1). The **primary structure** is represented by the sequence of amino acids that make up the protein. The **secondary structure**

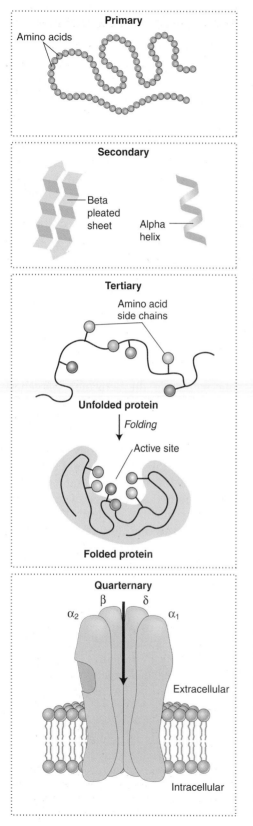

is determined by hydrogen bonding occurring between nearby amino acids to form α-helices and β-sheets. The **tertiary structure** represents a highly organized, three-dimensional shape with a distinct inside and outside. The three-dimensional shape also creates several pockets or **binding sites** (also called active sites) where molecules of appropriate structure may bind. Many proteins self-associate into assemblies composed of two to six individual polypeptide chains or subunits; this represents the **quaternary** structure of proteins. For example, the acetylcholine receptor, a membrane protein of critical importance in skeletal muscle contraction, has five distinct subunits that form a channel in the membrane of the muscle cell for entry of sodium ions. Only one final folded structure of the protein is functional.

In general, drugs act by interacting with four types of regulatory protein targets (Fig. 2.2):

- **Receptor proteins:** Receptors receive and process signals from other cells. An example of a drug that targets receptors is the antiallergy drug cetirizine (Zyrtec®), which interacts with and blocks the histamine H_1 receptor.
- **Ion channel proteins:** Channel proteins control passage of solutes and ions into and out of cells. The local anesthetic procaine (Novocain®) binds to and blocks sodium ion channel

Figure 2.1. An illustration depicting the four levels of protein structure. Note that that the primary and secondary structures do not have a unique binding site. Such a site is created when the protein folds in a specific way or assembles with other protein subunits. Panel D depicts the longitudinal view of the acetylcholine receptor–ion channel complex with one of the five subunits removed. The remaining subunits are shown creating an internal channel. Spans of α-helices with slightly bowed structures form the perimeter of the channel.

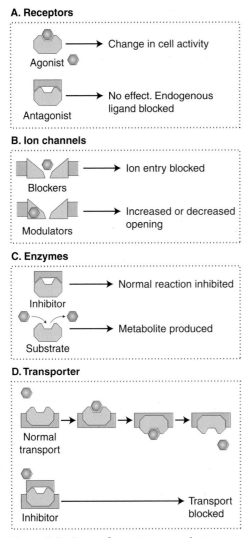

A. Receptors

Agonist → Change in cell activity

Antagonist → No effect. Endogenous ligand blocked

B. Ion channels

Blockers → Ion entry blocked

Modulators → Increased or decreased opening

C. Enzymes

Inhibitor → Normal reaction inhibited

Substrate → Metabolite produced

D. Transporter

Normal transport

Inhibitor → Transport blocked

Figure 2.2. Types of protein targets that can interact with drugs.

proteins to prevent transmission of pain signals.

- Enzymes: Enzymes catalyze biochemical and metabolic reactions. The drug celecoxib (Celebrex®) binds to and inhibits the COX2 (cyclooxygenase 2) enzyme to prevent synthesis of substances associated with pain and inflammation.
- Transporters: Transporters bring materials into and out of a cell. Fluoxetine (Prozac®) inhibits the serotonin transporter in the brain, an effect that triggers a series of changes in cells that ultimately leads to relief of depression.

Protein–Ligand Interactions

The proteins that are typically chosen for drug targets perform their cellular functions by interacting with chemical messenger molecules called ligands. A ligand is an ion or a molecule that binds to the protein to form a complex. This complex ultimately causes a target response. Ligands may be endogenous (already present in the body), or introduced into the body as drugs; examples of endogenous ligands include neurotransmitters and hormones. Most drugs are designed to take the place of endogenous ligands in exerting their action. For example, morphine uses the same receptors in the brain used by endorphins, compounds produced by the body to control pain.

The primary concept behind protein–ligand binding is that of complementarity, or "fit," between the ligand and the active site on the protein. The ligand must fit into a very specific site on the protein in order to produce a response. This matching between a protein and ligand depends not only on their shape but also the attraction between them. Weak, reversible bonds must bring and hold the complex together. Complementary shape and orientation of functional groups allow hydrogen bond donors to line up with acceptors, hydrophobic groups to position with other hydrophobic groups, and positive charges to be adjacent to negative charges (Fig. 2.3).

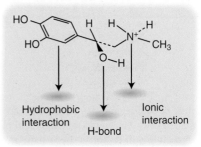

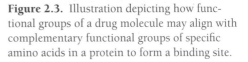

Figure 2.3. Illustration depicting how functional groups of a drug molecule may align with complementary functional groups of specific amino acids in a protein to form a binding site.

Binding to the Target

Given that there are endogenous ligands for many of the targets of interest for drug development, we have a starting point from which to determine the chemical and physical characteristics that a drug must have in order to bind to a target. The pharmacophore represents the simplest structure that will bind to the target. However, most drug molecules are more complex than the pharmacophore because we also need to address the issues associated with overcoming barriers or potential toxicities. The general concept of drug structure has various components (Fig. 2.4). Vector groups play a vital role in directing the drug to its site of action and may also aid in minimizing toxicity but may not be involved in binding to the target. Vector groups may be classified further as carrier groups and vulnerable groups. Carrier groups control ionization and lipophilicity of the molecule and consequently influence absorption, distribution, and excretion of the drug. Vulnerable groups are susceptible to enzymatic action and are responsible for determining the drug's metabolism.

Pharmacophore

The pharmacophore describes the features of the molecule that interact with the target protein or receptor; a change in this portion of the molecule will alter biological activity. The pharmacophore and the target must have physicochemical and stereochemical complementarity. That is, their size, shape and charges must allow them to fit together. Several parts of the molecule can together make up the pharmacophore. As we will see in the following text, altering a portion of the pharmacophore can alter the ability of the drug to bind to a particular receptor or alter the biological response it produces because different targets or receptors have different three-dimensional shapes.

Once the pharmacophore is established, several analogs are synthesized. An analog is a compound with the same or similar pharmacophore as the lead, but with differences in other parts of the molecule. If analogs differ in structure by a simple and constant increase in one part of the molecule (such as the length of an alkyl chain), they are part of a homologous series. The objective of making analogs is to retain pharmacological activity but to minimize or eliminate unwanted properties. Analogs are then tested in the laboratory to select the compound that will proceed to animal testing and ultimately into human clinical trials.

Complementarity

The two types of complementarity for us to consider are physicochemical complementarity, i.e., the presence of several physicochemical bonding interactions between the two molecules, and steric complementarity, i.e., whether the shape of the ligand fits the shape of the active site. Both determine the strength of the type of interaction.

Physicochemical Complementarity

Covalent bonds are not routinely formed between a protein and ligand during normal cellular processes. Therefore, several types of weaker noncovalent bonds

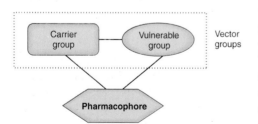

Figure 2.4. Typical components of the general structure of a drug candidate. The pharmacophore is needed for binding to the target and producing a biological response. The vector groups define the physicochemical properties of the molecule; the carrier groups control absorption, distribution, and excretion; vulnerable groups determine metabolism.

are necessary to attract and keep the two molecules together as a complex. In most cases, the initial attraction between the protein and the ligand is provided by a long-range force such as an ionic interaction between opposite charges on the protein binding site and the ligand. As the ligand approaches the protein, short-range forces such as hydrogen bonds provide additional attractive and orienting forces. Finally, van der Waals forces and hydrophobic interactions come into play to further orient and stabilize the complex. Thus, most protein–ligand interactions rely on many different molecular forces to form the final complex. Of the various physicochemical interactions involved in protein–ligand binding, ionic and hydrophobic interactions are probably the most important.

Because the initial interaction between a ligand and protein is often ionic, the ionization state of weak acid and base drugs is very important. Charged atoms (from ionized amino acids) often line the protein active site, imparting a localized charge in specific regions of the pocket. Opposite charges on the active site and ligand will attract each other, beginning the process of forming the complex. *Electrostatic complementarity* is important in preventing inappropriate molecules from binding to the active site, as the ligand must contain correctly placed complementary charged atoms for the interaction to occur.

Another critical force for ligand–protein binding is *hydrophobic interaction*. Nearly two-thirds of the body is water, and this aqueous environment surrounds all our cells. For a ligand and protein to interact, there must be a driving force that compels the ligand to leave water and bind to the protein; hydrophobic portions of the ligand are able to accomplish this. Thus the lipophilicity of the ligand is also an important factor in protein–ligand binding.

Consider the pharmacophore for two distinct proteins, alpha (α)- and beta (β)-

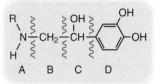

Figure 2.5. Pharmacophore for drugs acting at alpha- and beta-adrenergic receptors.

adrenergic receptors (Fig. 2.5). These receptors are located on several different tissues and organs and each receptor, when activated, produces different effects at these sites. In this example, we have divided the structure of the molecule into four distinct regions labeled A, B, C, and D and will examine how each region plays a role in binding.

Region A—The Amine Function. At physiological pH (7.4), the amine function is predominantly protonated (carries a positive charge) and is capable of forming an ionic bond to a negative site on the target protein. The anionic or negative site on the receptor is a carboxylic acid. Ionic bond formation is absolutely critical for α receptor binding.

Region A—The R Group. As the size of the R group is increased, α receptor binding decreases and there is a corresponding increase in β receptor binding. For example, if R is changed from a hydrogen to an isopropyl group, the overall effect is to change the drug from one that can bind α and β receptors to one that binds only to β receptors. The size of the R group on the amine and the ability of the amine to ionize dictates binding to the α or β receptor. By increasing the size of the R group, hydrophobic binding increases. Hydrophobic binding is most important for β receptor binding and activation, whereas ionic bonding is most important for α receptor binding and activation. Clinically, useful β agonists such as albuterol (Proventil®) will usually have an isopropyl or *t*-butyl group on the amine group.

Region D—The Catechol Function. The catechol group represents another hydrophobic region of the molecule and is attracted to the hydrophobic region of the active or binding site. Removing either of the hydroxyl groups or replacing the phenyl ring with a less hydrophobic group diminishes the ability of the molecule to bind to α and β receptors.

Region B—The α Carbon. Inserting a methyl group at this position will decrease α and β receptor binding and activation. The methyl group produces steric hindrance to ionic bond formation and hydrophobic bonding. That is, the methyl group physically interferes with the ability of the amine to bind to its complementary site on the target or receptor. Also notable is that the presence of this α methyl group produces steric hindrance to the binding of the drug to enzymes in the liver responsible for metabolism and inactivation of this drug.

Steric Complementarity

Although physicochemical complementarity is important for the initial attraction between ligand and protein, the ligand must also have stereochemical complementarity to sustain the ligand–protein complex. This means that the ligand must have a defined three-dimensional shape and size that fits well with the active site. Below is a brief review of the basic concepts of stereochemistry as they pertain to stereochemical complementarity in protein–ligand binding. Undergraduate textbooks in chemistry are good resources for a more thorough discussion of stereochemistry.

Stereoisomers are molecules that have the same molecular formula and sequence of bonds but different spatial arrangements; the only difference between them is the three-dimensional orientation of atoms or functional groups in space. Despite having identical chemical formulas and bonding, stereoisomers can have dramatically different chemical, physical, and biological properties. There are two main types of stereoisomers of interest in understanding stereocomplementarity: enantiomers and geometric isomers.

Enantiomers and Chirality. Chirality is the geometric property of a rigid object (like a molecule or drug) not being superimposable with its mirror image. A molecule that cannot be superimposed on its mirror image is said to be chiral (the Greek word for "handed"). This is in contrast to *achiral* molecules, which can be superimposed on their mirror images.

Chirality is analogous to our right and left hands—they are mirror images but are not superimposable. The two mirror images of a chiral molecule are termed enantiomers. Like hands, enantiomers come in pairs. Chirality usually occurs when a compound contains at least one asymmetric or chiral center in its structure. A chiral center is an atom at which the interchange of any two substituents attached to it creates a new stereoisomer. Various nomenclature systems have been used for enantiomers, the most common ones designate the two forms in the pair as L- and D-, or as R- and S-.

Chirality is a property found in many biologically important molecules such as amino acids, carbohydrates, and lipids. For example, the natural amino acids share a common stereochemistry, they are all L-amino acids. Our bodies use only D-sugars; DNA and RNA are made up of D-sugars, resulting in a right-handed DNA double helix. Consequently, most cellular targets are chiral and can recognize differences between enantiomers of a chiral ligand. Our receptors, such as the taste receptors in our tongue, can distinguish between stereoisomers of a ligand; for example, one isomer of leucine tastes sweet and the other tastes bitter. Chemicals with different enantiomeric forms can smell different also. One isomer of limonene smells of oranges, the other of lemons.

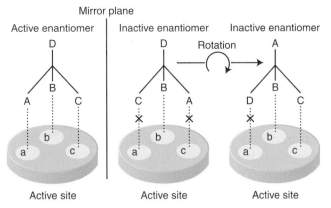

Figure 2.6. Binding of two hypothetical enantiomers of a drug to a receptor active site. The active enantiomer has a three-dimensional structure that allows drug domain **A** to interact with active site domain a, **B** to interact with b, and **C** to interact with c. All three binding interactions are necessary. In contrast, the inactive enantiomer cannot be aligned to have the same three interactions with the binding site simultaneously. The difference in three-dimensional structure allows the active enantiomer to bind and have a biological effect, whereas this is not possible for the inactive enantiomer.

Enantiomeric pairs have identical physicochemical properties, such as boiling point, melting point, density, and solubility. Enantiomers, however, can have marked differences in their interaction with proteins such as enzymes and receptors, and can behave very differently in biological systems as a result of their different three-dimensional shape. Figure 2.6 illustrates the binding of two hypothetical enantiomers of a drug to a receptor active site. In other words, the R enantiomer of a drug will not necessarily behave the same way as the S enantiomer of the same drug when taken by a patient. In essence, the two enantiomers of a chiral drug should be considered different drugs. The ability of biomolecules to distinguish between the various steric forms of a ligand or drug is called chiral recognition or *chiral discrimination*.

Region C—The Chiral Center. The carbon in region C has a chiral center (Fig. 2.7). The R isomer can present the hydroxyl in an orientation that allows it

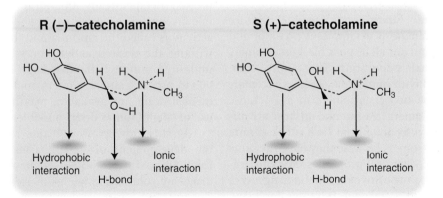

Figure 2.7. Illustration depicting how the orientation of the chiral center allows the R isomer to form three bonds to the active site on the receptor and the S isomer to form only two bonds.

to form a hydrogen bond with the target. This provides for greater attraction to the binding site and allows formation of a more stable drug–receptor complex. The R isomer is 25 times more potent than the S isomer. That is, the amount needed to produce an effect with the R isomer is 25 times less than that needed to produce an effect with the S isomer. The S isomer is equipotent to an identical molecule lacking the hydroxyl group in region C.

Geometric Isomers. Geometric isomers (or *cis–trans* isomerism) occur because of restricted rotation around a bond such as a carbon–carbon double bond, or in a ring such as cyclohexane. The *cis* and *trans* configurations are not mirror images of each other, and the two forms show significant differences in their physicochemical properties, such as ionization and lipophilicity, and in their biological activity.

Geometric *cis* and *trans* isomers can be isolated as pure substances, and mixtures of isomers are not commonly seen. However, the two trans isomers in a cyclic compound can exist as an enantiomeric pair. Differences in biological activity between *cis* and *trans* isomers may, therefore, be caused by either nonspecific physicochemical effects or stereoselectivity of receptor binding. Figure 2.8 illustrates geometric isomerism and how geometric isomers can bind differently to a target protein.

Racemic Mixtures. A racemic mixture or racemate is a sample of a compound that contains all its possible stereoisomers in equal proportions. Thus, for a compound with one chiral center, a racemate has the two enantiomers in a 1:1 ratio. Enantiomers in a racemic mixture are difficult to separate from each other as pure stereoisomers because they have the same physicochemical properties. For this reason, the majority of synthetic drugs were produced as racemic mixtures for many years, and the properties of the individual stereoisomers were not known. More

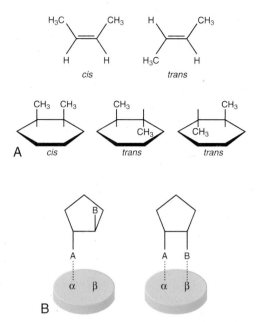

Figure 2.8. A. Geometric isomerism as a result of *cis–trans* orientation across a double bond or in a ring. B. Binding of geometric isomers to a target. On the left, the *trans* isomer does not have the B group in proper configuration for effective binding. On the right, the *cis* isomer has both the functional groups in a favorable orientation for binding to the receptor.

than 500 currently useful drugs are racemic mixtures containing an active drug and its enantiomer in equal proportions.

It is now clear that stereoisomers can have significantly different biological properties, and that a single stereoisomer is often therapeutically superior to a racemic mixture. The isomer with the desired activity is called the **eutomer** and the one without the desired activity or with an undesired activity is the **distomer**. Methods to produce single isomers on a commercial scale are available, making the use of single isomer drugs possible.

Chirality now plays a major role in the development of new pharmaceuticals; approximately 30% of marketed drugs are sold as a single isomeric form. The anti-inflammatory drug naproxen is marketed as the S isomer, because the R form is a liver toxin. Similarly, L-DOPA has anti-Parkinsonian activity, whereas D-DOPA exhibits none of the desired anti-Parkinsonian activity and can cause granulocytopenia (loss of white blood cells that leaves patients prone to infections). There are other examples such as penicillamine, used to treat arthritis, in which the S enantiomer is active while the R form is extremely toxic. The (S, S) form of the antituberculosis drug ethambutol is active while the (R, R) form causes optical neuritis that can lead to blindness.

An example of *cis–trans* isomerism in drugs is found in *trans*-diethylstilbestrol, which has estrogenic activity, and *cis*-diethylstilbestrol, which has only 7% of the estrogenic activity of *trans*-diethylstilbestrol.

Physicochemical Properties of Drugs

After identifying the basic structural requirements for a drug to bind to the target, structural changes are often needed to circumvent other problems or, in some cases, to further enhance biological activity. Issues such as solubility, ability to distribute to appropriate areas of the body, susceptibility to metabolism, enhancing potency or reducing toxicity may need to be addressed. The challenge, therefore, is to make changes that improve one property of the drug without changing other properties.

Bioisosterism

Chemical isosterism is the similarity in physicochemical properties of ions, compounds, or elements because of similarities in their electronic structures. This concept was first introduced for atoms: elements in the same vertical row of the periodic table have similar outer shells of electrons, giving them the same electronic properties. In these rows, atoms with the same size and mass also have similar physicochemical properties. A similar trend is seen for neighboring atoms in horizontal rows of the periodic table.

Thus, if one atom or group of atoms in a molecule is replaced with its *isostere*, the physicochemical properties of the compound do not change significantly. Chemical isosteric equivalents can be used to synthesize different compounds with the *same* physicochemical properties.

Bioisosterism is the application of isosterism to biological systems and guides molecular modification of drugs to produce desired changes in either the drug's physicochemical properties or biological actions. The underlying principle is that if a modified compound is to interact with the same target as the pharmacophore, then the modification cannot be too drastic. Small structural changes may be achieved by replacing specific atoms or groups of atoms with their bioisosteres. The reasons for making bioisosteric modifications is to synthesize similar compounds that (1) retain biological activity, but have improved physicochemical properties and better pharmacokinetic behavior or (2) retain these physicochemical properties while enhancing or refining the biological effects. This approach is widely used in the synthesis of improved drugs based on the pharmacophore.

Bioisosteric Equivalents

Bioisosteric equivalents may be subdivided into categories such that atoms or functional groups within a category are interchangeable with one another.

1. Atoms or groups of atoms that have the same number of total electrons. The following are considered bioisosteres because each has a total of eight electrons: O, NH, and CH_2. The pharmacophore for agents with antiseizure activity is shown in Figure 2.9A. The biological activity is retained if X = either O, NH or CH_2.
2. Atoms having the same number of electrons in the outer most shell. Halogens are in the same vertical row as hydrogen and are, therefore, isosteric. In the

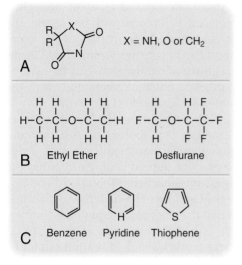

Figure 2.9. A. Pharmacophore for drugs possessing antiseizure activity. B. Chemical structures of ethyl ether and desflurane. Both agents can cause general anesthesia. C. Three different heterocyclics that have similar shapes and sizes.

case of inhalation anesthetics (Fig. 2.9B), substituting fluorine atoms for hydrogen retains the biological activity of inducing sleep and also provides the benefits of decreasing the flammability and increasing the potency of these agents compared to nonhalogenated hydrocarbons such as ethyl ether.

3. Atoms and groups of atoms having the same size and shape. The hydrogen atom is similar in size to fluorine atom; chlorine atom is similar in size to CF_3. The benzene ring is bioisosteric with pyridine and thiophene ring systems because the C = C bond is similar in size and presents bond angles similar to and C = N bond and the sulfur atom (Fig. 2.9C).

Bioisosteric Applications

In drug development, chemists will make bioisosteric modifications to a pharmacophore or to a drug currently on the market to produce a new drug that interacts with a newly identified target or to improve upon an established drug. Below

are examples of bioisosteric changes that alter the physicochemical properties of the drug or its actions at a target.

Lipid Solubility: Propranolol and pindolol are β-adrenergic receptor blockers used in the treatment of cardiovascular disease (Fig. 2.10A). Propranolol has high lipid solubility and gains access to the brain, a characteristic that is not always needed to treat cardiovascular diseases in certain patients. Pindolol, because of a bioisosteric modification to the ring structure, is less lipid soluble and does not enter the brain to the same extent as propranolol and therefore has fewer effects in the central nervous system.

Enzyme Inhibition: The compound para-aminobenzoic acid (PABA) is essential for the growth of bacteria; it is a substrate for the enzyme dihydropteroate synthetase and is required for the synthesis of folic acid. Sulfacetamide (Fig. 2.10B), an antibiotic used to treat bacterial infections, is structurally similar to PABA and can bind to the same site on the enzyme as PABA. Sulfacetamide, however, is not a substrate or perfect match for the enzyme and acts to inhibit the enzyme and prevent the synthesis of folic acid.

Receptor Blockade: Histamine is the endogenous ligand for histamine receptors located in the GI tract. When histamine binds to the receptor, it elicits a change in the receptor to cause release of gastric acid. The ring system in the H_2 blocker ranitidine is bioisosteric to the ring system in histamine which allows them to bind to the same target but other elements of ranitidine's structure do not allow it to activate the receptor (Fig. 2.10C). Therefore, ranitidine's action is to bind to the target and thereby prevent histamine from acting at the target to cause acid release.

Receptor Selectivity: The pharmacophore shown in Figure 2.10D, as discussed earlier, can activate α and β receptors. Clonidine, while appearing structurally different from the pharmacophore, fulfills the steric and electronic requirements of the receptor.

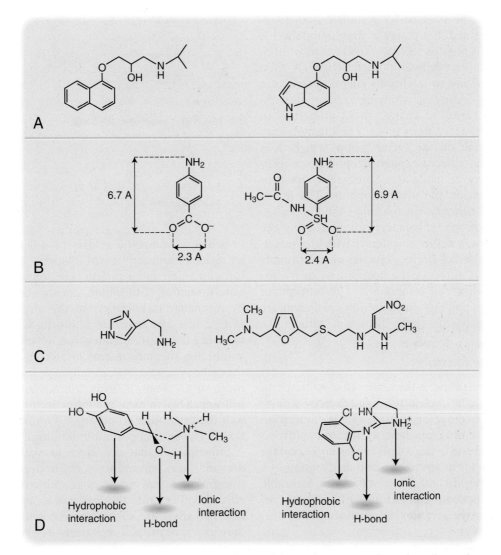

Figure 2.10. Examples of bioisosteres. In each pair of drugs, the compounds on the right are drugs designed using bioisosteric modifications.

Other features of the molecule (substituting Cl atoms for hydroxyls and the addition of an imidazole ring) limit the drug's ability to bind to all α and β receptors; it selectively binds to a small subset of receptors designated as α₂ receptors.

Lipophilic–Hydrophilic Balance

To be a successful drug, a compound has to be somewhat soluble in polar environments such as water, and also in nonpolar environments such as lipids. Aqueous solubility is necessary because most of the body is made up of water; thus a drug must dissolve in these aqueous environments to enter and travel through the body. Lipid solubility is needed because cells and tissues contain lipids, and most drugs need to first dissolve in these lipids to reach the site of action. Therefore, most drug molecules have a combination of hydrophilic (water-loving) and lipophilic (lipid-loving) properties.

The effect of various chemical substituents on lipophilicity and hydrophilicity

has been extensively studied and documented. If a potential drug compound is
too high or too low with regard to lipophilicity or hydrophilicity, chemists often
attempt to modify its chemical structure
by adding or removing appropriate substituents to change these properties in
a predictable manner. The changes may
occur on the vector group, which does
not alter the pharmacophore, or they
may be made as a bioisosteric substitu-
tion on the pharmacophore. The intent
in either case is to change the lipophilic–
hydrophilic balance without altering the
drug's ability to interact with the target.
Table 2.1 shows examples of substituents
that influence the lipophilicity or hydrophilicity of compounds. The concepts of
lipophilicity and partition coefficient are
discussed in more detail in Chapter 4.

Ionization

Ionization is the ability of a molecule to
gain or lose electrons and thereby acquire
a negative or positive charge. Ionization
of a drug can be critical to its ability to
bind to a target and is also an important
factor in absorption and distribution of a
drug. Two of the most common ionizable
functional groups found in drugs are carboxylic acids and aliphatic amines.

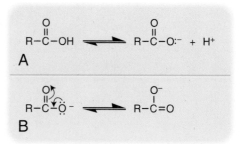

Figure 2.11. A. Ionization of the general
structure of a carboxylic acid. B. Resonance
structures of a carboxylic acid.

When a carboxylic acid is placed in
an aqueous solution, it will dissociate to
form an anion and a proton. The ionization (formation of the anion) is enhanced
by resonance stabilization of the anion
(Fig. 2.11). The structure of a drug can
influence the degree of ionization. That is,
by altering the substituents located near
the carboxylic acid, we can influence how
much of the anion is formed in aqueous
solution. This, in turn, can influence how
well the drug binds to its target if ionization or charge is important to binding.

Substituents that are electron withdrawing (also referred to as electronega-
tive groups or having negative inductive
effects) will enhance the degree of ionization of carboxylic acids. Electron withdrawing groups pull electrons toward
themselves making ionization more likely
because the bond (the shared pair of electrons between O and H) is pulled toward
the oxygen. In contrast, substituents that
are electron repelling will decrease the
degree of ionization of carboxylic acids.
These groups tend to push the electrons
away from themselves and force the electron pair toward the hydrogen atom making it more available to the hydrogen and
less likely for the hydrogen to dissociate
from the carboxyl group.

When an amine is placed in an aqueous solution, it has a free pair of electrons
that allows it to bind to a proton and
form a cation (Fig. 2.12). As seen with
the carboxylic acids, certain substituents

TABLE 2.1. Substituents That Influence the Lipophilic–Hydrophilic Balance	
Substituent	Structure
Substituents that increase lipophilicity	
Alkyl	$-CH_3$, $-CH_2-$, and so on
Aryl	$-C_6H_5$
Sulfur-containing groups	$-S-$, $-SCH_3$
Halogens	$-Cl$, $-Br$, $-I$
Substituents that decrease lipophilicity	
Hydroxyl	$-OH$
Carboxyl	$-COOH$
Carbonyl	$-C\neq O$
Amino	$-NH_2$, $-NH-R$
Ether	$-O-$

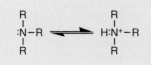

Figure 2.12. Ionization of the general structure of an aliphatic amine.

near the amine function can influence the degree of ionization. The effect of these substituents on the ionization of amines, however, is opposite to that of carboxylic acids. That is, electron repelling groups increase the degree of ionization of amines by pushing the electrons away from themselves and toward the amine making the free pair of electrons more available to bind with a proton to form a cation. Electron withdrawing groups pull the electrons toward themselves and away from the amine making the electrons less available to bind with a proton. As a result, electron withdrawing groups decrease the degree of ionization of amines. Examples of electron withdrawing groups are halogens, aromatic ring systems and nitro groups. Electron repelling groups include alkyls and nonaromatic ring systems. Quantitative measures and factors affecting ionization are discussed in more detail in Chapter 3.

Structure–Activity Relationships

A structure–activity relationship (SAR) is the relationship of the molecular structure of a compound with a biological property. The basic assumption behind these relationships is that different structures must give different activities or different degrees of the same activity. Relationships between structure and behavior can be found from a drug's pharmaceutical properties (solubility, stability, dissolution), its pharmacokinetic properties (absorption, distribution, metabolism, and excretion), or its pharmacodynamic properties (interaction

between drug and target). These correlations may be qualitative (simple SAR) or quantitative (quantitative SAR, or QSAR). In general, they are a set of rules that predict whether a compound will be active, and to what extent. SARs can then be used to predict which analogs will have the most desirable properties.

Qualitative predictions are based on a comparison of the properties of one or more analogs with the compound of interest. For example, terms such as "similarly active," "less active," or "more active" would be used in a qualitative SAR assessment for the biological activity of a series of analogs compared with the lead compound. An example is the SAR for analogs of the antipsychotic drug chlorpromazine (Fig. 2.13).

Quantitative predictions, on the other hand, are usually in the form of an equation that relates some property of the compound to specific structural features of the compound. They also give some estimation of the degree of biological activity expected. Researchers have attempted for many years to develop drugs based on QSAR, and there have been numerous attempts to mathematically correlate drug structure with biological activity. Many parameters enter into the development

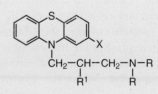

Figure 2.13. The structure–activity relationship (SAR) of the antipsychotic chlorpromazine. Three carbon atoms must separate the ring nitrogen from the side chain nitrogen for optimal antipsychotic. If two carbon atoms separate the two nitrogens, then antihistamine action predominates. The substituent at position X must be an electron withdrawing group such as a halogen or CF_3. If X is replaced by H, there is a drastic reduction in activity. If X is moved to another position, activity is lost. If R′ = hydroxyl or heterocyclic, then all activity is lost.

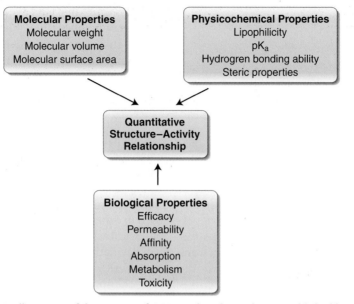

Figure 2.14. An illustration of the concept of QSARs. The relationship is established by correlating molecular or physicochemical properties of a drug with its biological or pharmacological behavior.

of a QSAR as illustrated in Figure 2.14. Classic QSAR analyses consider only two-dimensional structures, whereas the newer three-dimensional QSAR approach is much more complex and takes into account three-dimensional properties.

Equations have been developed to correlate activity with physicochemical properties such as partition coefficient, pK_a, hydrogen bonding ability, or other structural features such as steric effects and electronic properties of the drug. These properties may be determined experimentally, but are increasingly being calculated by computational methods.

Developing a QSAR is difficult. Molecules are typically flexible, and it is possible to compute many possibly useful properties that might relate to activity. For the method to work efficiently, compounds selected to define the equation should be diverse. Once the relationship is defined, it can be used to aid in prediction of new or unknown molecules. QSAR has been surpassed by rational drug design as a technique for lead identification, but it continues to be an important tool for lead modification and optimization to predict structures that have better ADME properties than the lead compound.

Key Concepts

- Proteins perform their biological function by binding to endogenous compounds called ligands.
- Drugs work by binding to targets, usually receptor or enzyme proteins, and thus influencing protein–ligand binding in some way.

- The binding of a ligand or drug to target sites requires physicochemical and steric complementarity.
- Principles of bioisosterism and SAR are used to modify the structure of the pharmacophore to provide suitable physicochemical properties and biological activity.

Review Questions

1. What is meant by the term drug target?
2. What are some major functions of proteins and how does a drug's actions relate to these functions?
3. Explain the concept of pharmacophores. What are vector groups and how do they relate to the pharmacophore?
4. What is meant by complementarity? Discuss the two types of complementarity.
5. Explain why chiral recognition is important in the binding of small molecule ligands to targets.
6. What is a racemic mixture? Discuss the advantages and disadvantages of using single isomers of drugs instead of racemic mixtures.
7. Explain the term bioisosterism. What is the intent of or what is to be gained from using bioisosteric equivalents?
8. Why is ionization important for protein–ligand interactions?
9. Explain how **SAR**s can predict the biological activity of a compound.

Practice Problems

1. How many optical isomers are possible for the following compounds?
   a. 2-pentanol
   b. 2,8-dimethyl-5-nonanol
2. Is *cis–trans* isomerism possible for either of the following compounds? Do either of them have optical isomers?
   a. 1,2,3-trichlororcyclopropane
   b.

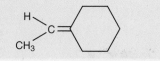

3. Write the structural formula for phenylephrine. What structural modifications can be made to this compound to increase its ability to bind to β-receptors?
4. Design a hypothetical receptor site for the compound shown below. Your answer should include a diagram that shows chemical links between the compound and the receptor with all bonds labeled. You may assume the ionizable groups are in the ionized state.

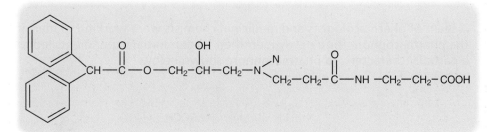

5. Label the acidic protons on the compound below and identify the one with the greatest degree of ionization.

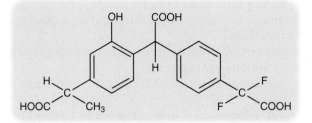

6. The structures below are classified as benzodiazepines, drugs used to treat anxiety and insomnia. Structure I represents the pharmacophore for this chemical class. Changing the lipophilicity of the molecule can alter the ability of the drug to enter the brain and therefore, how fast the drug can produce its effects.

   a. For structures II, III, and IV, compare each to structure I and determine which of the pair is more lipophilic.

   b. Which of the changes would be considered bioisosteric?

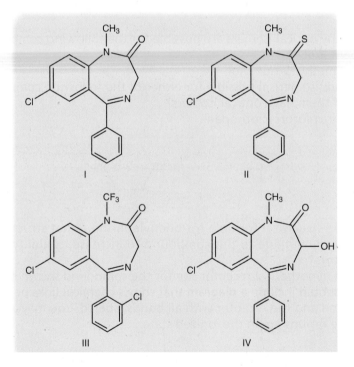

7. A team of pharmacologists and medicinal chemists were working to identify the pharmacophore for a newly identified target. Initial experiments led to a partially characterized pharmacophore shown below.

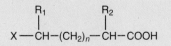

Additional experiments using the principles of SARs provided the following information.

X	R_1	$(CH_2)_n$	R_2	Activity
Phenyl	H	$n = 2$	H	+
Thiophene	H	$n = 2$	H	+
Cyclohexane	H	$n = 2$	H	−
Phenyl	OH	$n = 2$	H	+
Phenyl	OH	$n = 2$	H	+
Phenyl	OH	$n = 2$	H	+
Phenyl	OH	$n = 3$	H	+
Phenyl	OH	$n = 3$	CH_3	−
Phenyl	OH	$n = 3$	Cl	++
Phenyl	OH	$n = 4$	H	−
Phenyl	OH	$n = 4$	CH3	−
Phenyl	OH	$N = 4$	Cl	+

a. Using the information in the table above, identify the structural requirements for activity and draw a more specific pharmacophore for this target. Explain your rationale.

b. Are there additional structures you would need to test to make a more informed decision? If so, which series?

c. Can you make a case for testing enantiomers?

Additional Readings

Chan JN, Nislow C, Emili A. Recent advances and method development for drug target identification. Trends Pharmacol Sci 2010;31(2):82–88.

Lemke T, Williams D (eds). Foye's Principles of Medicinal Chemistry, 6th ed. Lippincott Williams and Wilkins, 2008.

Nelson D, Cox M. Lehninger Principles of Biochemistry, 5th ed. W.H. Freeman, 2009.

Rang H, Dale M, Ritter J, Flower R. Rang and Dale's Pharmacology, 6th ed. Elsevier, 2007.

Van Drie J. Monty Kier and the origin of the pharmacophore concept. Internet Electron J Mol Des 2007;6(9):271–279.

CHAPTER 3

Ionization of Drugs

As discussed in Chapter 2, a drug's behavior and action are ultimately determined by its chemical structure. The structure determines its physicochemical properties, which in turn play a major role in physical, chemical, and biological performance. A critical physicochemical property is ionization: a process by which a neutral molecule gains or loses a proton and thereby acquires a positive or negative electrical charge. The charged species formed are called ions.

Electrolytes and Nonelectrolytes

Ions can conduct an electrical current, and so substances that form ions in solution are called electrolytes. One way of classifying compounds is based on whether, and how much, they ionize in aqueous solutions.

A nonelectrolyte is a compound that does not ionize when dissolved in water, and exists solely as the neutral, uncharged species. Common examples of such compounds are ethanol, dextrose, and some steroids. Many drug compounds do not ionize under physiological conditions and are considered to be nonelectrolytes. Compounds with the following functional groups do not generally ionize in aqueous solution:

- Alcohols and sugars
- Ethers
- Esters
- Ketones
- Aldehydes
- Most amides

Figure 3.1 shows the structures of common nonelectrolyte functional groups found in drug molecules.

A strong electrolyte ionizes completely when dissolved in water, and exists *solely* in the form of positive and negative ions in solution. An example is NaCl, which ionizes to form Na^+ and Cl^- in aqueous solution. A few drugs are strong electrolytes; examples are KCl (as a potassium supplement) and Li_2CO_3 (in the treatment of manic depression).

A weak electrolyte is ionizable, but ionizes *partially*; a fraction of dissolved molecules remain un-ionized, while others acquire a positive or negative charge. Simple examples of weak electrolytes are acetic acid and ammonia. Many drugs and other pharmaceutically important compounds are weak electrolytes. We focus on the ionization of weak electrolytes in this chapter.

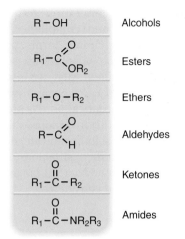

R – OH	Alcohols
R₁–C(=O)–OR₂	Esters
R₁ – O – R₂	Ethers
R–C(=O)–H	Aldehydes
R₁–C(=O)–R₂	Ketones
R₁–C(=O)–NR₂R₃	Amides

Figure 3.1. Structures of some common non-electrolyte functional groups.

Importance of Ionization of Weak Electrolytes

The properties of ionized (charged) and un-ionized (uncharged) forms of a drug or biologically active compound are dramatically different from each other, even though the only change in structure is the gain or loss of a proton, and the presence or absence of a charge. The charged and uncharged forms will be absorbed and distributed differently, will bind to receptors differently, and may be metabolized and eliminated differently. Thus, for a drug that can ionize, the proportion of ionized and un-ionized forms in the body is critical in determining its behavior. Ionization of drugs in the drug product is also important, influencing route of administration and shelf life of the drug product.

Indomethacin, an oral anti-inflammatory drug, provides a good example of the importance of ionization in drug design. On administration, indomethacin (a weak electrolyte) must first dissolve in aqueous contents of the gastrointestinal tract. The ionized form of the drug dissolves more rapidly and to a greater extent than the un-ionized form. To enter the bloodstream, however, it needs to cross lipophilic cell barriers, which requires at least some molecules to be in the un-ionized form in the intestines. Once indomethacin has reached its site of action, only the ionized form binds to the receptor. Thus, both ionized and un-ionized forms are important for different aspects of ADME (absorption, distribution, metabolism, excretion) and pharmacodynamics of indomethacin.

Water as a Solvent

According to the *Bronsted–Lowry* theory of acids and bases, an acid is a compound that can donate a proton and a base is one that can accept a proton. Therefore, there has to be another compound present to receive the proton from the acid, or to provide a proton to the base. In almost all situations we will deal with, this other compound is water, the solvent and medium for all living organisms. Water is also a reactant in many pharmaceutical reactions of interest. In addition, water is critical in determining the configuration of proteins and other biological macromolecules that are important in drug action.

Water is a remarkable solvent because it can behave as both an acid and a base. Compounds with this dual property are said to be amphoteric and are often called ampholytes. The water molecule possesses a dipole (two electric charges of equal magnitude but opposite sign, separated by a small distance), giving it the ability to accept or donate a positively charged proton. Water accepts a proton in the following equilibrium:

$$H^+ + H_2O \rightleftharpoons H_3O^+ \quad \text{(Eq. 3.1)}$$

The species H_3O^+ is called the hydronium ion. Water can also donate a proton as follows:

$$H_2O \rightleftharpoons H^+ + OH \quad \text{(Eq. 3.2)}$$

The ionization product constant of water is K_w, given by the following equation:

$$K_w = [H^+][OH^-] \quad \text{(Eq. 3.3)}$$

This relationship says that the product of protons and hydroxide ions in an aqueous solution is always constant. The value of K_w at 25°C is 10^{-14}.

Concept of pH

The pH value is a convenient way to express the acidity of a solution and is defined as follows:

$$pH = -\log[H^+] \quad \text{(Eq. 3.4)}$$

The symbol p is an operator that converts a number into its negative logarithm. The pH scale has a range from 0 to 14. Seven is considered neutral pH where the concentration of hydrogen ions is equal to the concentration of hydroxide ions. A solution pH below 7 means that the solution is acidic and the concentration of hydrogen ions exceeds the concentration of hydroxide ions. If the concentration of hydroxide ions is greater than that of hydrogen ions, the solution is basic or alkaline and has a pH greater than 7.

pH of Pharmaceutical Systems

The pH of body fluids ranges between 1 and approximately 8. The stomach is the most acidic region of the body with a pH that varies between 1 and 3. The normal pH of intestinal fluids is approximately 6 to 7. The pH of blood is 7.4, which corresponds to a $[H^+]$ of approximately 40 nM. This value can only vary from 37 to 43 nM without serious metabolic consequences. Local pH in various tissues depends on composition and function of each tissue, and rarely exceeds 8. Thus, a drug can be expected to encounter physiological environments that vary between pH 1 and 8, which makes ionization in this pH range of greatest interest. If a drug does not have a functional group that ionizes in this pH region, it behaves as a nonelectrolyte and remains un-ionized over the entire physiological pH range.

From a formulation perspective, it is important to control pH of a product to minimize drug degradation, to improve patient comfort and compliance, or to improve delivery. Dosage forms, particularly liquids (such as solutions, suspensions, and emulsions), may have pH values outside the pH 1 to 8 range. Higher pH values of pharmaceutical liquids are often required to make the drug more soluble, or to maintain good stability and an adequate shelf life. Thus, in these situations, ionization behavior over a wider pH range has to be understood and considered.

Strong Acids and Bases

Let us first examine the behavior of strong acids and bases, so that we can distinguish them from weak acids and bases. Strong acids such as HCl and H_2SO_4 dissociate completely in water and exist entirely in their ionized form, making them strong electrolytes.

$$HCl \rightarrow H^+ + Cl^- \quad \text{(Eq. 3.5)}$$

$$H_2SO_4 \rightarrow 2H^+ + SO_4^{-2} \quad \text{(Eq. 3.6)}$$

The H^+ ion formed will react with a water molecule to produce the hydronium ion (see Eq. 3.1), although for convenience we usually do not write the complete reaction. Thus, when a strong acid is added to water, hydrogen ion concentration in solution increases and pH decreases.

Because a strong acid dissociates completely, the molar concentration of H^+ is equal to the molar concentration of acid added for a monoprotic acid (HCl), and twice the molar acid concentration for a diprotic acid (H_2SO_4).

Similarly, a strong base like NaOH dissociates completely in water and exists entirely in its ionized form:

$$NaOH \rightarrow Na^+ + OH^- \quad \text{(Eq. 3.7)}$$

The actual base here is hydroxide ion, OH^-, which will react with H^+ in water (in the reverse reaction shown in Eq. 3.2).

Consequently, the concentration of H^+ will decrease and the solution pH will increase. The molar decrease in H^+ concentration will be equal to the molar concentration of NaOH added.

Although strong acids and bases are often used in pharmaceutical products to adjust the pH of liquids, there are no strong acids or strong base drugs.

Weak Acids and Bases

Many drugs can be classified as weak acids or weak bases. Like strong acids and bases, these compounds can also dissociate in water and donate or accept protons. The main difference is that weak acids and bases are only *partially* dissociated in water because of their diminished ability to donate or accept protons.

When a weak acid is added to water, solution pH decreases, but only a fraction of acid molecules dissociate to donate protons to water. The rest of the weak acid molecules remain un-ionized. Therefore, weak acids exist in solution in two forms—the uncharged, un-ionized species and negatively charged ions. Similarly, when a weak base is dissolved in water, only a fraction of molecules accept protons. Weak bases also exist in solution in two forms—the uncharged, un-ionized species and positively charged ions.

Typical weak acids have the following functionalities:

- Carboxylic acids
- Sulfonic acids
- Phenols
- Thiols
- Imides

Figure 3.2 shows the structures of weak acid functional groups.

Most weak bases fall into the following categories:

- Aliphatic amines (primary, secondary, or tertiary)

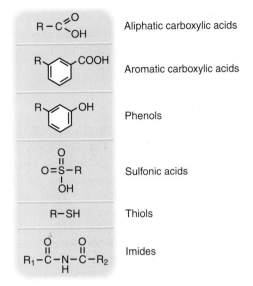

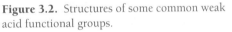

Figure 3.2. Structures of some common weak acid functional groups.

- Aromatic amines (primary, secondary, or tertiary)
- N-heterocycles (pyridine, imidazole)

Figure 3.3 shows the general structures of weak base functional groups.

A few drug compounds are quaternary ammonium salts—analogues of ammonium

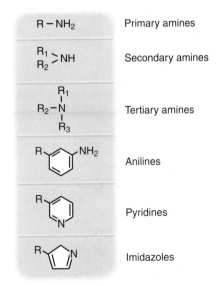

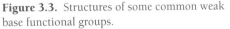

Figure 3.3. Structures of some common weak base functional groups.

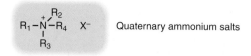

Figure 3.4. General structure of quaternary ammonium salts.

salts in which all four hydrogens of the ammonium cation are substituted for with alkyl, aryl, or aralkyl groups (Fig. 3.4). Quaternary ammonium compounds are strong electrolytes, neither acidic nor basic, and dissociate completely in water. Examples of drugs that are quaternary ammonium salts are ipratropium bromide (Atrovent®) and trospium chloride (Sanctura®).

Ionization of Weak Acids and Bases

Weak Acids

Consider the ionization of a weak acid such as acetylsalicylic acid, or aspirin, which has one carboxylic acid group. Its dissociation can be represented by the equilibrium shown in Figure 3.5. In this equilibrium, acetylsalicylic acid is a weak acid because it donates a proton, and the acetylsalicylate ion is a weak base because it accepts a proton. An acid and base that can be represented by an equilibrium in which the two species differ only by a proton is called a conjugate acid–base pair.

K_a is called the acid dissociation constant. A simplified way of representing dissociation of any weak acid, denoted as HA for convenience, is as follows:

$$HA \xrightleftharpoons{K_a} A^- + H^+ \quad \text{(Eq. 3.8)}$$

where A$^-$ is the conjugate base of the acid HA.

Weak Bases

The ionization of the weak base benzocaine with one amino group is shown in Figure 3.6. A simplified way of representing ionization equilibrium for any base B is as follows:

$$B + H^+ \rightleftharpoons BH^+ \quad \text{(Eq. 3.9)}$$

Here, BH$^+$ is the conjugate acid of the base B. By convention, we write Equation 3.9 in the reverse form:

$$BH^+ \xrightleftharpoons{K_a} B + H^+ \quad \text{(Eq. 3.10)}$$

The equilibrium is now expressed as the dissociation of the conjugate acid of the weak base, with K_a as the corresponding acid dissociation constant.

Generalizations

In summary, the dissociation equilibria for acidic forms of conjugate acid–base pairs of a weak acid or base are written as follows:

$$HA \xrightleftharpoons{K_a} A^- + H^+ \quad \text{(Eq. 3.11)}$$

$$BH^+ \xrightleftharpoons{K_a} B + H^+ \quad \text{(Eq. 3.12)}$$

Note that the charge is on the conjugate base form (A$^-$) of an un-ionized weak acid HA, and on the conjugate acid form (BH$^+$) of a weak un-ionized base B. Because ions behave differently from uncharged molecules, we are interested

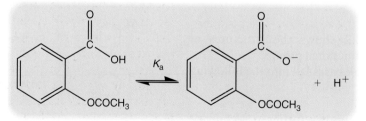

Figure 3.5. Ionization of the weak acid, acetylsalicylic acid (aspirin) in aqueous solution.

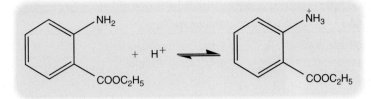

Figure 3.6. Ionization of the weak base benzocaine in aqueous solution.

in what proportion of a weak acid or weak base is un-ionized or ionized in a given situation; this will help us understand and predict its behavior.

Strength of Weak Acids and Bases

The law of mass action describes the dissociation of a weak acid and of the conjugate acid of a weak base. It states that at equilibrium the product of the concentrations on one side of an equation, when divided by the product of concentrations on the other side of the equation, is a constant regardless of the individual concentrations. Therefore, for a weak acid:

$$\frac{[H^+][A^-]}{[HA]} = K_a \quad \text{(Eq. 3.13)}$$

A large value of K_a means that the acid favors giving up protons and dissociates extensively. Consequently, the reverse reaction is not favored; the conjugate base A^- is stable and does not have a high propensity to accept protons. The larger the K_a, the stronger the acid HA, and the weaker its conjugate base A^-. Therefore, K_a is a property of the conjugate acid–base pair and gives us information about the strengths of both forms.

Similarly, we can define K_a for the conjugate acid of a weak base as:

$$\frac{[H^+][B]}{[BH^+]} = K_a \quad \text{(Eq. 3.14)}$$

The larger the value of K_a, the more BH^+ dissociates to donate protons. There-

fore, the larger the K_a, the stronger the conjugate acid BH^+ is, and the weaker the base B.

pK_a Value

The negative logarithm of K_a is referred to as the pK_a, giving the following relationship:

$$pK_a = -\log K_a \quad \text{(Eq. 3.15)}$$

The symbol p is an operator that converts a number into its negative logarithm. This manipulation makes pK_a smaller as K_a gets larger. In other words, weak acids (or conjugate acids of weak bases) with a large K_a have a small pK_a, whereas weak acids with a small K_a have a large pK_a.

The pK_a value itself does not tell us whether a drug is a weak acid or base. For example, if a drug has a pK_a value of 5, it could be either a weak acid or a weak base. One way to tell is to examine the structure of the molecule and identify functional groups that are known to be acidic or basic. Another way is to see the types of salts that the compound forms; we shall discuss this below.

The pK_a is a convenient parameter for comparing the strengths of acids or bases. The lower the pK_a of a compound, the stronger is the acidic form of the conjugate acid–base pair. As an example, a weak acid with a pK_a of 3 is a stronger acid than a weak acid with a pK_a of 4. Conversely, the higher the pK_a of a compound, the stronger is the basic form of the conjugate acid–base pair. A weak base of pK_a 8 is a stronger base than a weak base of pK_a 7.

TABLE 3.1. The Relative Strengths of Some Conjugate Acid–Base Pairs

Conjugate Acid	Conjugate Base	pK_a
C_6H_5COOH (benzoic acid)	$C_6H_5COO^-$ (benzoate ion)	4.20
CH_3COOH (acetic acid)	CH_3COO^- (acetate ion)	4.76
$C_6H_5NH_3^+$ (anilinium ion)	$C_6H_5NH_2$ (aniline)	4.70
NH_4^+ (ammonium ion)	NH_3 (ammonia)	9.25
$CH_3NH_3^+$ (methylammonium ion)	CH_3NH_2 (methylamine)	10.6

Acetic acid and benzoic acid are weak acids. Ammonia, methylamine, and aniline are weak bases. Benzoic acid, with a lower pK_a, is a stronger acid than acetic acid. Conversely, acetate ion, with a higher pK_a, is a stronger base than benzoate ion. Methylamine, with the highest pK_a, is a stronger base than ammonia, which is in turn much stronger than aniline. Conversely, anilinium ion is a much stronger acid than ammonium ion, which is stronger than methylammonium ion. Acetic acid and anilinium ion have about the same strength as weak acids, with anilinium ion being a slightly stronger acid because its pK_a is lower.

Each ionizable group on a drug molecule has a pK_a value that conveys its relative strength as a conjugate acid–base pair. Remember that pK_a is always defined for the conjugate acid donating a proton. Therefore, for weak acids, pK_a is defined for the *un-ionized* acid donating a proton to form the *negatively charged* conjugate base. However, the pK_a of a weak base is defined for its *positively charged* conjugate acid donating a proton to give the *un-ionized* base. Table 3.1 shows the relative strengths of some conjugate acid–base pairs. Table 3.2 lists the pK_a ranges for various types of weak acids and bases,

while Table 3.3 shows the pK_a values of some common weak acid (HA) and weak base (BH$^+$) drugs.

Salts of Weak Acids and Bases

Weak acid and base drugs are frequently available as their salts. For example, the weak acid drug naproxen is also available as its sodium salt, sodium naproxen. The weak base drug clonidine is also available in its salt form, clonidine hydrochloride. The salt of a weak acid is usually obtained by reacting it with a strong base such as NaOH, which gives the sodium salt. The salt of a weak base is obtained by reacting it with a strong

TABLE 3.2. pK_a Ranges of Weak Acids and Weak Bases

Weak Acids	
Type of Compound	pK_a Range
Carboxylic acids ($RCOOH$)	2–6
Sulfonic acids (RSO_3H)	−1 to 1
Phenols ($ArOH$)	7–11
Thiols (RSH)	7–10
Imides (—$CONHCO$—)	8–11
Sulfonamides ($RNHSO_2R$)	6–8
Weak Bases	
Type of Compound	pK_a Range
Aliphatic amines	8–11
Anilines	3–5
Pyridines	4–6
Saturated nitrogen heterocycles	9–11

TABLE 3.3. pK_a Values of Some Weak Acid and Weak Base Drugs

Drug	pK_a Values	
	HA	BH$^+$
Penicillin G	2.8	
Aspirin	3.5	
Warfarin	5.1	
Phenytoin	8.3	
Phenothiazine		2.5
Oxycodone		8.5
Scopolamine		7.6
Morphine		8.0

Note that for bases, the pK_a value reflects that of the conjugate acid (BH$^+$) form.

acid such as HCl, which gives the hydro-chloride salt. Some drug salts are also made by combining weak acids with weak bases. An example is chlorpheniramine maleate, a salt of the weak base drug chlorpheniramine with a weak acid, maleic acid.

Salt names can give us information about whether a drug in its un-ionized form is a weak acid or base. Weak un-ionized acids form salts with strong bases, such as NaOH, KOH, and Ca(OH)$_2$, to give sodium, potassium, or calcium salts of the weak acid. Conversely, weak un-ionized bases form salts with strong acids such as HCl, H$_2$SO$_4$, and HNO$_3$, to give hydrochloride, sulfate, or nitrate salts.

Salts themselves are strong electrolytes, in that they dissociate completely into their constituent ions in water. However, the ions generated do not remain com-pletely ionized if one of the components of the salt is a weak acid or base.

Consider the hydrochloride salt of a weak base (e.g., RNH$_3^+$Cl$^-$, also written as RNH$_2\cdot$HCl), which dissociates completely to release the conjugate acid BH$^+$:

$$BH^+Cl^- \rightarrow BH^+ + Cl^- \quad \text{(Eq. 3.16)}$$

The conjugate acid BH$^+$ is a weak acid, so it dissociates further as dictated by its pK_a:

$$BH^+ \rightleftharpoons B + H^+ \quad \text{(Eq. 3.17)}$$

Making a weak base drug into a salt does not change its pK_a.

Salts of weak acids will behave analo-gously. For example, the sodium salt of a weak acid (RCOO$^-$Na$^+$) will dissociate completely in water, and then participate in an acid–base equilibrium according to its pK_a. Making a weak acid drug into a salt does not change its pK_a.

$$Na^+A^- \rightarrow Na^+ + A^- \quad \text{(Eq. 3.18)}$$

$$A^- + H^+ \rightleftharpoons HA \quad \text{(Eq. 3.19)}$$

Therefore, salts of weak acids and bases behave like weak electrolytes, in that the proportion of ionized and un-ionized forms of the weak acid or base is deter-mined in part by the pK_a.

Pharmaceutical companies often develop the salt form of a drug rather than the original weak acid or base form for sev-eral reasons. Salts can be more readily crystallized into stable, easy to manufac-ture crystals. They dissolve faster in aque-ous solutions, are more stable on storage, and are easier to handle during process-ing. In particular, salts of amine drugs are preferred over the weak base form. Many amines are volatile and unstable, and have a short shelf life as solids. Stability and shelf life improve dramatically if an amine is converted to the hydrochloride salt, for example.

Ionization and pH

We saw that weak electrolytes (weak acids and weak bases and their salts) can exist as both the ionized and un-ionized forms in aqueous solution. The relative concentrations of the ionized and un-ionized forms depend not only on the pK_a of the weak acid or base, but also on the pH of the aqueous solution in which it is dissolved.

The Henderson–Hasselbalch Equation

Equations 3.13 or 3.14 can be used to find the relationship between pK_a, pH, and concentration of drug in its acid and base forms. Taking logarithms of both sides of the equations, and rearranging appropri-ately, gives the Henderson–Hasselbalch equation. Whether we start with Equa-tion 3.13 or 3.14, we get:

$$pH = pK_a + \log\frac{[base]}{[acid]} \quad \text{(Eq. 3.20)}$$

where *[base]* is the concentration of the basic form of the drug, and *[acid]* is the concentration of the acidic form of the drug. It is very important to remember that for a weak acid drug, [acid] is the concentration of the un-ionized HA and [base] is the concentration of the ion A⁻, while, for a weak base, [acid] is the concentration of the ion BH⁺ and [base] is the concentration of the un-ionized B.

The Henderson-Hasselbalch equation may be written in various forms, obtained by rearranging Equation 3.20 in different ways, as shown below.

$$pH = pK_a - \log \frac{[acid]}{[base]} \quad \text{(Eq. 3.21)}$$

$$pK_a = pH + \log \frac{[acid]}{[base]} \quad \text{(Eq. 3.22)}$$

$$pK_a = pH - \log \frac{[base]}{[acid]} \quad \text{(Eq. 3.23)}$$

All of these equations give the same information.

The Henderson–Hasselbalch equation allows us to calculate the *ratio* between acidic and basic forms of a drug if pK_a of the drug and pH of the solution are known. From this ratio we can determine the *fraction* or *percentage* of drug that is in its acidic or basic form in various pH environments.

Buffered Solutions

A buffered solution is one that resists changes in its pH when small amounts of acid or base are added, or when the solution is diluted. Buffer solutions contain an acid to react with added OH⁻ and a base to react with added H⁺. These can be any weak acid–weak base pair, but are usually a conjugate acid–conjugate base pair. The pH of the buffer depends on the pK_a of the buffering substance and on the relative concentrations of conjugate acid and base, and can be calculated using the Henderson–Hasselbalch equation.

Acidic buffer solutions (pH <7) are commonly made from a weak acid and one of its salts—often a sodium salt. An exam-

ple is a solution of acetic acid ($pK_a = 4.75$) and sodium acetate. If the solution contains equimolar concentrations of the acid and salt, it will have a pH of 4.75. The following equilibrium describes this system:

$$CH_3COOH \underset{}{\overset{K_a}{\rightleftharpoons}} CH_3COO^- + H^+$$

$$\text{(Eq. 3.24)}$$

If additional hydrogen ions are added to this solution, they are consumed in the reaction with CH_3COO^-, and the equilibrium shifts to the left. If additional hydroxide ions enter, they react with CH_3COOH, producing CH_3COO^-, and shift the equilibrium to the right. In this way, the [H⁺] and thus the pH of the solution remain constant.

An alkaline buffer solution (pH >7) is commonly made from a weak base and one of its salts. An example is a solution of ammonia ($pK_a = 9.25$) and ammonium chloride. If these are mixed in equimolar proportions, the solution has a pH of 9.25.

Buffer Capacity

The ability of a buffer to maintain constant pH is known as its buffer capacity. It is defined as the amount of acid or base that can be added to a given volume of the buffer solution before pH changes to an appreciable degree. A buffer system is most useful at a solution pH at or close to its pK_a, because there are adequate concentrations of both the conjugate acid and base forms of the buffer to neutralize added acid or base. Thus, the most effective buffers (with a large buffer capacity) contain the acid and base in large and equal amounts. Pharmaceutical formulations are often buffered to control pH and thus help to minimize drug degradation, improve patient comfort and compliance, or allow delivery of a sufficient drug dose.

Biological Buffers

The pH of body fluids can vary from 8 in pancreatic fluid to 1 in the stomach. The average pH of blood is 7.4, and of cells is 7.0 to 7.3. Although there is great variation in pH between fluids in the body, there is little variation within each system. For example, blood pH only varies between 7.35 and 7.45 in a healthy individual. Proteins are the most important buffers in the body, because their amino and carboxylic acid groups act as proton acceptors or donors as hydrogen ions are added or removed from the environment.

The phosphate buffer system is also important in maintaining pH of intracellular fluid. This buffer system consists of dihydrogen phosphate ions ($H_2PO_4^-$) as proton donor (acid) and hydrogen phosphate ions (HPO_4^{2-}) as proton acceptor (base). These two ions are in equilibrium with each other as indicated by the equation below:

$$H_2PO_4^- \rightleftharpoons HPO_4^{2-} + H^+$$

(Eq. 3.25)

If additional hydrogen ions enter, they are consumed in the reaction with HPO_4^{2-}, and if additional hydroxide ions enter, they react with $H_2PO_4^-$, producing HPO_4^{2-}. Thus, the pH of cellular fluid is kept constant.

pH–Ionization Profiles

When an acidic or basic drug or its salt is added to a properly buffered solution, the pH of the solution does not change. Rather, the concentrations of un-ionized and ionized drug adjust appropriately to obey the Henderson–Hasselbalch equation. The percentage of drug ionized and un-ionized is of interest because charged and uncharged drug molecules behave and react differently in drug products as well as in the body. Remember that for weak acids (and their salts), the *conjugate base* carries a negative charge, whereas for weak bases (and their salts), it is the *conjugate acid* that carries a positive charge. Once we know how much of the drug is ionized and un-ionized in the fluid of interest, e.g., a drug product, blood, urine, tissue, or cell, we can explain or anticipate some of the drug's behavior, as we will learn in the following chapters.

Figure 3.7 shows the percentage of [*acid*] and [*base*] forms as a function of pH for a weak acid of $pK_a = 4$. Figure 3.8 shows a similar profile for a weak base of $pK_a = 8$. These graphs are based on the Henderson–Hasselbalch equation, which allows us to calculate the ratio of [*acid*]/[*base*] at any pH value if we know the

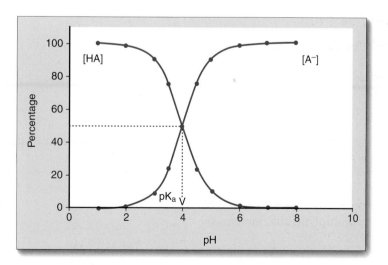

Figure 3.7. Percentage of un-ionized [HA] and ionized [A⁻] forms as a function of pH for a weak acid with $pK_a = 4$. At pH = pK_a, the weak acid is 50% ionized and 50% un-ionized.

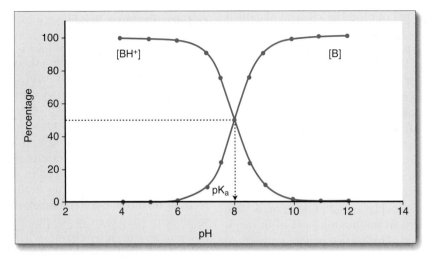

Figure 3.8. Percentage of un-ionized [B] and ionized [BH⁺] forms as a function of pH for a weak base with $pK_a = 8$. At $pH = pK_a$, the weak base is 50% ionized and 50% un-ionized.

pK_a. From this ratio, the percentage (or fraction) of each form can be determined. For example, if $[acid]/[base] = 0.1$, then the fraction of the acid form = $0.1/(1 + 0.1) = 0.0909$ (or 9.09%).

A more direct way of calculating the fraction (f) of ionized and un-ionized forms is using the following equations, derived from the Henderson–Hasselbalch equation:

For a weak acid HA:

$$f_{HA} = \frac{10^{-pH}}{10^{-pH} + 10^{-pK_a}} \quad (Eq.\ 3.26)$$

$$f_{A^-} = \frac{10^{-pK_a}}{10^{-pH} + 10^{-pK_a}} \quad (Eq.\ 3.27)$$

For a weak base B:

$$f_{BH^+} = \frac{10^{-pH}}{10^{-pH} + 10^{-pK_a}} \quad (Eq.\ 3.28)$$

$$f_{B} = \frac{10^{-pK_a}}{10^{-pH} + 10^{-pK_a}} \quad (Eq.\ 3.29)$$

The corresponding percentages may be calculated by multiplying the fractions by 100.

Table 3.4 shows how the degree of ionization of a weak acid or weak base changes with the relative values of pH and pK_a. Overall, the following generalizations can be made:

- A weak acid will be more ionized (negatively charged) when the pH is

TABLE 3.4. Dependence of Percent Ionization on the pH and the pK_a of a Weak Acid or Weak Base		
pH–pK_a	Percentage (Conjugate Acid Form)	Percentage (Conjugate Base Form)
−4	99.99	0.01
−3	99.9	0.10
−2	99.0	1.00
−1	90.9	9.10
−0.8	86.3	13.7
−0.6	79.9	20.1
−0.4	71.5	28.5
−0.2	61.3	38.7
0	50.0	50.0
0.2	38.7	61.3
0.4	28.5	71.5
0.6	20.1	79.9
0.8	13.7	86.3
1	9.10	90.9
2	1.00	99.0
3	0.10	99.9
4	0.01	99.99

above its pK_a, whereas a weak base will be more ionized (positively charged) when the pH is below its pK_a.

- Small changes in pH (within 2 pH units) near the pK_a of the compound result in large changes in the percentage ionized and un-ionized.
- Changes in pH away (more than 2 pH units) from the pK_a of the compound result in small changes in the degree of ionization.
- A weak acid is almost completely un-ionized when the pH is 4 units below its pK_a, and completely ionized when the pH is 4 units above its pK_a.
- A weak base is almost completely un-ionized when the pH is 4 units above its pK_a, and completely ionized when the pH is 4 units below its pK_a.

Ionization in Unbuffered Solutions

Ionization of weak electrolyte drugs in an unbuffered solution (e.g., pure water) is more complex, because pH does not remain constant as the drug dissolves. Consider a weak acid, such as RCOOH, and its basic sodium salt, RCOO⁻Na⁺. When RCOOH is dissolved in water, we are adding an *acid* to water and the pH will decrease. If RCOONa is dissolved in water, we are adding a *base* (RCOO⁻) to water and the pH will increase. In both the cases, equilibrium will be established between the acid and conjugate base forms in accordance with the Henderson–Hasselbalch equation. The proportion of ionized or un-ionized drug in each case will depend on pK_a of the weak acid, and the final solution pH. Thus, the fraction ionized or un-ionized in these two cases will be different because the final pH of the two solutions will be different.

Similarly, if we add a weak base (RNH₂) to water the pH will increase, and if we dissolve the acidic salt of the weak base (e.g., a salt such as RNH₃⁺Cl⁻, also written as RNH₂·HCl) in water, the pH will decrease. In both the cases, there will be equilibrium between RNH_3^+ and RNH_2 in solution, but the relative amounts of ionized and un-ionized drug will be different in the two solutions, because the final pH of the two solutions will be different.

To determine the proportion of ionized to un-ionized forms in these situations, it is important to determine how the pH will change when a weak acid or weak base is added to water, or any unbuffered solution.

pH of Unbuffered Solutions

The pH of an unbuffered solution containing a weak acid or base depends on the pK_a of the weak acid or base, and its concentration in solution. Consider the example of a weak acid HA added to water. An approximate expression relating the $[H^+]$ concentration with the pK_a and concentration is obtained using the assumption that $[H^+]$ is much less than the total concentration of the acid $[HA]_t$ (i.e., the acid is "very weak"). It can be used, however, to estimate the hydrogen ion concentration in the solution of the weak acid.

$$[H^+] \approx \sqrt{K_a[HA]_t} \quad \text{(Eq. 3.30)}$$

where $[HA]_t$ is the total concentration of weak acid added to the solution. This equation can also be written to directly give the pH:

$$pH = \frac{pK_a}{2} - \frac{\log[HA]_t}{2} \quad \text{(Eq. 3.31)}$$

This equation shows that a large K_a (small pK_a) and a large HA concentration result in a more acidic solution. When a salt of a weak base is added to water, it is similar to adding a weak acid to water, and the pH will be given by Equation 3.31.

Similarly, the $[H^+]$ of a solution after a base B is added to water is approximated by the following equation:

$$[H^+] = \frac{K_w}{[OH^-]} \approx \frac{\sqrt{K_w K_a}}{[B]_t}$$

$$\text{(Eq. 3.32)}$$

where $[B]_t$ is the total concentration of base added, and K_w is 10^{-14} at 25°C. This equation can be modified to give the pH of the solution:

$$pH = \frac{pK_w}{2} + \frac{pK_a}{2} + \frac{\log[B]_t}{2}$$

(Eq. 3.33)

pK_w ($-\log K_w$) is 14 at 25°C. This expression also gives the acidity of a solution made with the salt of a weak acid.

Once the pH of an unbuffered solution is calculated, the Henderson–Hasselbalch equation can be used to determine the fraction of a weak acid or weak base drug ionized or un-ionized at that pH. Again, note that these fractions will depend on how much drug was dissolved.

Compounds with Multiple Ionizable Groups

Many drugs and natural substances contain several ionizable groups in the same molecule, resulting in complex ionization patterns. Although a detailed discussion of such compounds is outside the scope of this book, let us examine them briefly.

Amphoteric Compounds

A compound with both acidic and basic groups on the same molecule is called an amphoteric compound or an ampholyte,

and has a pK_a for each ionizable group. Such compounds can behave as both weak acids and weak bases in aqueous solution.

Consider an ampholyte with one weak acid group HA and one weak base group B. Its ionization can be divided into two general cases as shown in Figure 3.9.

In both the cases, the ionization scheme involves a positively charged species at low pH, a net neutral species at intermediate pH, and a negatively charged species at high pH. The difference is that ordinary ampholytes form true neutral species at intermediate pH, whereas zwitterionic ampholytes form zwitterions, defined as a molecule with both a positive and a negative charge. Zwitterions have a net charge of zero, are electrically neutral, and behave as nonelectrolytes. The pH where the net charge is zero is known as the molecule's isoelectric point, and is the mean of the two pK_a values: $pK_{a(HA)}$ and $pK_{a(BH+)}$.

Whether an amphoteric compound is ordinary or zwitterionic depends on the values of the two pK_as; in other word, on whether HA or BH⁺ dissociates first as pH is increased from low to high.

- Ordinary ampholytes: If the pK_a of the acidic group, $pK_{a(HA)}$, is higher than that of the basic group, $pK_{a(BH+)}$, the first group that loses its proton as the pH is increased is BH⁺, and the neutral species has no charge.
- Zwitterionic ampholytes: If the pK_a of the acidic group, $pK_{a(HA)}$, is lower than that of the basic group, $pK_{a(BH+)}$, the first

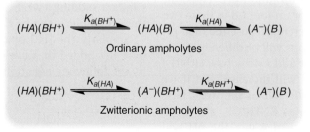

Figure 3.9. Ionization schemes for ampholytes.

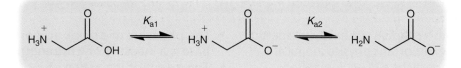

Figure 3.10. Ionization scheme of the amino acid glycine, a zwitterionic ampholyte.

group that loses its proton as the pH is increased is the acidic group, and the neutral species is a zwitterion. The most common examples are amino acids.

For illustration, consider the amino acid glycine whose ionization is described by two equilibria as shown in Figure 3.10.

K_{a1} is the acid dissociation constant for the carboxylic acid and K_{a2} is the acid dissociation constant for the protonated amine. The pK_a of the acid is 2.34 and that of the protonated amine is 9.34. Thus, glycine exists as a zwitterion at intermediate pHs. The isoelectric point of glycine is 5.84. Since the two pK_as are well separated, glycine exists completely in the zwitterionic form at and around its isoelectric point. However, many drugs have pK_a values that are close enough to each other that they overlap, making acid–base calculations more complicated.

Polyprotic Acids and Bases

Amphoteric compounds have one acidic and one basic group. Compounds that have more than one acidic group and can donate more than one proton are called polyprotic acids. Analogously, bases that can accept more than one proton are called polyprotic bases. Polyprotic acids and bases also have multiple pK_a values, one for each ionizable group. The ionization of these compounds occurs in a successive manner. If the pK_as are widely separated (e.g., by at least 4 pH units) they can be treated individually to calculate the fraction ionized or un-ionized.

A familiar polyprotic acid is phosphoric acid with three ionizable protons and three pK_a values ($pK_{a1} = 2.15$, $pK_{a2} = 7.2$, $pK_{a3} = 12.15$). These three values are separated well enough that we can treat each one independently. However, many polyprotic acid and base drugs have overlapping pK_a values; i.e., the pK_as are closer than 4 units. The ionization profiles of such drugs are complex, and outside the scope of our discussion. Table 3.5 lists the observed pK_a values of some amphoteric and polyprotic drugs.

TABLE 3.5. pK_a Values of Some Amphoteric and Polyprotic Drugs

Drug	pK_a Values HA	pK_a Values BH⁺
Amphoteric Drugs		
Amphotericin B	5.5	10.0
Apomorphine	8.9	7.0
Ampicillin	2.5	7.2
Baclofen	5.4	9.5
Ciprofloxacin	6.0	8.8
Enalapril	3.0	5.5
Lorazepam	11.5	1.3
Nystatin	8.9	5.1
Pyridoxine	8.9	5.0
Rifampin	1.7	7.9
Polyprotic Drugs		
Brompheniramine		3.6, 9.8
Fluorouracil	8.0, 13.0	
Doxorubicin		8.2, 10.2
Hydrochlorothiazide	7.0, 9.2	
Novobiocin	4.3, 9.1	
Prochlorperazine		3.7, 8.1
Quinidine		4.2, 7.9

Key Concepts

In this chapter, we have considered one important physicochemical property of a drug, ionization.

- When dissolved in water, a strong electrolyte dissociates completely, a weak electrolyte dissociates partially, and a nonelectrolyte does not dissociate.
- Many drugs are weak electrolytes (weak acids, weak bases or their salts).

- The pK_a value of a weak acid or base is a measure of its strength.
- The extent of ionization of a weak electrolyte depends on its pK_a and the pH of the medium, and can be calculated using the Henderson–Hasselbalch equation.
- Weak acid–weak base systems are useful as buffers, and are most effective at a pH near the pK_a of the system.

Review Questions

1. Compare and contrast the ionization behavior of nonelectrolytes, weak electrolytes, and strong electrolytes when they are dissolved in water.
2. Describe what is meant by weak acid, weak base, strong acid, and strong base.
3. List the functional groups that have weak acid, weak base, and nonelectrolyte properties in the physiological pH range.
4. Explain what is meant by conjugate acid–base pair. Which form of the pair, the conjugate acid or conjugate base, is charged for a weak acid? A weak base? Is this charge positive or negative?
5. How do the equilibrium acid dissociation constant, K_a, and the pK_a give you information about the strength of a weak acid or base?
6. Explain the difference between a buffered and an unbuffered solution. How does the pH of an unbuffered solution change when an acid or base is added to it? When a salt of a weak acid or weak base is added to it?
7. Discuss the use of the Henderson--Hasselbalch equation in making buffers and in determining percentage of drugs ionized at different pH values.
8. Explain what is meant by an amphoteric compound. How do ordinary ampholytes differ from zwitterionic ampholytes?

Practice Problems

1. The K_a for the dissociation of acetic acid is 1.74×10^{-5}. What is its pK_a? ($pK_a = -\log K_a = 4.76$)
2. The pK_a of propranolol (Inderal®) is 9.5. What is its K_a?
3. Glyburide (Micronase®) is a weak acid drug used in the treatment of diabetes. It has a $pK_a = 6.8$.
   a. What is the K_a of glyburide?
   b. Which form of the conjugate acid–base pair is charged, and what charge (positive or negative) does it bear?
   c. What percentage of glyburide is ionized in the small intestines (pH = 6)? In the blood (pH = 7.4)?

4. Naproxen (Aleve®) is an anti-inflammatory drug with a molecular weight of 230 and a $pK_a = 4.2$. It has the following structure:

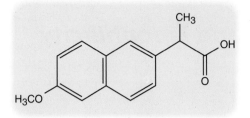

a. Is naproxen a weak acid or a weak base?
b. At what buffer pH will the concentration of the conjugate acid and conjugate base be equal?
c. When naproxen is added to an unbuffered solution, will the pH of the solution go up or down? Why?
d. What fraction of naproxen is ionized in a buffer at pH 3 and a buffer at pH 6?
e. In a 25 mg/mL solution of naproxen in a pH 6 buffer, what is the molar concentration of the drug in its ionized and un-ionized forms?
f. Naproxen is also available as its sodium salt. When naproxen sodium is added to an unbuffered solution, will the pH of the solution go up or down? Why?

5. Cimetidine (Tagamet®) is a drug used to treat duodenal ulcers to reduce excessive secretion of gastric acid. The drug has a $pK_a = 6.8$ and is also available as its hydrochloride salt.
a. Is cimetidine a weak acid or a weak base?
b. What fraction of cimetidine is un-ionized in the stomach (pH = 1), small intestines (pH = 6), and blood (pH = 7.4)?
c. When cimetidine hydrochloride is added to an unbuffered solution, will the pH of the solution go up or down? Why?

Additional Readings

Amiji M, Sandmann BJ. Applied Physical Pharmacy, 1st ed. McGraw-Hill/Appleton & Lange, 2003.

Connors KA, Mecozzi S. Thermodynamics of Pharmaceutical Systems—An Introduction to Theory and Applications, 2nd ed. Wiley Interscience, 2010.

Florence AT, Attwood D. Physicochemical Principles of Pharmacy, 4th ed. Pharmaceutical Press, 2006.

Sinko PJ. Martin's Physical Pharmacy and Pharmaceutical Sciences, 5th ed. Lippincott Williams & Wilkins, 2006.

CHAPTER 4

Solubility and Lipophilicity

Solubility is the property of a compound (solute) that enables it to dissolve in a liquid (solvent) to form a homogeneous solution. In Chapter 2, you were introduced to the concept that most drug molecules have a combination of hydrophilic (water-loving) and lipophilic (lipid-loving) properties. Therefore, drug structures are often optimized to make compounds somewhat soluble in polar environments such as water, and in nonpolar environments such as lipids.

The solubility properties of a drug are also important when it comes to designing a liquid dosage form, such as an injectable or ophthalmic solution. The solvent chosen must be able to dissolve the drug at an appropriate concentration for convenient dosing to the patient.

Solubility Principles

Solubility is an equilibrium relationship between the solid and dissolved states of a solute at saturation. The numerical value of solubility is the concentration (expressed as mole/L or mg/mL, etc.) of a saturated solution of the solute, in a given solvent, under a fixed set of conditions (temperature, pressure, pH, etc.).

Equilibrium solubility of a solute in a solvent is the net result of solute–solute, solvent–solvent and solute–solvent interactions. The process by which a solid solute dissolves in a solvent can be broken down into three steps and is illustrated in Figure 4.1. Although these steps occur simultaneously and not in sequence, it is useful to break them up as shown to understand the role of each interaction.

- Step 1: Removal of a solute molecule from solid solute; requires energy to break solute–solute bonds.
- Step 2: Separation of solvent molecules to create cavity for solute; requires energy to break solvent–solvent bonds (hydrogen bonds in the case of water).
- Step 3: Insertion of solute molecule into the cavity created in the solvent; releases energy due to formation of new solute–solvent bonds.

The energy needed in step 1 depends on the solid-state structure of the solute, and the intermolecular attractive forces holding solute molecules together. A solute whose molecules are very tightly held in the solid state will not dissolve readily regardless of the solvent. Thus, the solid state structure of a compound plays a role in its solubility.

Step 1

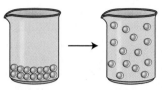

Separation of solute molecules

Step 2

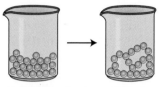

Separation of solvent molecules

Step 3

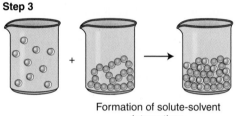

Formation of solute-solvent
interactions

Figure 4.1. The process by which a solid solute dissolves in a solvent can be broken down into three steps as shown.

The energy required for step 2 will depend on the size and shape of the cavity that needs to be created in the solvent to accommodate the solute molecule, and the strength of solvent–solvent bonds. For water, this requires breaking hydrogen bonds between water molecules.

In order for a solute to go into solution, the energy released in step 3 must compensate for energy needed for steps 1 and 2. This is where the attractive forces between the solute and the solvent come into play; strong and numerous solute–solvent interactions will favor solubility.

The solute's molecular size also affects solubility. The larger the molecule (higher its molecular weight), the less soluble the substance is, in general. Larger molecules are more difficult to surround with solvent molecules during the solvation step.

Solid-state Structure of the Drug

Solubility depends partly on the solid-state structure of the solute, because it represents an equilibrium condition between the solute in the solid and solution phases. Many drug substances can exist in more than one solid form with different spatial arrangement of molecules or ions, and thus different intermolecular forces.

Crystalline and Amorphous Drugs

Most drugs are crystalline, in which molecules or ions are arranged in a regular, repetitive pattern called a crystal lattice. Crystalline solids show a definite melting point, converting rather sharply from solid to liquid state over a narrow temperature range. The melting point is an indication of the strength of the crystal lattice; the stronger the lattice, the higher the melting point.

A few drugs are amorphous, with disordered arrangements of molecules and no distinguishable crystal lattice. These materials do not have a characteristic melting temperature but soften over a very wide temperature range, generally lower than the melting points of the crystalline forms of the same compound.

A given drug may exist in several crystalline forms as well as in an amorphous form. For example, chloramphenicol-3-palmitate, a broad-spectrum antibiotic, is known to exist in one amorphous form and at least three different crystalline forms. The crystal lattice of a drug has to be disrupted (step 1, Fig. 4.1) before the drug can dissolve. If the molecules of a drug are held together tightly in the crystal lattice, the driving force for the drug to dissolve is lower. Hence, crystalline drugs have lower intrinsic solubility compared with the same drug in its amorphous form.

A practical illustration of the importance of the solid state structure of the drug is found in insulin, which is available in both amorphous and crystalline forms. The amorphous form has a higher solubility, dissolves faster, and enters the bloodstream rapidly after injection. Thus, it is used when a rapid lowering of blood glucose is needed. The crystalline form has a lower solubility, slower dissolution rate, and enters the blood more gradually. It, therefore, is most appropriate in situations where a slower but more prolonged effect on blood glucose is desired.

Polymorphs

A drug can be crystallized in more than one crystal form; this property is known as polymorphism, and the individual crystal forms are called polymorphs. Different polymorphs arise from differences in the crystallization process during manufacture of the drug. Polymorphs, although chemically identical, generally have different crystal lattice energies, melting points, and solubilities. The polymorph with the lowest melting point usually has the highest solubility. Many pharmaceuticals, such as the barbiturates, sulfonamides, and steroids, exhibit extensive polymorphism.

The different aqueous solubilities of polymorphic forms of a given drug may lead to differences in the rate at which the drug is absorbed into the body after administration. The desire to achieve fast absorption may point to the use of the lower melting polymorph, or an amorphous form, in a drug product. These forms, however, have a tendency to crystallize into the stable, lower solubility form at any stage of the "life cycle" of a pharmaceutical product, i.e., during manufacturing, packaging, distribution, and storage, leading to unexpected changes in behavior. The polymorphic behavior of drugs is a major concern of the pharmaceutical industry because it has considerable implications on formulation design and therapeutic performance.

A classic example of the importance of polymorphism is the drug ritonavir (Norvir®), a protease inhibitor used to treat patients infected with HIV-1. During early development, ritonavir was thought to exist in only one crystalline form. This form, now called Form I, was poorly absorbed after oral administration, requiring formulation as a soft-gelatin capsule filled with an ethanol–water solution of drug. Two years after marketing, several batches of Norvir® capsules were found to be dissolving much slower than expected. Evaluation of failed batches revealed that a second polymorphic form of ritonavir (Form II) had precipitated in the capsules during storage. Form II was only half as soluble as Form I, resulting in the lower rate of dissolution observed. To ensure continuous supply of this life-saving drug, an oral suspension had to be developed until the issue of polymorphic forms was resolved. Substantial time and effort went into identifying and correcting the polymorphism problem, and a new soft-gelatin capsule with Form II was subsequently developed and introduced onto the market.

The Solvent

In order to dissolve in a solvent, the solute molecule needs functional groups that can favorably interact and bond with solvent molecules. Compounds are more likely to dissolve in solvents with similar chemical properties to themselves, a rule of thumb often expressed in the maxim 'like dissolves like.'

Solvent Polarity

Pharmaceutical solvents may be classified as polar, nonpolar or semipolar. Molecules with large dipole moments and high dielectric constants are considered polar. Those with low dipole moments and small dielectric constants are classified as nonpolar, and semipolar solvents fall somewhere in between. The water molecule has a large dipole moment which makes it a polar solvent. Examples of nonpolar solvents are hydrocarbons, oils and lipids. In general, solvents that are miscible with water are polar or semipolar, while those that are not miscible with water are nonpolar.

Water as a Solvent

Water is the most important solvent for us to consider. It is a polar solvent that can interact with many types of functional groups by forming temporary (noncovalent) bonds. Molecules that can interact with water in this way are considered polar, or hydrophilic. The primary interactions that allow solutes to dissolve in water are ones we have discussed earlier, and are listed here.

- *Ion–dipole interaction*: Ion–dipole bonds are formed between an ion and an uncharged polar molecule with a permanent dipole moment, like water. This interaction is very strong and makes water an excellent solvent for ions.
- *Van der Waals Forces*: The attractive forces between electrically neutral molecules are collectively called van der Waals forces. These intermolecular forces are quite weak, and operate only when molecules are fairly close to each other.
- *Dipole–dipole interaction*: Polar molecules with permanent dipole moments but no charge can interact with each other at close distances. Thus, water can interact with drug molecules that have dipoles, even if they are not charged. This interaction is usually weaker than the ion–dipole bond.
- *Dipole-induced dipole interaction*: A polar molecule with a permanent dipole can temporarily induce a dipole in a nonpolar molecule, resulting in an attractive force that brings the two molecules

together. Thus, water can induce a dipole in a nonpolar drug molecule. Obviously, this interaction is very weak and does not contribute significantly to water solubility.

- *Hydrogen bonds*: Hydrogen bonds contribute significantly to aqueous solubility of drugs because water is both a H-bond donor and acceptor. Once one H-bond forms, the probability of a second one forming may be increased, leading to an increased probability of a third forming, and so on. This can lead to a very strong and stable interaction, even though it is made up of individually weak hydrogen bonds.

Ions are very hydrophilic because of the strong ion-dipole interaction. Compounds that can form several hydrogen bonds with water are also very hydrophilic. The polarity ranking of various functional groups is shown in Figure 4.2. In general, hydrophilic compounds dissolve readily in water.

If the solute has several polar functional groups, aqueous solubility will be high because energy released when these groups are solvated more than compensates for energy needed in step 2 (Fig. 4.1). Conversely, water cannot dissolve hydrocarbons because the attraction between water and the hydrocarbon is much less than that between two water molecules. In general, it is the balance between polar and nonpolar groups on the solute that determines the overall balance between steps 2 and 3. As the number of nonpolar groups on a molecule increases (e.g., as alkyl groups are added), aqueous solubility decreases. Drug molecules are complex and most contain several functional groups. It is

Amide > Acid > Alcohol > Ketone ~ Aldehyde > Amine > Ester > Ether > Alkane

Figure 4.2. Order of polarity of common functional groups found on drug molecules, starting with the most polar (amide) and ending with the most nonpolar (alkane).

the relative proportion of polar and non-polar parts of a compound that determines its overall polarity.

Nonpolar Solvents

A nonpolar solvent is one whose molecules do not have a dipole moment, and which has a low dielectric constant. Nonpolar solvents, such as hydrocarbons and lipids, can use only weak van der Waals forces to interact with solutes. These forces are not strong enough to overcome the polar and/or ionic forces that hold electrolyte and weak electrolyte solid solutes together. Consequently, nonpolar solvents are poor solvents for strong electrolytes and ions because they cannot reduce attractive forces between ions. These solvents also cannot break covalent bonds to make weak electrolytes ionize. However, nonpolar solutes that are held together by weak van der Waals forces in the solid state are able to dissolve in nonpolar solvents quite well because of induced dipole interactions.

Molecules that do not have appropriate functional groups to interact with water are considered hydrophobic or nonpolar. In the ranking of functional groups above, ethers and esters are somewhat hydrophobic, with alkanes being the most hydrophobic. Hydrophobic compounds will not dissolve in water to any significant extent, and will actually repel water. This phenomenon is called the hydrophobic effect, the tendency of nonpolar groups or nonpolar compounds to cluster so as to shield themselves from contact with water.

Nonpolar compounds will not dissolve in water but may dissolve in non-polar solvents, such as hydrocarbons, oils, and lipids. Compounds that dissolve in nonpolar solvents are termed lipophilic. A hydrophobic compound is usually lipophilic, but it is possible for a compound to be both hydrophobic and lipophilic, i.e., it does not dissolve in either polar or nonpolar solvents.

Semipolar Solvents

Certain pharmaceutical solvents have properties that fall somewhere between water and lipids. Such solvents, e.g. alcohols and ketones, are miscible with both water and with some lipids. In pharmaceutical products, these liquids are used as cosolvents, along with water, to dissolve nonpolar drugs. They may also be used to make oils and water miscible with one another.

Water Solubility

When a drug product is administered to the body, it usually encounters an aqueous environment in which the drug must dissolve. For example, an orally administered drug must dissolve in gastric fluids. If a drug is not sufficiently water soluble and has trouble dissolving, all of it may not be available to the body. Thus, adequate aqueous solubility is a very important property for a drug.

Intrinsic Aqueous Solubility

For simplicity, first consider a nonelectrolyte drug dissolved in water. Its aqueous solubility is the concentration of a saturated solution of the compound in water at a given temperature. In a saturated solution, the solid form of the drug is in equilibrium with drug in solution, as follows:

$$\text{Drug}_{\text{solid}} \rightleftharpoons \text{Drug}_{\text{solution}} \qquad \text{(Eq. 4.1)}$$

This means further addition of solid drug will not change the solution concentration because no more can dissolve. The equilibrium constant K is given by

$$K = \frac{[\text{Drug}]_{\text{solution}}}{[\text{Drug}]_{\text{solid}}} \qquad \text{(Eq. 4.2)}$$

The numerator of Equation 4.2 is the concentration of drug dissolved in the saturated solution. The denominator is, by convention, set equal to 1. The constant K is called the intrinsic solubility (S_0) of the nonelectrolyte drug in water at the temperature of the experiment; in other words, S_0 is the concentration of the saturated solution of drug, as shown in Equation 4.3:

$$S_0 = K = [\text{Drug}]_{\text{solution}} \quad \text{(Eq. 4.3)}$$

Intrinsic water solubility depends on the drug's chemical and solid-state structures, and on the temperature. The intrinsic solubility of most compounds increases as temperature increases, so solubility is always stated along with the temperature of measurement. The temperatures of interest for pharmaceutical application are normal body temperature (37°C) and controlled room temperature (15–30°C).

Solubility of Weak Acids and Bases

Ionization of weak acids and bases in water complicates the solubility equation. For drugs that ionize, observed solubility depends not only on the intrinsic solubility of the un-ionized drug but on the extent of ionization as well. In general, aqueous solubility of ions is much greater than solubility of the corresponding un-ionized form, because of the ability of water to form additional ion–dipole bonds with ionized drug. Therefore, it is the intrinsic solubility (solubility of the un-ionized form) that limits the overall solubility of a weak electrolyte.

When a solid weak electrolyte drug (weak acid or weak base) is added to an aqueous medium, it will dissolve to the extent of the intrinsic solubility of the un-ionized form. The dissolved drug will ionize in accordance with the Henderson–Hasselbalch equation and pH of the aqueous medium. As the drug ionizes, more solid drug will dissolve to maintain a saturated solution of the un-ionized form of drug. This process will continue until both the solubility equilibrium and ionization equilibrium are satisfied.

We can write the following equations to describe how a weak acid or weak base dissolves and ionizes in a buffered solution:

$$\text{HA}_{\text{solid}} \rightleftharpoons \text{HA}_{\text{solution}} \rightleftharpoons \text{H}^+ + \text{A}^- \quad \text{(Eq. 4.4)}$$

$$\text{B}_{\text{solid}} \rightleftharpoons \text{B}_{\text{solution}} + \text{H}^+ \rightleftharpoons \text{BH}^+ \quad \text{(Eq. 4.5)}$$

The saturated solutions of weak acids and bases will contain some ionized and some un-ionized forms of the drug, depending on the pH of the buffer. The observed solubility, S_t, therefore, is the total concentration of drug (ionized and un-ionized) in solution, as shown by the following equations:

$$\text{Weak acid}: S_t = [\text{HA}]_{\text{solution}} + [\text{A}^-] \quad \text{(Eq. 4.6)}$$

$$\text{Weak base}: S_t = [\text{B}]_{\text{solution}} + [\text{BH}^+] \quad \text{(Eq. 4.7)}$$

The concentration of un-ionized drug in the saturated solution is always equal to the intrinsic solubility of the drug, S_0. Therefore, we can rewrite Equations 4.6 and 4.7 as follows:

$$\text{Weak acid}: S_t = S_{0(\text{HA})} + [\text{A}^-] \quad \text{(Eq. 4.8)}$$

$$\text{Weak base}: S_t = S_{0(\text{B})} + [\text{BH}^+] \quad \text{(Eq. 4.9)}$$

Knowing the concentration of the un-ionized form, the pK_a of the drug, and the pH of the medium, allows us to calculate the concentration of the ionized forms using the Henderson–Hasselbalch equation. After incorporating these relationships into Equations 4.8 and 4.9, simplifying and converting into a more convenient logarithmic form, we get the following general equations:

$$\text{Weak acid}: \ S_t = S_0(1 + 10^{(\text{pH} - pK_a)})$$
$$\text{(Eq. 4.10)}$$

$$\text{Weak base}: \ S_t = S_0(1 + 10^{(pK_a - \text{pH})})$$
$$\text{(Eq. 4.11)}$$

These equations can be used to calculate the total solubility of a drug at any pH if the pK_a and intrinsic solubility are known. Conversely, if pK_a and total solubility at a given pH are known, the intrinsic solubility may be calculated. By inspection of Equations 4.10 and 4.11, we can see that the total solubility of a weak acid or base changes (increases or decreases) by a factor of 10 for every 1 unit change in pH.

pH–Solubility Profiles

Figure 4.3 shows a graphical representation of the pH–solubility profiles for a weak acid and a weak base. The graphs show that if the pH of the solution allows ionization of a weak electrolyte drug, total solubility will be greater than intrinsic solubility. As the degree of ionization increases, total solubility of the drug also increases. If the pH of the solution keeps the drug essentially un-ionized, total solubility is equal to intrinsic solubility of the drug. A weak base will show higher solubility at a low pH and a lower solubility at a high pH. A weak acid will show a higher solubility at a high pH and a lower solubility at a low pH. The terms "low" and "high" are always relative to the pK_a of the drug.

Solubility of Drug Salts

Many weak acid and weak base drugs are available as their salts. The physical properties of salts (crystal structure, melting point, and so forth) are usually very different from those of their parent weak acid or weak base. However, salt formation does not change the pK_a or the intrinsic solubility of a weak acid or weak base. Therefore, in a *buffered* solution, total solubility of a weak acid and its salt (or a weak base and its salt) is usually the same and will be represented by the pH–solubility profiles shown in Figure 4.3.

Solubility in Unbuffered Solutions

We have seen that when weak acids, bases, or their salts are dissolved in an *unbuffered*

solution, the pH of the solution changes. When a weak acid is dissolved in water to make a saturated solution, the pH of the solution becomes lower than the pK_a of the acid, resulting in a low solubility. Conversely, when a *salt* of a weak acid is dissolved in water to make a saturated solution, the solution pH increases above the pK_a, resulting in a higher solubility. Analogous behavior is seen with weak bases and their salts.

One may generalize and say that solutions of salts in unbuffered solutions promote a pH that is on the ionized side of the pK_a of the drug. Therefore, salts appear to have a higher solubility in water than their parent weak acid or base, primarily due to a change in solution pH. If the pH of the solution were to be measured, the total solubility of a weak electrolyte or its salt will be as shown in Figure 4.3.

Solubility Product of Salts

Equations 4.8 and 4.9 predict that total solubility will increase infinitely as extent of ionization increases. However, the solubility of the ionized form of drug is actually limited by the type and concentration of the counter-ions present in solution. For example, for a completely ionized weak acid in solution, solubility is generally higher if the counter-ions in solution are Na^+, rather than Ca^+-. In other words, the calcium salt of the weak acid may be less soluble than the sodium salt. In the solid state, salts exist as ionic crystals with ions occupying crystal lattice points. In general, more stable lattices are formed by cations and anions that are relatively close in size, thus making such salts less soluble.

Thus, at pH values where the weak acid is almost completely ionized, the total solubility is determined by the type of salt (e.g., Na or Ca) that can be formed in solution. A more stable, less soluble salt may precipitate out in this situation if the concentration of counter-ions is large enough. The solubility of salts is characterized by a special constant called

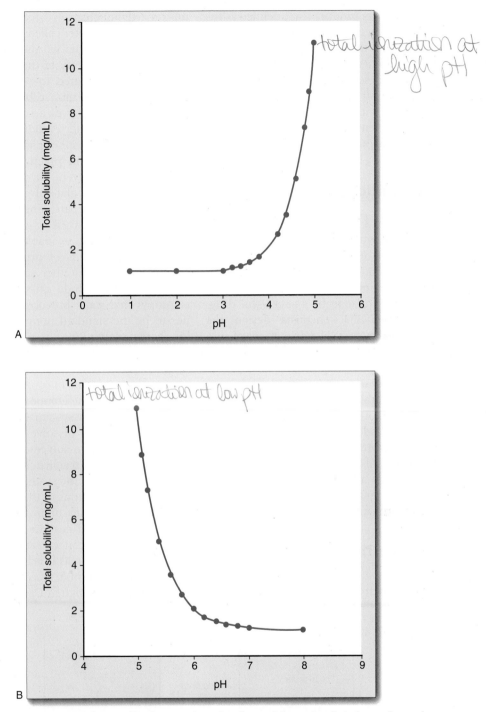

total ionization at high pH

total ionization at low pH

Figure 4.3. The pH–solubility profiles for a weak acid and a weak base. Graph A shows the total solubility as a function of pH for a weak acid of $pK_a = 4$. Graph B shows the total solubility as a function of pH for a weak base of $pK_a = 6$. Both compounds have an intrinsic solubility of 1 mg/mL.

the solubility product (K_{sp}), defined as the equilibrium constant of the dissociation reaction of the salt in a saturated solution. A discussion of solubility product is outside the scope of this book. The main point to note is that salts of weak acids and bases with different counter-ions will have different solubilities at pHs where the drug is predominantly ionized.

Lipophilicity

In Chapter 2, we learned that drugs need to be somewhat lipophilic to bind to their targets and to cross cell membranes. In fact, a compound must have an appropriate balance of hydrophilic and lipophilic properties for it to be a successful drug. Thus, medicinal chemists design the chemical structure of a drug to make sure the molecule is somewhat compatible with both aqueous and lipid environments.

Rather than characterizing lipophilicity or lipid solubility per se, a more important consideration is the *relative* affinity of a drug for lipid and aqueous environments. In other words, we are most interested in the ability of a drug to dissolve in a lipid phase when an aqueous phase is present, and vice versa, because this mimics typical situations found in the body.

The Partition Coefficient

The balance between lipophilicity and hydrophilicity of a compound in its un-ionized, nonelectrolyte form is characterized by a parameter called its partition coefficient P. In other words, P is a measure of relative affinity of the compound for lipids as compared to water. In the laboratory, P is determined by measuring the relative solubility of a compound in water and in a lipid. Although biological lipids (e.g., phospholipids) would be most appropriate, in practice we use a model nonpolar solvent for convenience. The choice of nonpolar solvent has been subject to much debate. The most commonly used solvent is n-octanol, and extensive data are available for partitioning of thousands of drugs between octanol and water. Other solvents used more recently include chloroform and isopropyl myristate, but octanol continues to be the standard nonpolar solvent for characterizing P.

Water and octanol are immiscible with each other. Determination of P involves placing these solvents in contact with one other and adding the compound of interest to this two-phase system. Molecules of the compound will dissolve and distribute between the two solvents, or phases, until equilibrium is reached, as illustrated in Figure 4.4. After the system is at equilibrium, concentrations of the compound in each phase are measured.

If the compound is more hydrophilic than lipophilic, its concentration in water will be higher, whereas if it is more lipophilic than hydrophilic, its concentration in octanol will be higher. Denoting C_o as

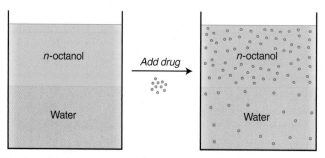

Figure 4.4. Partitioning of a drug compound between octanol and water. In this example, more drug is in the octanol phase than in the aqueous phase at equilibrium.

the concentration in octanol and C_w as the concentration in water, the partition coefficient (P) is defined as

$$P = \frac{C_o}{C_w} \qquad \text{(Eq. 4.12)}$$

Thus, P provides a measure of the relative affinity of a compound for octanol and water. A compound with $P = 1$ has equal affinity for octanol and water. A P value greater than one implies the compound is lipophilic; the larger the value of P, the greater its lipophilicity. A P value less than one implies a compound is hydrophilic; the smaller the value, the lower its lipophilicity. In general, the amount of compound added during the experiment has no effect on the measured P.

Remember that partition coefficient is defined only for the *un-ionized* form of a drug. For a weak electrolyte, this means that P is measured at a pH at which the compound is entirely un-ionized. In this respect, partition coefficient is analogous to the intrinsic solubility of a compound; both are dependent on the chemical structure of the drug, but without the complication of ionization. Later, we will examine the effect of ionization of a compound on its partitioning behavior.

The Log P Value

Partition coefficient is often stated as a logarithmic value ($\log P$) for convenience. The log P of thousands of drugs and potential drugs has been measured over the years. We can make some generalizations about the viability of a compound as a drug based on this large data set.

A compound with $\log P < 0$ (or $P < 1$) is usually considered too hydrophilic to be a suitable drug candidate, particularly if it must cross lipophilic biological membranes to reach its site of action. At the other extreme, compounds with $\log P > 3.5$ (or $P > 3000$) are usually too lipophilic to be good drugs because they tend to be poorly

soluble in aqueous biological fluids, or tend to concentrate in lipid environments. However, some successful drugs have log P values that lie outside the desirable range of $0 < \log P < 3.5$, showing that the body is more complex than simple physicochemical approximations make it out to be. Nevertheless, the partition coefficient is still useful as a simple in vitro parameter to help predict the behavior of a drug in the body, and select a promising drug candidate from a large pool of compounds.

Apparent Partition Coefficient

The definition of partition coefficient applies to only the un-ionized form of the compound. Ionization of an electrolyte complicates partitioning behavior. The apparent partition coefficient (P_{app}) of a compound is defined as the ratio of the sum of the concentrations of *all* forms of the compound (ionized plus un-ionized) between octanol and the aqueous phase, and is given by

$$P_{app} = \frac{(C_i)_o + (C_u)_o}{(C_i)_w + (C_u)_w} \qquad \text{(Eq. 4.13)}$$

Here, C_i and C_u are the concentrations of the ionized and un-ionized forms, respectively. Weak acids and bases ionize to some extent in water, depending on their pK_a and the pH of the aqueous phase. Electrolytes cannot ionize in lipids or octanol because these nonpolar solvents cannot stabilize ionic charge. In other words, the ionized form of a drug can be present in the aqueous phase, but cannot partition into octanol. Therefore, $C_i \sim 0$ and Equation 4.13 can be simplified as follows:

$$P_{app} = \frac{C_o}{(C_i + C_u)_w} \qquad \text{(Eq. 4.14)}$$

When the influence of pH on partitioning is studied, a buffer is used to maintain the pH of the aqueous phase at the desired value. Two equilibrium conditions have to be satisfied in these situations:

- The ratio of ionized to un-ionized drug in the aqueous phase must obey the Henderson–Hasselbalch equation.
- The un-ionized form has to partition between the two phases as governed by its partition coefficient.

Consequently, ionization in the aqueous phase decreases the amount of un-ionized form available to distribute into octanol.

If the buffered aqueous phase pH causes practically all the drug to be in its un-ionized form, then $C_i = 0$ and Equation 4.14 can be written as follows:

$$P_{app} = \frac{C_o}{(C_u)_w} = P \qquad \text{(Eq. 4.15)}$$

Therefore, the apparent partition coefficient P_{app} is equal to the partition coefficient P when the drug is completely un-ionized. Performing a partition coefficient measurement at an aqueous pH at which ionization is negligible is one way of determining the P of weak acid and base drugs. Figures 4.5 and 4.6 illustrate partitioning equilibria of a weak acid and weak base between octanol and a buffer.

If the aqueous phase pH allows some drug molecules to ionize, $P_{app} < P$. In such cases, P_{app} can be related to P if the fraction (α) of drug ionized in the aqueous phase is known. The value of α is easily determined using the Henderson–Hasselbalch equation if pK_a of the drug and pH of the aqueous phase are known. Inasmuch as only un-ionized drug can partition into octanol

$$P = \frac{P_{app}}{(1-\alpha)} \qquad \text{(Eq. 4.16)}$$

This equation applies if $\alpha < 1$. If pH is such that the entire drug is ionized and

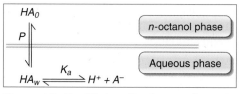

Figure 4.5. Equilibrium distribution of a weak acid between octanol and water. The extent of ionization in the aqueous phase depends on the pK_a of the acid and the pH of the aqueous phase. Only the un-ionized form HA (partition coefficient = P) can distribute into n-octanol. This system must obey the following relationships at equilibrium:

$$\log \frac{[HA]_w}{[A^-]_w} = pK_a - pH$$

$$\frac{[HA]_o}{[HA]_w} = P$$

The apparent partition coefficient P_{app} of the weak acid between octanol and aqueous phases is given by

$$P_{app} = \frac{[HA]_o}{[HA]_w + [A^-]_w}$$

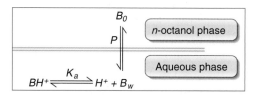

Figure 4.6. Equilibrium distribution of a weak base between octanol and water. The extent of ionization in the aqueous phase depends on the pK_a of the base and the pH of the aqueous solution. Only the un-ionized form B (partition coefficient = P) can distribute into n-octanol. The following relationships must be obeyed by this system at equilibrium:

$$\log \frac{[BH^+]_w}{[B]_w} = pK_a - pH$$

$$\frac{[B]_o}{[B]_w} = P$$

The apparent partition coefficient P_{app} of the weak base between octanol and aqueous phases is given by

$$P_{app} = \frac{[B]_o}{[B]_w + [BH^+]_w}$$

$\alpha = 1$, then there is no un-ionized drug in the aqueous phase to distribute into octanol, and $P_{app} = 0$.

A more convenient way of calculating P_{app} when the pH and pK_a are known is by using the following equations:

$$\text{Weak acid: } P_{app} = \frac{P}{1 + 10^{(pH - pK_a)}}$$

(Eq. 4.17)

$$\text{Weak base: } P_{app} = \frac{P}{1 + 10^{(pK_a - pH)}}$$

(Eq. 4.18)

Therefore, a drug with a large partition coefficient may be so extensively ionized in aqueous body fluids that very little drug is able to cross into the lipid phase. The apparent partition coefficient of the drug will be close to zero under these conditions. This concept is important because biological membranes contain lipids, and the ability of drugs to penetrate into these membranes will depend not only on the P and pK_a of the drug but also on the pH of surrounding fluids.

Importance of Partition Coefficient

The apparent partition coefficient of a drug has a strong influence on the ADME behavior of a drug. For rapid and complete dissolution, a drug must be sufficiently hydrophilic. For efficient absorption, the drug needs to cross lipid membranes of cells. If it is too lipophilic, it will accumulate in the lipid membranes and will not partition out again. Therefore, the apparent partition coefficient controls the rate of absorption and distribution of a drug. Distribution patterns, in turn, play a role in how rapidly a drug is metabolized and excreted.

The hydrophobic effect, or the affinity of hydrophobic compounds for each other,

is an important driving force for binding of drugs to proteins and for drug–target interactions. However, very lipophilic drugs also tend to be more toxic. Thus, an appropriate balance of hydrophilic and lipophilic properties is important for almost all aspects of a drugs disposition and action.

Amphiphilicity

As we have discussed, compounds that have both hydrophilic and lipophilic groups on the molecule can dissolve to some extent in both lipids and in water. The relative affinity for water and lipid is characterized by the partition coefficient of the molecule. Some molecules have their hydrophilic functional groups located at one end of the molecule and their hydrophobic functional groups at the other end. Such molecules, which have distinct hydrophilic and lipophilic regions, are amphipathic and are called amphiphiles. Examples of amphiphiles include soaps and detergents, fatty acids, and phospholipids. Some drugs also show amphiphilic properties; examples are amiodarone (Cordarone®), imipramine (Tofranil®), and promethazine (Phenergan®).

The lipophilic group (called the *tail*) in amphiphilic compounds is typically a long chain hydrocarbon moiety, such as $-CH_2(CH_2)_n-$, with $n > 4$. The hydrophilic or polar group (called the *head*) can be one or more of the following:

- Uncharged, such as an alcohol or glycol.
- Anionic, such as a phosphate, sulfate, carboxylate or sulfonate.
- Cationic, such as a protonated amine, or quaternary ammonium group.

Again, the relative proportion of hydrophobic and hydrophilic groups determines whether the amphiphile is more soluble in water or lipids.

Effect on Surface Tension

Rather than simply partitioning between lipids and water, amphiphiles are able to orient themselves at the lipid–water interface such that the tails are in the lipid and the head groups are in the aqueous phase, forming a monolayer at the interface. This property of amphiphiles is useful in stabilizing emulsions of oil and water, and amphiphilic compounds are often used as inert ingredients (excipients) in pharmaceutical products.

Amphiphiles, when dissolved in water, can also form monolayers at the air–water interface. This spontaneous behavior occurs because the head groups are attracted to water, whereas the tails are repelled and try to remove themselves from water, toward air. This behavior, driven by the exclusion of nonpolar sections or residues of a molecule from water, is called a hydrophobic interaction. Orientation of an amphiphile at the air–water interface results in lowering of the surface tension of water. We see an application of this behavior in the sudsing of soaps solutions and the formation of foams. In Chapter 2, we saw that such hydrophobic interactions between the nonpolar groups of a drug and its target are also important in protein–ligand binding.

Monolayers of an amphiphile can also form at the interface between an amphiphile solution and a hydrophobic solid. Thus, amphiphiles are used as *wetting agents*, allowing water to maintain contact with a hydrophobic solid. Amphiphilic excipients are used in many suspensions and solid dosage forms. Monolayer formation of amphiphiles is illustrated in Figure 4.7.

Micelle Formation

Monolayer formation is possible at fairly low concentrations of the amphiphile. At higher concentrations, amphiphiles can

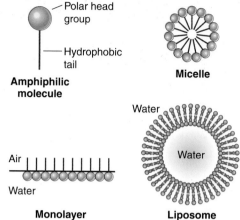

Figure 4.7. Organization of amphiphilic molecules into monolayers, bilayers, micelles, and liposomes (*not to scale*).

also form unique, organized structures when exposed to water, as illustrated in Figure 4.7. Hydrophobic bonding may cause some amphiphiles to aggregate into structures known as micelles, in which the hydrophobic tails are in the interior, away from water, and polar heads form the outer surface. By gathering hydrophobic groups together in the center of the micelle, disruption of the hydrogen-bonded structure of liquid water is minimized. Polar head groups extend into the surrounding water where they can participate in hydrogen bonding. Micelles, which can be made up of 50 or more molecules, are often spherical in shape, but may also assume cylindrical or other shapes.

Certain amphiphilic molecules organize into stable sheet-like structures called bilayers more readily than they form micelles; e.g. phospholipids that form the lipid bilayer of cell membranes. Bilayers can also form small vesicle-like structures termed vesicles or liposomes, which have been used as specialized drug delivery systems.

Key Concepts

Hydrophilicity Versus Lipophilicity of Drugs

- Aqueous solubility is a measure of hydrophilicity, and partition coefficient is a measure of lipophilicity of a drug.
- A high partition coefficient often goes hand-in-hand with poor intrinsic solubility; i.e., functional groups that enhance water solubility make a drug less lipid soluble, and vice versa.
- Ionization behavior of a drug molecule has a strong impact on total water solubility and apparent partition coefficient.

General Principles of Aqueous Drug Solubility

- The intrinsic solubility depends on the polarity of the drug molecule and the structure of the solid state.
- Intrinsic solubility does not depend on pH of the aqueous medium.

Solubility of Weak Acid Drugs

- Total solubility increases as pH increases (and the drug ionizes).
- The lowest solubility will be reached at pH values about 3 units below the pK_a; this will be the intrinsic solubility of the weak acid.

Solubility of Weak Base Drugs

- Total solubility increases as pH decreases (and the drug ionizes).
- The lowest solubility will be reached at pH values 3 units above the pK_a; this will be the intrinsic solubility of the weak base.

Solubility of Salts of Weak Acids and Bases

- Solubility of salts in buffered solutions is the same as the solubility of the parent weak acid or base.
- Solubility of salts in unbuffered solutions is higher than the corresponding weak acid or base because the pH changes to favor ionization of the drug.

General Principles for Partitioning of Drugs

- The partition coefficient of a drug depends on its chemical structure.
- The partition coefficient is defined for the un-ionized drug and does not vary with pH.
- The *apparent* partition coefficient of weak acids and bases changes with pH of the aqueous phase.
- The apparent partition coefficient of a weak acid decreases as pH increases.
- The apparent partition coefficient of a weak base decreases as pH decreases.

Review Questions

1. Why does a drug need to have both hydrophilic and lipophilic properties?
2. What determines the intrinsic solubility of a weak acid or weak base?
3. What is polymorphism? How does it affect intrinsic solubility?

4. Describe the change in total solubility of a weak acid and weak base as the pH *decreases* below the pK_a.

5. Describe the change in total solubility of a weak acid and weak base as the pH *increases* above the pK_a.

6. Why do salts of weak acids and bases appear to have a higher water solubility than the parent acid or base?

7. What is meant by the partition coefficient of a compound? How is it measured?

8. What is meant by log *P*? What is the approximate range of desirable log *P* values for a drug? What is the problem if the log *P* value is outside this range?

9. Describe the change in apparent partition coefficient of a weak acid and weak base as the pH *decreases* below the pK_a.

10. Describe the change in apparent partition coefficient of a weak acid and weak base as the pH *increases* above the pK_a.

Practice Problems

1. Consult the information about naproxen given in Problem 4 of Chapter 2.
   a. A saturated solution of naproxen is made in a buffer at pH 3, and a buffer at pH 6. Which solution will have a higher concentration, and why?
   b. If the intrinsic solubility of naproxen is 0.0001 M, calculate the total solubility when naproxen is dissolved in a buffer of pH 4.2. Express the solubility in units of mg/mL.

2. Consult the information about cimetidine given in Problem 5 of Chapter 2.
   a. Is cimetidine more soluble in stomach fluids or in small intestinal fluids?
   b. Cimetidine and cimetidine hydrochloride are allowed to dissolve in water (unbuffered) until the solutions are saturated. Which solution will have a higher concentration? Why?
   c. Cimetidine and cimetidine hydrochloride are allowed to dissolve in a pH 7 buffer until the solutions are saturated. Which solution will have a higher concentration? Why?

3. A new drug is a sodium salt of a carboxylic acid. It has a molecular weight = 150, a pK_a = 5, and an intrinsic solubility = 0.002 M. What is the maximum concentration of drug that can be dissolved in a buffer at pH 6? Give the concentration in both molar and mg/mL units.

4. A partition coefficient experiment was carried out with a nonelectrolyte drug. Drug was added to an *n*-octanol–water system that contained 100 mL of each solvent and allowed to equilibrate. At equilibrium, the concentration of drug in the octanol phase was 0.52 M and in the aqueous phase was 0.33 M.
   a. What is the partition coefficient of the drug?
   b. What is the log *P*?
   c. Will the partition coefficient change if the pH of the aqueous phase is changed?

5. Diphenhydramine (Benadryl®) is an antihistamine and has the following structure:

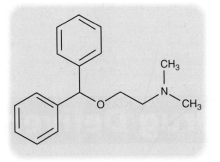

The *n*-octanol–water partition coefficient of diphenhydramine is 3500, and its $pK_a = 9.0$.

a. What is the log *P* value of diphenhydramine? Would you call this drug more hydrophilic or lipophilic?

b. Will the apparent partition coefficient of diphenhydramine be greater at pH 7 or at pH 9? Calculate the apparent partition coefficient at pH 7 and at pH 9.

c. Will the aqueous solubility of diphenhydramine be greater in a buffer of pH 7 or a buffer of pH 9?

d. If you wanted to make a salt of diphenhydramine, would you react it with an acid or a base?

6. Warfarin (Coumadin®) is an anticoagulant drug. It is a weak acid with a $pK_a = 5.1$ and a log *P* = 0.9.

a. Calculate the partition coefficient of warfarin.

b. Will warfarin be more ionized at pH 2 or pH 7? Calculate the fraction ionized at each of these pH values.

c. Will the apparent partition coefficient be higher at pH 2 or at pH 7? Calculate these apparent partition coefficient values.

d. If 100 mg of warfarin is added to an *n*-octanol–buffer experiment, calculate the total milligrams in the octanol phase and in the buffer phase at pH 2 and at pH 7.

e. Will warfarin be more water soluble at pH 2 or pH 7?

Additional Readings

Amiji M, Sandmann BJ. Applied Physical Pharmacy, 1st ed. McGraw-Hill/Appleton & Lange, 2003.

Florence AT, Attwood D. Physicochemical Principles of Pharmacy, 4th ed. Pharmaceutical Press, 2006.

Martin AN, Bustamante P. Physical Pharmacy—Physical Chemical Principles in the Pharmaceutical Sciences, 4th ed. Lippincott Williams & Wilkins, 1993.

Sinko, PJ. Martin's Physical Pharmacy and Pharmaceutical Sciences, 5th ed. Lippincott Williams & Wilkins, 2006.

Drug Delivery

> Nothing can be more incorrect
> than the assumption one
> sometimes meets with, that
> physics has one method,
> chemistry another, and
> biology a third.
> —Thomas Henry Huxley

Chapter 5   Transport Across Biological Barriers

Chapter 6   Drug Absorption

Chapter 7   Drug Delivery Systems

Transport Across Biological Barriers

A chemical compound is not a drug unless it affects the human body in some way. In earlier chapters, we examined important physicochemical properties of drugs and gained an understanding of how drugs interact with their targets to exert a biological response. For most drugs, the targets are some distance away from the site of administration. The effectiveness of a drug, at least in part, depends on how much and how rapidly it reaches its site of action. Thousands of compounds may show biological activity in test tubes, but few are viable drugs because most cannot withstand our body's biological barriers and reach their targets.

In this chapter, we will examine the different mechanisms by which drug molecules (and other molecules in the body) move in and out of cells, and travel from tissue to tissue. In subsequent chapters, we will integrate this biological information with the drug's physicochemical and kinetic properties to gain insight into drug action and behavior.

The cell is the smallest fundamental structural and functional unit in our body. Everything between the cell membrane and the nucleus is the cytoplasm. It is composed of the *cytosol* (primarily water with dissolved salts, nutrients, gases, enzymes, and proteins), components of the *cytoskel-eton*, and various *organelles* (such as ribosomes, endoplasmic reticulum, and Golgi apparatus). The cytosol is often called the intracellular fluid, separated from the extracellular fluid (the aqueous region outside the cell) by the cell membrane. The target for a drug may be inside the cell, somewhere in or on the cell membrane or in the extracellular fluid. Depending on its size, structure and physicochemical properties, a drug may or may not be able to enter a particular cell.

Cells are often arranged into groups called tissues, representing the next level of organization in the body. Cells in a tissue have similar structural and functional characteristics and, together, can impart additional properties. The four main types of tissues are muscle tissue, nervous tissue, connective tissue, and epithelial tissue. The latter is of particular interest to us, because it functions as the barrier that controls movement of drugs into, within, and out of the body. Such multicellular tissue barriers are often called *functional membranes.*

A drug may have to cross several types of epithelial tissues to reach its site of action, and eventually, its target. For example, when a drug is administered orally, it must cross the intestinal lining before it can enter the bloodstream. From the bloodstream, the drug must leave capillaries through the capillary wall and enter various organs and tissues, including the site of action. Many endogenous ligands must also travel from their site of synthesis to reach their targets; this may involve crossing the capillary wall and other tissues. Depending on its size, structure, and physicochemical properties, a molecule may or may not be able to cross a particular functional membrane.

In this chapter, we will first learn about the different mechanisms by which a molecule can cross the cell membrane. Then we will use these concepts to further explore how a molecule can cross a functional membrane such as an epithelial membrane.

Transport Across the Cell Membrane

The cell membrane or plasma membrane is the outermost layer of a cell. Its major functions are to

- hold together the aqueous cell contents (*structure*)
- separate cellular contents from the aqueous external fluid (*barrier*)
- respond to the environment (*sensitivity*)
- control transport of substances in and out of the cell (*regulation*)

This chapter will focus on the regulation function of the cell membrane; the different mechanisms by which the cell membrane controls transport and movement of molecules and ions between extracellular and intracellular fluids. To understand how a cell membrane regulates transport, we first need to review its structure.

Components of Cell Membranes

The primary constituents of the cell membrane are lipids, proteins, and carbohydrates attached to these lipids and proteins. A brief review of these biomol-

ecules is presented here. More complete discussions of the structure and properties of lipids, proteins, and carbohydrates can be found in introductory biochemistry textbooks; suggestions are included at the end of this chapter.

Lipids are a wide variety of structurally diverse biomolecules primarily made up of nonpolar groups. As a result of their hydrophobic character, lipids typically dissolve more readily in nonpolar solvents than in water. The hydrophobicity of lipid molecules drives them out of contact with water and causes them to cluster into structures such as the bilayer of the cell membrane. Lipids can link covalently with carbohydrates to form glycolipids and with proteins to form lipoproteins.

Proteins are macromolecular chains built from amino acids, which coil or fold to adopt a characteristic three-dimensional structure. This overall structural organization gives each protein its unique three-dimensional configuration and determines its properties. The tertiary and quaternary folded structure of a protein depends on the surrounding environment. A protein will fold spontaneously to adopt and preserve a conformation most compatible with its surroundings.

Carbohydrates are compounds named for their characteristic content of carbon, hydrogen, and oxygen, which occur in the ratio of 1:2:1. They are very important as our body's fuel and energy stores, and form the structural framework of DNA and RNA. Short chains containing three to seven carbons are called monosaccharides or sugars, the individual building blocks of carbohydrates. Monosaccharides in the ring form can link together through a glycoside bond to form oligosaccharides or, in greater numbers, polysaccharides.

A glycoconjugate is a complex hybrid molecule made up of a carbohydrate and a noncarbohydrate portion. The two major types of glycoconjugates of interest in cell membranes are glycoproteins and glycolipids. The carbohydrate confers specific biological functions on the proteins and lipids carrying them. When embedded in the cell membrane, they cover the cell surface with specific oligosaccharide structures that are often crucial to cell function.

The Lipid Bilayer

The *fluid mosaic model* provides a good, simple description of cell membrane structure. It proposes that the basic structural unit of almost all cell membranes is the lipid bilayer in which a variety of proteins are embedded. It also depicts the cell membrane as a fluid structure in which many of the constituent molecules are free to diffuse in the plane of the membrane.

Phospholipids. The primary lipids of biological membranes are phospholipids, a group of phosphate-containing molecules. Glycerol forms the backbone of most common phospholipids, with one hydroxyl

linked to a phosphate group. The two other hydroxyl groups are esterified with carboxyl groups of two fatty acids, which can be either saturated or unsaturated. Fatty acids of phospholipids usually contain an even number of carbons, e.g., myristic acid (14 carbons), palmitic acid (16 carbons), and arachidonic acid (20 carbons).

The other end of the phosphate bridge links to an alcohol, most commonly a nitrogen-containing alcohol such as *choline*. Other alcohols that may link at this position include ethanolamine, serine, threonine, and inositol; the alcohol gives the phospholipid its name (e.g., *phosphatidylcholine, phosphatidylserine*). Phosphatidylcholine is a major component of most cellular membranes. Each phospholipid is actually a family of closely related molecules because different fatty acids may bind at the 1- and 2-carbons of the glycerol residue. Figure 5.1 illustrates the structure of a typical phospholipid molecule.

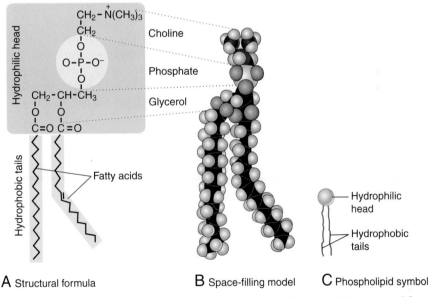

Figure 5.1. Structure of a typical phospholipid, phosphatidylcholine. A and B. Structural formula and space-filling model of phosphatidylcholine. Note that the fatty acids (one of which is unsaturated) make up the hydrophobic portion, whereas the hydrophilic portion includes glycerol, phosphate, and the alcohol (choline in this case). Note further that the hydrophilic head is zwitterionic because phosphate is negatively charged and choline is ionized and positively charged at physiological pH. C. Cartoon of phospholipid molecules as shown in diagrams of cell membranes.

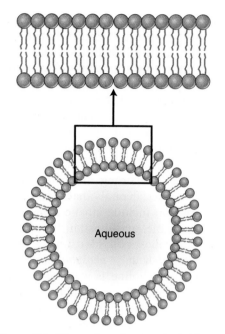

Figure 5.2. Illustration of a phospholipid bilayer. Note that the bilayer is composed of two layers of phospholipid molecules with their polar head groups facing outward. The bilayer forms closed structures with aqueous inner and outer compartments.

The phosphate group on the phospholipid molecule carries a negative charge, whereas the alcohol may be positively charged because of ionization of the amine group. Thus, a phospholipid may be either negatively charged or zwitterionic (no net charge) at physiological pH.

Phospholipids are amphiphilic lipids; recall that amphiphilic molecules have a hydrophobic part and a hydrophilic part, enabling them to organize into various structures such as micelles and bilayers as a result of hydrophobic bonding. In the phospholipid molecule, fatty acids make up the hydrophobic "tail" whereas the polar alcohol end makes up the polar "head group." Thus, phospholipids can spontaneously assemble to form a *lipid bilayer*, as illustrated in Figure 5.2.

Characteristics of the Bilayer. The bilayer is a sheet-like structure composed of two layers of phospholipid molecules whose polar alcohol head groups face the surrounding water and whose fatty acid chains form a continuous hydrophobic interior. The bilayer is closed, separating intracellular and extracellular aqueous compartments of the cell. It is held together by hydrophobic and van der Waals interactions between fatty acid chains of phospholipid molecules and hydrogen bonding and electrostatic interactions between polar head groups and water molecules.

Other amphiphilic or lipophilic molecules such as steroids (e.g., cholesterol), fatty acids, and so forth are interspersed in the bilayer. These compounds are present in different amounts in different types of cells in our body. The unique lipid composition of each membrane contributes to the fluidity or rigidity of the membrane. The melting temperature of this complex lipid mixture is below normal body temperature, making the bilayer mobile, like a viscous fluid. Thermal motion allows phospholipids and other molecules in the bilayer to rotate freely around their long axes and to diffuse sideways within the membrane.

The hydrophobic interior of the lipid bilayer restricts movement of molecules; ions and other polar compounds pass very slowly or not at all through the bilayer, whereas small lipophilic compounds can cross the bilayer readily.

Cellular Proteins

Although the lipid bilayer provides the framework of the cell membrane, other types of molecules, such as proteins, are also present. The presence of these proteins modifies the properties of the bilayer considerably.

Soluble Proteins. Soluble proteins, such as plasma proteins and enzymes, are found in aqueous environments in the body (intracellular and extracellular fluids) and adopt specific confirmations compatible with water. The interior of the folded protein molecule contains a high proportion of hydrophobic amino acids, which tend to cluster and exclude water. The exterior of the folded protein is primarily composed of hydrophilic amino acids that are charged or able to hydrogen bond with water, making the protein water soluble. Soluble proteins are usually globular and tightly packed.

Membrane Proteins. Membrane proteins are located in or near the hydrophobic region of the lipid bilayer of cell membranes. Proteins that sit on the inner or outer surface of the cell membrane (extrinsic or *peripheral* proteins) are folded such that a large percentage of their hydrophobic amino acids are close to or anchored within the membrane lipids. Amino acids facing aqueous environments of the cytoplasm or extracellular fluid are mostly hydrophilic, allowing the protein to be compatible with water.

Proteins embedded in the lipid bilayer are called intrinsic or *integral* proteins; most of these have a portion that extends out into the aqueous environment on the outer or inner surface of the bilayer. The portion of the protein that resides in the bilayer is composed of hydrophobic amino acid residues, whereas the portion exposed to water is largely hydrophilic. Many integral membrane proteins extend through the bilayer (*transmembrane* proteins) and have portions extending onto both the inner and outer bilayer surfaces.

Figure 5.3 shows the cell membrane with its lipid bilayer and the location of peripheral and integral proteins. Although proteins are mobile within the bilayer, their large size makes them diffuse much more slowly than the membrane lipids.

Membrane proteins play a variety of roles and are often named on the basis of their function.

- Marker proteins identify cells to each other. The immune system uses these proteins to identify foreign invaders.
- Receptor proteins are involved with the passage of information between the extracellular and intracellular regions of cells.
- Transport proteins regulate transport of materials in and out of cells. Transport proteins can be classified into two types: channel proteins and carrier proteins.
  - Channel proteins are usually transmembrane proteins that create a water-filled pore or channel through which ions and some small hydrophilic molecules can pass. In general, channels are quite specific for the type of solute or ion they will allow to pass. Many channels are gated, meaning that they can be opened or closed according to the needs of the cell.
  - Carrier proteins are transmembrane proteins that have one or more sites

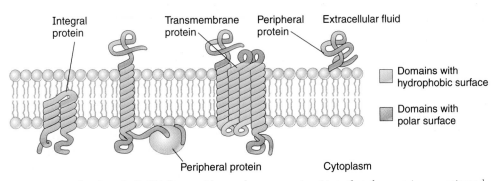

Figure 5.3. The phospholipid bilayer with membrane proteins. Note that the proteins are oriented so that their hydrophobic domains reside in the lipid bilayer, whereas their hydrophilic regions are exposed to the aqueous cytoplasm or extracellular fluid.

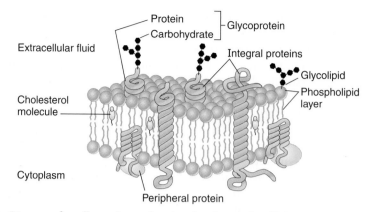

Figure 5.4. Diagram of a cell membrane showing the phospholipid bilayer and the various types of membrane proteins, glycoproteins, and glycolipids.

at which a substrate (e.g., an ion or molecule) can bind. The carrier protein then transports the substrate into or out of the cell.

As discussed in Chapter 2, many of these proteins are targets for various endogenous ligands and drugs.

Like lipids, many proteins are covalently bonded to carbohydrates to form glycoproteins (see Figure 5.4), which play an important role in cell–cell interactions. An important example for us is P-glycoprotein (P-gp), which is important in the transport of drugs and other substrates in and out of cells. We will discuss P-gp in more detail later in the chapter.

Most glycoproteins and glycolipids in cell membranes have their carbohydrate chains almost exclusively on the external surface of the cell. The negative charge on the external surface of most cell membranes is ascribed to the negatively charged sialic acid, a carbohydrate attached to many glycoproteins and glycolipids.

Mechanisms of Transport

Cell membranes are *semipermeable or selectively permeable* in that they allow certain types of molecules to cross and restrict or limit the transport of others.

The three primary mechanisms for transport of a substance across a cell membrane are as follows:

1. Passive diffusion
2. Carrier-mediated transport
3. Endocytosis and exocytosis

These processes exist to transport substances necessary for the cell's survival. Drugs and other molecules that are similar in structure or properties to these substances can also use these transport mechanisms. The targets of some drugs are located inside the cell, so the drug must enter the cell to exert its action. Other drugs may have their targets located on the cell membrane, but may be able to enter cells, also. The ability to enter and leave cells enables a drug to be absorbed and reach its site of action, as we will see later in the chapter.

The rate of transport depends on both the composition of each specific cell membrane, and the properties of the solute (size, lipophilicity, charge, etc.). Passive diffusion allows some small molecular weight solutes (such as drugs) to cross a cell membrane. Carrier-mediated mechanisms will transport both small and large molecules of the appropriate properties. Depending on the specific conditions, passive diffusion and carrier-mediated mechanisms can transport materials either into the cell or out of the cell.

Endocytosis and exocytosis are the primary mechanisms for transport of macromolecules (such as proteins) and small particles (such as viruses and bacteria). Endocytosis allows materials to enter the cell, while exocytosis transports materials out of cells.

Passive Diffusion

Diffusion is the natural tendency of molecules to move from a region of higher concentration to a region of lower concentration until the two regions reach the same concentration. It is a process by which a system tries to achieve equilibrium, and is a result of the random kinetic movement of molecules in a medium. Passive diffusion describes a diffusion process that is not energy-dependent; i.e., a source of energy is not required for diffusion to occur. Passive diffusion proceeds as long as there is a concentration difference, or *concentration gradient*, between the two regions. When the concentrations in the two regions become equal and equilibrium is reached, there is no further *net* change in concentration of the two regions. Exchange of molecules between the two regions continues at equilibrium, but at the same rates.

A barrier such as a cell membrane may separate these regions of high and low solute concentration. For diffusion to occur, the membrane must be permeable to the diffusing solute; i.e., it must allow the solute to cross. Diffusion will not occur if the membrane is impermeable to the solute, even if a concentration gradient is present.

The diffusion coefficient (D) is a constant that measures how fast a molecule can diffuse in a particular medium. It is defined as amount of substance diffusing through a unit area across a unit concentration gradient in unit time. D depends on size (or molecular weight) of the molecule, the viscosity of the medium

in which it is diffusing, and temperature. The larger the molecular weight of a solute, or the higher the viscosity of the medium, the lower the diffusion coefficient. The higher the temperature, the higher the diffusion coefficient. The units of D are $cm^2 s^{-1}$.

Consider passive diffusion of a solute with diffusion coefficient D diffusing in or out of a cell. The two regions (intracellular fluid and extracellular fluid) are separated by the cell membrane. The concentration on one side of the membrane is C_1 and on the other side of the membrane is C_2 (assume $C_1 > C_2$). If the membrane is permeable to the solute, transport will occur from the side with high concentration (the *donor* side) to the side with lower concentration (the *receiver* side); the magnitude of the concentration gradient $(C_1 - C_2)$ is considered the driving force for passive diffusion.

Fick's law of diffusion is a mathematical expression that describes the passive diffusion process. It states that the rate of passive diffusion (called *flux*, or change in donor side concentration with time, with units of concentration/time, e.g., mg/s) is

- directly proportional to concentration gradient $(C_1 - C_2)$ of solute (mg/mL)
- directly proportional to surface area (A) of membrane exposed to solute (cm^2)
- directly proportional to diffusion coefficient (D) of solute (cm^2/s)
- inversely proportional to thickness (h) of membrane (cm)

$$\frac{dC}{dt} \propto -\frac{A \cdot D(C_1 - C_2)}{h} \quad \text{(Eq. 5.1)}$$

Recall that cell membranes are composed of a lipid bilayer with embedded peripheral and transmembrane proteins. A solute, depending on its polarity, may cross the cell membrane by diffusion through the lipid bilayer of the membrane, or through hydrophilic pores created by transmembrane channel proteins.

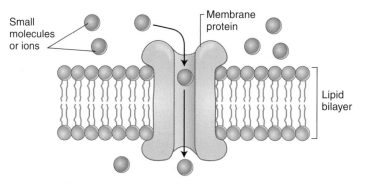

Figure 5.5. Illustration of the transport of very small solutes and ions through aqueous protein pores in the lipid bilayer of a cell membrane. Transport may be driven by a concentration or electrochemical gradient.

Passive Diffusion Through Hydrophilic Pores. The lipid bilayer contains nonspecific aqueous "holes," or pores, created by the hydrophilic centers of membrane proteins. These aqueous pores allow small molecules (such as water) and small dissolved solutes to diffuse through if they are smaller than the pore diameter (~0.5 nm), as illustrated in Figure 5.5. Transport is by passive diffusion, driven by a concentration gradient between intracellular and extracellular regions; no energy is required.

Most drugs and endogenous ligand molecules are too large to be transported through these narrow aqueous pores in the cell membrane. Thus, passive diffusion through hydrophilic protein pores is not an important pathway for ligand or drug transport in and out of cells.

Passive Diffusion Through the Lipid Bilayer. The cell membrane is permeable to molecules that are able to dissolve in the lipid bilayer. The solute partitions into the lipid bilayer on one side of the membrane, diffuses through the bilayer, and partitions out of the lipid bilayer on the other side. If extracellular solute concentration is higher, solute will be transported into the cell, whereas if intracellular concentration is higher, it will be transported out of the cell. The appropriate balance of hydrophilicity and lipophilicity is essential for this type of transport. Molecules with log $P < 0$ do not have enough lipophilicity to partition into bilayer lipids; molecules with a log $P > 3.5$ will tend to remain in the lipids and not partition out into the aqueous intracellular or extracellular fluids.

Uncharged molecules with an appropriate partition coefficient are able to diffuse through the lipid bilayer. Hydrophilic molecules, including ions, are not soluble in the lipid bilayer to any significant extent. Therefore, the lipid bilayer is not permeable to ionized forms of weak acid and weak base drugs, and these cannot cross cell membranes by passive diffusion. Only nonelectrolyte drugs and the un-ionized forms of weak acid and weak base drugs can diffuse passively through cell membranes. This is analogous to partitioning of compounds between *n*-octanol and water—only un-ionized neutral forms can partition from the aqueous phase into *n*-octanol.

Passive diffusion through the lipid bilayer is the primary mode of transport of most drugs into and out of cells. This is because drug molecules are intentionally designed to optimize the balance between hydrophilicity and lipophilicity and enable such transport.

Rate of Passive Diffusion Across the Lipid Bilayer. The rate at which a solute diffuses across the lipid bilayer of cell membranes will additionally depend

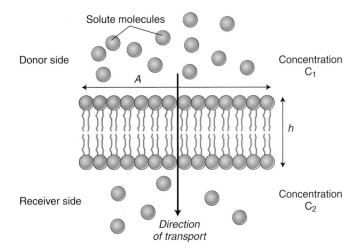

Figure 5.6. Schematic representation of passive diffusion of a solute across the lipid bilayer of a cell membrane. The direction of transport is from a region of high concentration (donor side) to a region of lower concentration (receiver side). The thickness of the membrane is h, and the area of membrane exposed to the drug is A.

on its partition coefficient between the lipid bilayer and water. Solutes that enter the bilayer readily will diffuse faster. In practice, we use the partition coefficient between n-octanol and water to approximate lipid–water partitioning, and a modified form of Fick's Law.

Figure 5.6 illustrates passive diffusion of a solute with partition coefficient P and diffusion coefficient D across a cell membrane of thickness h and exposed surface area A. Extracellular concentration of the neutral (un-ionized) form of the solute is C_1 and its intracellular concentration is C_2. The concentration of the neutral form rather than total concentration is appropriate because the lipid bilayer is permeable to the neutral form only.

Assume that $C_1 > C_2$, so that transport occurs from the extracellular donor side to the intracellular region receiver side. The rate of passive diffusion is given by

$$\frac{dC}{dt} = -\frac{P \cdot A \cdot D(C_1 - C_2)}{h} \qquad \text{(Eq. 5.2)}$$

The negative sign denotes a decrease in donor side concentration with time. In reality, molecules are continuously diffus-

ing both in and out of the cell. However, the diffusion rate into the cell is greater than diffusion rate out because of the higher extracellular concentration. The overall direction of transport is the net result of transport rates in and out of the cell.

Consider how transport rate is influenced by terms in Equation 5.2. If the solute is in contact with a large membrane surface area, A, transport will be faster. A large cell membrane thickness, h, makes the diffusion path longer and results in slower transport. If the solute diffusion coefficient D is large, the solute can move rapidly (smaller molecules have larger diffusion coefficients) resulting in a high transport rate.

Balance Between Lipophilicity and Hydrophilicity. If the solute partition coefficient P is large it means that the solute is very lipophilic, dissolves readily in the lipid bilayer, and Equation 5.2 predicts a high transport rate. Equation 5.2 also shows that transport rate is influenced by the concentration gradient $(C_1 - C_2)$. At the beginning of the transport process, $C_2 = 0$ and transport rate will be highest. If the solute is very water soluble, C_1 will be high and Equation 5.2 predicts a high transport rate. Therefore, a solute that can achieve higher concentrations on the donor side will be initially transported faster than one that attains lower concentrations. Because the medium on the donor and receiver sides is aqueous, polar solutes will be able to achieve higher concentrations and are predicted to be transported faster. This appears to contradict the prediction that solutes with greater lipophilicity will have a higher transport rate.

The reality is that both hydrophilicity and lipophilicity are important in drug transport, and good drugs need a balance between these properties. Transport depends on both P and C_1. Very polar molecules (usually with very low P) will partition slowly from water into lipids. If the receptor is in the membrane interior or inside the cell, this molecule will have a low probability of reaching it in the desired time. Conversely, very lipophilic molecules (with a very high P) will not attain the high intracellular or extracellular concentrations needed to drive the diffusion process. In addition, such molecules may be trapped in membrane lipids and will not exit and reach the desired target. Hence, drugs with a balance of hydrophilic and lipophilic characteristics are able to achieve optimum transport, where neither entry into nor departure from the lipid membrane is too slow.

Passive Diffusion of Nonelectrolytes. Consider a situation in which a nonelectrolyte solute of suitable P is initially present in extracellular fluid but not in intracellular fluid. Let C_1 = total solute concentration on the donor side and C_2 = total solute concentration on the receiver side. Initially, $C_2 = 0$ initially, and the concentration gradient = C_1.

Diffusion begins, and the solute is transported passively into the cell. As C_2 begins to increase, the concentration gradient ($C_1 - C_2$) progressively decreases, slowing diffusion. Eventually $C_1 = C_2$,

the concentration gradient becomes zero, and passive diffusion stops because equilibrium has been reached. The pH of the donor or receiver sides has no influence on the transport rate of nonelectrolytes, and the total concentration of the solute on the donor and receiver sides is equal at equilibrium. If the solute is consumed in the cell, or is somehow removed from the cell, C_2 may remain small and passive diffusion will continue.

Although we have considered transport *into* the cell, remember that passive diffusion can occur from the intracellular to the extracellular region if the concentration inside the cell is higher than that outside. In this case, the intracellular region is the donor and the extracellular region is the receiver.

Passive Diffusion of Weak Acids and Bases. The situation is somewhat different when the solute is either a weak acid or weak base. These solutes can ionize, with concentrations of ionized and un-ionized forms dependent on the pK_a of the compound and pH of donor and receiver fluids. The lipid bilayer is permeable to the un-ionized form but not to the ionized form; thus only the un-ionized form of a weak acids and bases can diffuse passively through cell membranes. Therefore, the driving force for diffusion of weak acids and bases through the lipid bilayer is the *concentration gradient of the un-ionized form*, as depicted in Figure 5.7.

Influence of pH and pK_a on Passive Diffusion. Consider a weak acid drug HA of pK_a 7. Initially, assume that total donor drug concentration $[HA]_{total}$ is 0.1 M, and that there is no drug on the receiver side. Also assume that the donor and receiver pH is 7. The drug on the donor side is 50% un-ionized (determined using the Henderson–Hasselbalch equation), so the un-ionized concentration [HA] is 0.05 M (Figure 5.8A). Because transport has not yet begun, the concentration gradient of [HA] is = (0.05 M − 0 M) = 0.05 M.

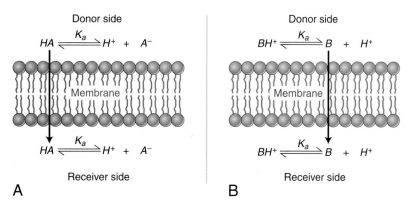

Figure 5.7. Passive diffusion of a weak acid (A) and a weak base (B) across a lipid bilayer from higher concentration (donor side) to lower concentration (receiver side). The concentration gradient of the un-ionized form (not the total concentration of drug) is the driving force for diffusion.

A driving force for diffusion is present, and HA will begin to diffuse passively through the lipid bilayer. Once some HA appears on the receiver side, it will ionize to satisfy the Henderson–Hasselbalch relationship. This means that any drug on the receiver side will be 50% ionized and 50% un-ionized. As long as there is a favorable concentration gradient of HA across the membrane, diffusion will continue but at a progressively slower rate, as the receiver side concentration increases.

Eventually, equilibrium will be reached when *the concentration gradient of the perme-* *ating species* (un-ionized HA) is zero, which is the same as saying that the concentration of un-ionized HA is equal on the donor and receiver sides. At the same time, the Henderson–Hasselbalch relationship must be satisfied on the donor and receiver sides; in this particular case, the drug on both sides has to be 50% ionized. This condition is satisfied when the concentrations of all the species are as shown in Figure 5.8B. A similar outcome would be achieved if the drug were a weak base.

This was a simple example in which the pK_a of the drug was the same as the pH of the extracellular and intracellular

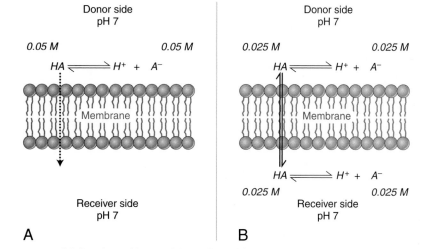

Figure 5.8. Initial (A) and equilibrium (B) conditions for the passive diffusion of a weak acid of $pK_a = 7$ across a cell membrane. The pH of the donor and receiver sides is 7.

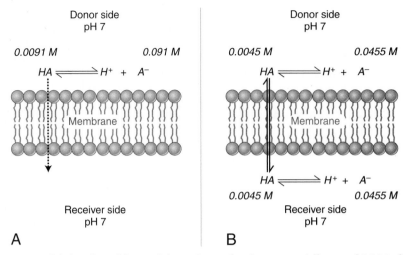

Figure 5.9. Initial (A) and equilibrium (B) conditions for the passive diffusion of 0.1 M of a weak acid HA of $pK_a = 6$, across a cell membrane. The pH of the donor and receiver sides is 7. Note that the initial concentration gradient is much smaller than that in Figure 8.6, so it will take longer for this system to reach equilibrium.

fluids. Figures 5.9 and 5.10 illustrate the situation in which the pK_a is not the same as the pH of the environment. Figure 5.9 shows the equilibrium state for passive diffusion of 0.1 M of a weak acid of pK_a 6 while Figure 5.10 shows it for 0.1 M of a weak base of pK_a 8.

For passive diffusion of a weak acid or base drug across a cell membrane when the pH of both the receiver and donor sides is the same, we can say that

- The drug is too large to diffuse through hydrophilic channels, and can only diffuse through the lipid bilayer.
- Rate of passive diffusion depends on the concentration gradient of the unionized form.

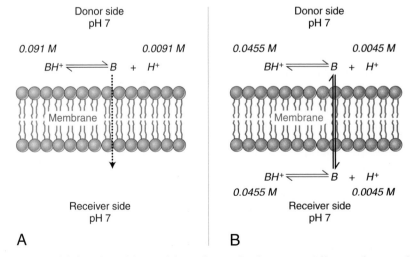

Figure 5.10. Initial (A) and equilibrium (B) conditions for the passive diffusion of 0.1 M of a weak base of $pK_a = 8$ across a cell membrane. The pH of the donor and receiver sides is 7.

- Concentration of the un-ionized form depends on the pH of the environment, the pK_a of the solute, and its total concentration.
- Concentration of the un-ionized form on the two sides will be the same at equilibrium.
- Concentration of the ionized form on the two sides will be the same at equilibrium.
- Total concentration of solute (ionized + un-ionized) on the two sides is the same at equilibrium.
- If either form of the solute is consumed in the cell, or is somehow removed from the cell, concentration gradient is maintained and passive diffusion will continue.

Ion Trapping. Understanding equilibrium across a semipermeable membrane is more complex when the pH of donor and receiver fluids is different. As before, equilibrium is reached when the concentration of *un-ionized* solute (the permeable species) is equal on both sides. However, the difference in pH between the donor and receiver sides means that the concentration of *ionized* solute will

be different on the two sides: higher on the side where the pH favors greater ionization. The total solute concentration is consequently higher on the side where the solute is more ionized, and the solute is said to be *trapped* on the side of greater ionization. In general, ion trapping causes weak bases to accumulate in acidic body fluids, and weak acids to accumulate in basic fluids.

Ion Trapping Equilbria. Consider a weak acid of pK_a 6 crossing a cell membrane by passive diffusion, from a donor side of pH 7 to a receiver side of pH 8 (Figure 5.11A). Initially, before diffusion starts, the situation on the donor side is the same as in Figure 5.9A. Once transport begins and some un-ionized HA diffuses to the receiver side, it is ionized to a greater extent on the receiver side because the pH is higher. Using the Henderson–Hasselbalch equation, the ratios of ionized and un-ionized forms on the two sides are as follows:

$$\frac{[A^-]_{donor}}{[HA]_{donor}} = 10 \quad \text{and} \quad \frac{[A^-]_{receiver}}{[HA]_{receiver}} = 100$$

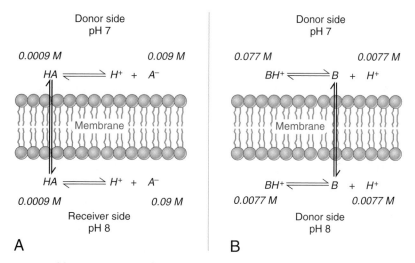

A

Donor side
pH 7

0.0009 M   0.009 M

$HA \rightleftharpoons H^+ + A^-$

Membrane

$HA \rightleftharpoons H^+ + A^-$

0.0009 M   0.09 M

Receiver side
pH 8

B

Donor side
pH 7

0.077 M   0.0077 M

$BH^+ \rightleftharpoons B + H^+$

Membrane

$BH^+ \rightleftharpoons B + H^+$

0.0077 M   0.0077 M

Donor side
pH 8

Figure 5.11. Equilibrium conditions for passive diffusion across a cell membrane when the pH of the donor and receiver sides is different. A. Ion trapping of a weak acid (pK_a = 6) on the receiver side. B. Ion trapping of a weak base (pK_a = 8) on the donor side.

What is the situation at equilibrium? If we designate $[HA]_{donor} = x$, then $[HA]_{receiver} = x$, by the definition of equilibrium. Simultaneously, to satisfy the Henderson–Hasselbalch equation, $[A^-]_{donor} = 10x$, and $[A^-]_{receiver} = 100x$. The total drug concentration in the system is 0.1 M; in other words

$$[HA]_{donor+receiver} + [A^-]_{donor+receiver} = 112x = 0.1 \text{ M}$$

Solving for x to determine the individual concentrations of all the species, we obtain x = approximately 0.0009 M. Thus, the *total* (un-ionized + ionized) drug concentration on the donor side is 0.0099 M, but there is 0.0909 M total drug on the receiver side (Figure 5.11B). In other words, most of the drug is on the receiver side after the passive diffusion process.

Clinical Consequences of Ion Trapping. An example of ion trapping is found in the treatment of human tumors with chemotherapeutic drugs. The extracellular pH (pH_e) in tumors is acidic while the intracellular pH (pH_i) is neutral-to-alkaline. Normal tissues generally have alkaline-outside pH gradients. Ion trapping predicts that weakly basic drugs such as anthracyclines, anthraquinones, and vinca alkaloids will be trapped in the extracellular tumor fluid and will be hindered from reaching their intracellular target. Meanwhile, the lower pH_e of tumors improves uptake of weak acids such as chlorambucil into the comparatively neutral intracellular fluid.

Another important illustration of ion trapping is placental transfer of weak base drugs such as local anesthetics from mother to fetus. The placental membrane serves as the interface between maternal and fetal circulation, and allows exchange of physiologically important substances. Fetal plasma pH is lower than maternal pH and results in basic drugs (such as local anesthetics) becoming more ionized when they reach fetal circulation. This effectively traps them on the fetal side of the circulation since ionized molecules cannot easily cross the placenta. This also maintains a continuous gradient for diffusion. Such ion trapping can be quite a significant effect especially during times of fetal distress, when fetal plasma pH gets even lower.

Ion trapping also occurs in intracellular organelles such as endosomes, lysosomes, and other intracellular particles. The pH of cytoplasm is around 7, whereas the pH in these organelles is lower, around 5. This acidity is maintained by proton pumps (an active transport mechanism) in the membranes surrounding the organelles, e.g., the endosomal membrane. When a weak base drug enters a cell, it will be concentrated in a ratio of approximately 100 to 1 inside organelles compared with the cytoplasm. Ion trapping in macrophage phagolysosomes is credited for the effectiveness of the basic antimalarial drug chloroquine.

It should be apparent from the earlier discussion that the pH of the donor and receiver sides is an important issue for ionizable drugs only. For drugs that do not ionize under physiological conditions, the pH has no effect on passive diffusion.

Carrier-Mediated Transport

The earlier discussion has treated the cell membrane as a simple semipermeable barrier that allows lipophilic solutes to diffuse passively through the lipid bilayer. However, many hydrophilic solutes, can cross the cell membrane and enter and leave cells, too. Because the aqueous pores in the cell membrane are too small to allow hydrophilic ligands or drugs to cross, other transport mechanisms have to be present that make this possible.

The body has specialized processes to transport a variety of important polar solutes that have difficulty crossing the lipid bilayer by passive diffusion. For example, glucose, an essential source of energy for most cells, cannot enter the cell by passive diffusion. One process by which polar solutes can cross the cell membrane is carrier-mediated transport in which the solute binds to and hitches a ride on a membrane protein called a carrier or transporter. Drugs with appropriate structures may also bind to and use these carriers to cross cell membranes.

Transporters. Transporters are integral membrane proteins with one or more active sites for its substrate, which may be a particular molecule or ion. The transporter binds to the substrate on one side of the cell membrane and transports it through the lipid bilayer to the other side. Recall that the cell membrane is fluid in nature and allows the movement of membrane proteins. Transporters have the ability to recognize (often through attached carbohydrates) and bind to particular substrates that they are designed to transport. Glucose, for instance, can be transported by a family of integral membrane proteins called GLUT transporters. Many transporters show specificity and stereoselectivity; e.g., D-glucose is transported by glucose transporters, but not L-glucose. Carrier-mediated transport does not require the substrate to be lipophilic;

both hydrophilic and lipophilic solutes may be transported in this manner.

Transporters, depending on their function, can carry molecules into or out of cells. A representation of carrier-mediated transport is shown in Figure 5.12. Cell membranes contain specific transporters to transport solutes needed for homeostasis. Drugs similar in structure to these natural substrates may also bind to and be transported by these transporters. Scientists have known for a while that transporters present in the kidney, liver, intestines, and other tissues play a role in elimination, distribution, and absorption of many drugs. However, only recently have some of these mechanisms been carefully examined and understood. Studies show that many drug transporters are somewhat nonselective, being able to transport drugs with diverse structures. In particular, transporters capable of binding to organic cations are important in transporting several amine drugs in their protonated forms. The total number of drug transporters is still unknown, and the functions of many known transporters have not yet been fully defined. Genetic variation of these transporters is also being shown to account for the variability among individuals in handling certain drugs.

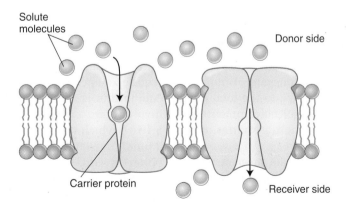

Figure 5.12. Representation of carrier-mediated transport. A solute molecule binds to the carrier on the donor side of the membrane. The drug then dissociates from the complex and is released on the receiver side. Carrier-mediated processes can transport drugs in or out of cells.

Transporters may also be good drug targets for certain diseases. Many pathogens depend on their hosts to provide essential nutrients such as amino acids and vitamins. Bacterial transport proteins are attractive targets in designing drugs that can prevent the transport of essential nutrients, resulting in death of the pathogen.

Rate of Carrier-Mediated Transport. After binding of the substrate to its transporter on the donor side of the membrane, the resulting substrate–transporter complex undergoes a change in conformation. This complex, which is now soluble in the lipid bilayer, diffuses to the receiver side and releases the substrate. The transporter then regains its original conformation and transports another substrate molecule to continue the carrier-mediated process.

The rate of carrier-mediated transport is governed by Michaelis–Menten kinetics. The Michaelis–Menten equation is written as follows:

$$V = \frac{V_{max}[S]}{K_m + [S]}$$ (Eq. 5.3)

V is the rate of transport, K_m is called the Michaelis–Menten constant, V_{max} is the maximum rate of transport, and $[S]$ is the concentration of the substrate being transported.

V_{max} and K_m together define the kinetic behavior of a transporter as a function of $[S]$. V_{max}, a measure of how fast the given amount of transporter can go at full speed, is the maximum rate of transport possible. V_{max} is related to the total number of transporter molecules present and to the mobility of the transporter in the cell membrane.

K_m is an approximate measure of the amount of substrate required to reach full speed. A low K_m implies a high affinity between transporter and substrate and a fast transport rate, and vice versa. K_m can be different on the two sides of the cell membrane, so that the substrate is easily released on the receiver side of the membrane. Such a difference in K_m also favors transport in one direction over the other.

The concentration of transporter available is usually fixed and limited. At low substrate concentrations ($<<K_m$), there are sufficient transporter molecules to bind with and transport all the substrate molecules, and the rate of transport depends directly on substrate concentration. At very high substrate concentration, all transporter molecules are occupied by substrate, and it is said to be saturated. An increase in substrate concentration beyond this saturation point will give no further increase in transport rate. At intermediate substrate concentrations, the transport rate still increases with substrate concentration, but not proportionately.

Types of Carrier-Mediated Transport. The two major types of carrier-mediated transport processes are facilitated diffusion and active transport. The difference between the two lies in the absence or presence of an external energy source.

Facilitated Diffusion. Facilitated diffusion is a carrier-mediated process that occurs only when there is a concentration gradient between the donor and receiver sides. In other words, the transporter can only transport substrate from a region of high concentration to a region of low concentration, in the direction of the concentration gradient. Like other diffusion processes, facilitated diffusion does not require an energy source and stops when equilibrium is reached. The transporters involved are called uniporters (Figure 5.13A), which transport one molecule at a time. An example of this type of transporter is GLUT1, a widely distributed glucose transporter that transports glucose either in or out of cells depending on the direction of the concentration gradient. Examples of drugs that use facilitated diffusion transporters in the body

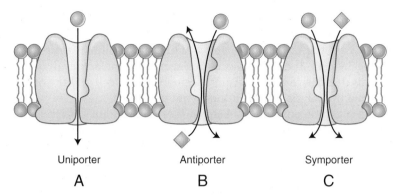

Uniporter
A

Antiporter
B

Symporter
C

Figure 5.13. Different types of transporters involved in carrier-mediated transport. A. Uniporters move one molecule at a time, and can be involved in either facilitated diffusion or active transport. B and C. Antiporters transport one solute across the membrane in one direction while simultaneously transporting a second solute across the membrane in the opposite direction. Symporters simultaneously transport two solutes across the membrane in the same direction. Both of these are active processes.

are penicillin, furosemide, morphine, and dopamine.

The rate at which a solute is transported by facilitated diffusion depends on

- Concentration gradient of the solute
- Concentration of transporter molecules in the membrane
- Affinity ($1/K_m$) between transporter and substrate.

In general, the rate of facilitated diffusion is greater than that of passive diffusion. At low substrate concentrations, increasing concentration on the donor side increases the concentration gradient and hence the transport rate. However, if substrate concentration on the donor side is sufficiently large, there may not be enough transporter molecules in the cell membrane to bind to the substrate. Increasing the concentration beyond this value exhibits no further increase in transport rate because the transporter is saturated.

Active Transport. Active transport is very similar to facilitated diffusion in that it requires a transporter, and can be saturated. However, active transport processes are able to transport a substrate against a concentration gradient, i.e., from a region of low concentration to a region of high concentration. This is not a simple diffusion process and requires a source of energy from the cell. This active involvement of the cell's energy resources in transport gives this process the name active transport.

In addition to uniporters, two other types of transporters are involved in active transport, as illustrated in Figure 5.13B and C. Antiporters transport one solute across the membrane in one direction while simultaneously transporting a second solute across the membrane in the opposite direction. Symporters simultaneously transport two solutes across the membrane in the same direction. Energy is required for both of these transporters to function. Substances called metabolic poisons can deplete the energy source, resulting in reduced active transport.

Examples of drugs that use active transport are 5-fluorouracil and some cardiac glycosides across the intestinal membrane, absorption of methyldopa into the brain, and secretion of certain drugs into the bile and urine.

Drug Efflux. Drug efflux (meaning *flowing out*) is a special term given to an active transport process that transports substrates only out of cells. The transporters are called efflux proteins or *efflux pumps*. The major mechanism of efflux relies on carrier proteins that derive their transport energy from the hydrolysis of ATP. Efflux can be viewed as a protective mechanism by which cells are able to rapidly remove undesirable materials. Efflux transporters provide a barrier to the uptake of xenobiotics, and promote their excretion into bile and urine. However, efflux pumps can also remove drugs from cells, and can reduce intracellular concentrations of drug below effective levels.

Multidrug efflux is a phenomenon in which a single type of transporter (multidrug resistance transporter, or MDR transporter) recognizes and pumps many drugs, with no apparent common structural similarity, out of cells. Many of these transporters belong to the ABC (ATP-binding cassette) superfamily of membrane transporters. MDR transporters are transmembrane proteins that detect and bind to substrates as they cross the lipid bilayer passively on their way into the cell. The substrate is then transported back out into the extracellular environment, thus preventing it from entering the cell (Figure 5.14). This restricts entry of certain substrates into cells, or at least slows their transport into the cell. The conse-

quence is a lower than expected intracellular concentration of the substrate. The actual intracellular drug concentration depends on the net result of passive diffusion into the cell and the opposing efflux out of the cell.

An important characteristic distinguishing MDR transporters from other mammalian transporters is their wide substrate specificity; unlike other selective (classic) transporters, MDR transporters recognize and handle a wide range of substrates. MDR transporters include the clinically significant multidrug resistance pump P-gp and the multidrug resistance protein (MRP). In humans, these efflux pumps are found in cells of the gastrointestinal tract, liver, and kidney, as well as the capillaries of the brain, testes, and ovaries.

In normal tissues, MDR transporters function as protective mechanisms against toxins and as transporters of metabolic byproducts out of cells. Related transporters are also found in a number of pathogenic bacteria and fungi, and in parasitic protozoa. Efflux pumps may become overexpressed in abnormal cells or resistant cells. Multiple drug resistance as a result of MDR transporter efflux is known to develop in bacterial and cancer cells. Drugs that were once effective become ineffective, presumably because cells that express more of the transporter survive and become more efficient at pumping out the drug.

Since efflux of chemotherapeutic and antimicrobial drugs is generally undesirable, inhibition of efflux transporters may be a way to improve efficacy of such treatments. Many currently available drugs (e.g., verapamil, quinine) have been found to inhibit MDR transporters, and therefore decrease efflux out of cells. For most of these drugs, the inhibitory activity is coincidental and not related to the drug's primary pharmacological use. For example, verapamil is used to treat cardiovascular diseases and was only later found to inhibit P-gp-mediated efflux. In

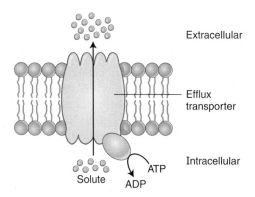

Figure 5.14. Illustration of multidrug efflux out of a cell via a membrane transporter protein. Note that energy from the cell (conversion of ATP to ADP) is required for this process.

principle, one of these efflux inhibitors could be dosed with anticancer or antimicrobial drugs to improve their effectiveness. However, the dose needed would be large and the side effects would be unacceptable.

Research continues to search for more effective inhibitors of MDR proteins to improve activity of existing antibiotics and anticancer drugs. These inhibitors would have a high affinity for binding to the MDR transporter protein. When administered along with an anticancer drug, for instance, the inhibitor will keep the transporter proteins occupied and allow the drug to reach effective concentrations inside the cells.

Endocytosis and Exocytosis

These are also called *vesicular transport* processes, in which substances (usually macromolecules such as proteins, polysaccharides, polynucleotides, and antibodies) are transported across cell membranes by the formation of vesicles. Substances can be taken into a cell by endocytosis, a process in which the cell membrane forms a vesicle to internalize extracellular materials into the cell. In exocytosis, a vesicle inside the cell fuses with the cell membrane and expels its contents into the extracellular fluid. Endocytosis and exocytosis can occur against a concentration gradient and require cellular energy like in active transport.

Endocytosis. Three primary mechanisms of endocytosis are exhibited by cells, shown in Figure 5.15. In *receptor-mediated endocytosis*, cells are able to take in large amounts of particular molecules that bind to receptor sites extending from the cell membrane into the extracellular fluid, along with smaller amounts of other extracellular material. A less specific mechanism of endocytosis is *pinocytosis*, in which a cell ingests a small portion of liquid from the extracellular fluid. All solutes found in the extracellular fluid

A. Phagocytosis

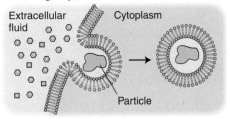

B. Pinocytosis

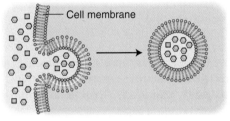

C. Receptor-mediated endocytosis

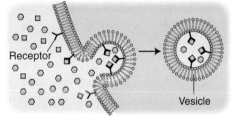

Figure 5.15. Three primary mechanisms of endocytosis. The cell membrane takes in extracellular material to form a vesicle in the cell.

become encased in these vesicles and transported into the cell along with the liquid.

Finally, *phagocytosis* is a form of endocytosis in which cells engulf large particles such as bacteria and viruses. Phagocytosis is mainly a cellular defense mechanism rather than a way to transport necessary substances into cells. For example, leukocytes take in protozoa, bacteria, dead cells, and similar materials by phagocytosis to help stave off infections.

Exocytosis. During exocytosis, a membrane-enclosed vesicle in the cell fuses with the plasma membrane and then opens and releases its contents into the extracellular fluid. Cells use exocytosis to expel proteins, secreted substances, and wastes from the cell. Many signaling molecules

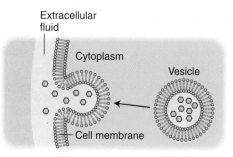

Figure 5.16. An illustration of exocytosis.

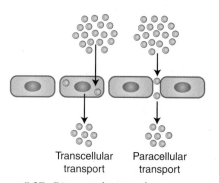

Figure 5.17. Diagram showing the two major transport routes of solutes across a multicellular (epithelial or endothelial) membrane. This membrane is composed of a single layer of cells. Paracellular transport occurs when the molecules travel between the cells, through cell junctions. Transcellular transport involves the drug molecules going through the cells, across the cell membrane.

secreted by cells, such as insulin secreted by the pancreas and neurotransmitters secreted by neurons, are released extracellularly by exocytosis. Exocytosis is illustrated in Figure 5.16.

Transport Across a Tissue

We have learned that cell membranes have many structural features designed to control the passage of molecules in and out of the cell, and have discussed different mechanism by which a molecule or particle can cross the cell membrane to enter or leave a cell. We also saw that some polar molecules (such as drugs in their ionized state, and very polar nonelectrolytes) may not be able to cross cell membranes by passive diffusion, and cannot enter a cell unless they are substrates for a specific carrier protein. Thus, many polar drugs cannot enter cells.

When a drug or other molecule encounters a layer of cells such as the epithelial tissue, it can hypothetically cross this functional membrane barrier by either diffusing through the aqueous space between the cells (paracellular transport) or by going through the cell (transcellular transport), as illustrated in Figure 5.17. Which of these two pathways are available to the drug depends on the characteristics of the molecule and the characteristics of the epithelial tissue in question.

Let us examine the structural features of epithelial tissue, particularly the components that regulate transport of substances across it.

Epithelial Tissue

The internal cavities and external surfaces of the body are lined with a tissue called the epithelial tissue, epithelial membrane or simply, the epithelium. Epithelial tissue serves as a protective barrier for the body. All materials that enter or leave the body do so through some type of epithelium. It also provides an interface between masses of cells on one side and a cavity or space (lumen) on the other. The surface of the cell exposed to the lumen is called its apical or lumenal surface; the sides and base of the cell are the basolateral or basal surface. Examples of epithelial tissue are the outer layers of skin, linings of body cavities exposed to the environment (e.g., the mouth, gastrointestinal tract, and respiratory tract), and the tissues that cover all internal organs.

Epithelial tissue may be composed of a single or multiple layers of cells, often arranged in sheets. The sheets rest on a connective tissue called the basement membrane, anchoring the cells and attaching them to other tissues. In certain organs, the basement membrane assumes major significance; e.g., the basement

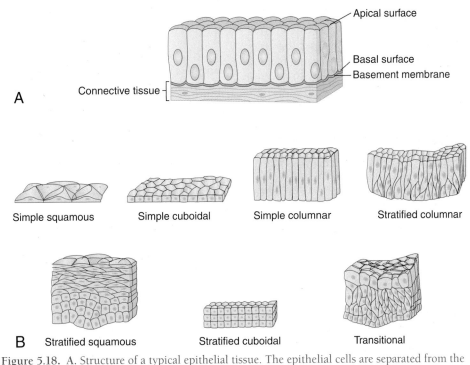

Figure 5.18. **A.** Structure of a typical epithelial tissue. The epithelial cells are separated from the underlying connective tissue by a basement membrane. The apical surface of cells is exposed to the environment, whereas the basal surface rests on the basement membrane. **B.** Types of epithelia based on number of layers and the shape of the cells. Simple epithelia consist of one cell layer, whereas stratified epithelia have multiple layers. Epithelial tissue is classified on the basis of cell shape as squamous (flat, scale-like), cuboidal (cube-shaped), columnar (tall and column-shaped), or transitional (columnar and squamous).

membrane in the kidney serves as a filter for plasma on its way to becoming urine. In other locations, the absence of a basement membrane is functionally important; the absence of a basement membrane in the liver permits plasma to come into direct contact with liver cells.

Epithelia may be described based on the shape of cells and number of cell layers. When classified by number, epithelial tissue is distinguished as simple (one layer) or stratified (more than one layer). When classified by shape, epithelial tissue may be squamous (flat, scale-like), cuboidal (cube-shaped), or columnar (tall and column-shaped). Some of the different types of epithelia are illustrated in Figure 5.18.

Epithelial cells often display surface specializations such as cilia (seen in cells lining the trachea) or microvilli (present in the epithelium of the small intestines). Cilia are motile, hair-like surface projections found on specialized cells and play a role in moving fluid or mucus over the surface of the epithelium. Microvilli are nonmotile, finger-like projections of the cell surface, commonly found in epithelial cells involved in absorption of materials from the lumenal side. Epithelial tissue can also exhibit down-growths, called glands, into the underlying connective tissue; glands are responsible for the secretion and excretion of a variety of substances.

Cell Junctions

If groups of cells are to come together to form a tissue or part of an organ, it is imperative that each cell be held in its proper place and be able to communicate with its neighbors. One important characteristic of tissues is that cells are closely packed, with specialized contacts or junctions between them. These contacts are a result of interactions between membrane proteins of adjoining cells. Cell junctions fall into three functional classes: anchoring junctions, gap junctions and tight junctions. These specialized cell junctions occur at many points of cell–cell and cell–matrix contact in all tissues, but they are particularly important and abundant in epithelia.

- Anchoring junctions provide cellular adhesion, holding cells together using membrane proteins. They provide structural cohesion and are most abundant in tissues that are subject to constant mechanical stress such as skin and heart.
- Gap junctions are communicating junctions that allow cells in a tissue to respond as an integrated unit. Proteins from adjoining cells join to form channels that permit substances and chemical information to be transmitted between cells, allowing the coordinated behavior of a group of cells.
- Tight junctions seal the space between adjacent cells to regulate substances from moving between cells through the intercellular space. Tight junctions are most important type of cell junction for

our discussion on paracellular transport across tissues.

Role of Tight Junctions

Tight junctions are formed when specific proteins on the cell membranes of neighboring epithelial cells make direct contact across the intercellular space, forming a complex, impenetrable network (Figure 5.19). This protein network "seals" adjacent cells in a narrow band just beneath their apical surface.

Tight junctions regulate the paracellular transport of substances across epithelial tissue; i.e., the movement of substances between cells from the lumenal side to the basolateral side, and vice versa. The diameter of a typical epithelial tight junction is less than 1 nm, so molecules with molecular weights greater than approximately 200 cannot diffuse paracellularly between cells. The more the contacts between membrane proteins of adjacent cells, the tighter the junction becomes. However, this seal between cells is not absolute or uniform. The tight junction is almost always impermeable to macromolecules, but its diameter, and therefore its permeability to small molecules, varies greatly in different epithelia. Epithelia are often classified as *tight* or *leaky*, depending on the size of molecules that are allowed to cross paracellularly.

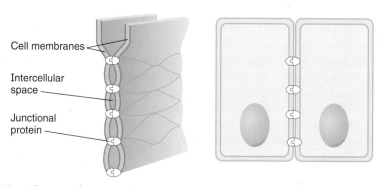

Cell membranes

Intercellular
space

Junctional
protein

Figure 5.19. A diagram showing tight junctions between epithelial cells. Tight junctions seal neighboring cells together and prevent movement of materials through the intercellular space.

Tight junctions are essential for the barrier function of epithelial tissue; their presence prevents potentially harmful molecules, especially macromolecules, from crossing the epithelium from the lumenal side to the basolateral side, and vice versa. This barrier is variable and physiologically regulated, and its disruption contributes to human diseases.

Drug Transport Across Epithelial Tissues

When a drug is administered by any route except by injection, it encounters an epithelium at the site of administration. In theory, the drug can cross this epithelial tissue either paracellularly or transcellularly. Based on our earlier discussion, we can conclude that most drug molecules will not be able to cross an epithelial membrane paracellularly because they are too large to diffuse through epithelial tight junctions. Only some minerals and metal ions (such as calcium and iron) are small enough to diffuse paracellularly through epithelia; e.g., during absorption from the gastrointestinal tract into the blood, through the intestinal epithelium.

The only pathway available to most drugs is to cross epithelia by a transcellular mechanism; i.e., by going through the cells. The drug molecule must cross cells in its path by successively moving into and out of each cell layer in its path. For a single layered epithelium, e.g., the intestinal epithelium, the drug must move in and out of the intestinal epithelial cell. For multilayered epithelia such as the skin, the drug must move in and out of several epidermal cells.

We have already discussed the various ways in which drugs can enter or leave cells (passive diffusion, carrier-mediated transport or endocytosis/exocytosis). These same mechanisms enable a drug to cross epithelial tissues, except that now the drug molecule must both enter and leave all the cells in its path. Which pathways a drug or other molecule can use to get across an

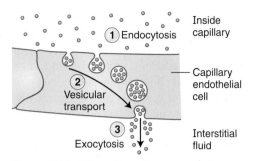

Figure 5.20. Illustration of transcytosis for transporting material through a cell. In this case, the substances are moving in vesicles through a capillary endothelial cell.

epithelium depends on its physicochemical properties (size, ionization state, partition coefficient), whether the membrane has transporters that recognize the drug, and whether the drug molecule has the appropriate properties to undergo transcytosis (endocytosis into the cell and subsequent exocytosis out of the cell; see Fig. 5.20).

Passive Transcellular Diffusion. The rate of passive transcellular transport across an epithelium is given by an equation familiar to us from transport across a cell membrane. The terms in the equation now have slightly different meanings than before:

$$\text{Rate} = -\frac{P \cdot A \cdot D(C_1 - C_2)}{h} \quad \text{(Eq. 5.4)}$$

In this context, A is the surface area of the *epithelium* exposed to the drug, $(C_1 - C_2)$ is the concentration gradient of the drug (in the un-ionized form) across the *epithelium* (one or several cell layers), and h is the thickness of the epithelium. The rate of transport still depends on P, the partition coefficient of the drug, because transport occurs through successive lipid bilayers.

Consider how transport rate is influenced by terms in Equation 5.4. If the drug is in contact with a large surface area of the epithelium, transport will be faster.

If the drug diffusion coefficient D is large, the solute can move rapidly through the epithelium (smaller molecules have larger diffusion coefficients), resulting in a high transport rate. If the solute partition coefficient P is large it means that the solute dissolves readily in the lipid bilayer, and will have a high transport rate. A thicker epithelium (large h) makes the diffusion path longer and results in slower transport.

The inherent ability of a given epithelial membrane to allow passage of a particular solute is called its permeability coefficient, given by

$$\text{Permeability coefficient} = \frac{P \cdot D}{h} \quad \text{(Eq. 5.5)}$$

The units of the permeability coefficient are cm/s. The permeability coefficient depends on both the properties of the solute (partition coefficient, and diffusion coefficient in the lipid bilayer) and on properties of the membrane (thickness). It is important to note that epithelia in various parts of the body have different compositions and characteristics, so that the permeability coefficient of a drug may be faster across one epithelium than another.

Carrier-Mediated Transport. The role of transport proteins is emerging rapidly and several drugs have been shown to be transported to some extent across functional membranes by these carriers. Clinical evidence is accumulating that shows that transport proteins play some role in the absorption, distribution, and excretion of drugs. For absorption across epithelia, P-gp efflux is well known to limit permeability of several drugs across the intestinal membrane. At the same time, many polar peptide-like drugs are shown to cross epithelia, presumably by a carrier-mediated process.

Although this is an important pathway for some drugs, it does not play a significant role for the vast majority of drugs.

Transcytosis. Transcytosis is a relatively slow process compared with other transport mechanisms we have discussed. Thus, transport by transcytosis is negligible for drugs that can be effectively transported by passive diffusion or carrier-mediated processes. However, transcytosis becomes important for materials that cannot cross the cell membrane by another mechanism. For example, many proteins (such as antigens, botulinus toxin, and oral vaccines) are able to enter the bloodstream after being orally ingested. Transcytosis through intestinal epithelial cells is presumed to be the mechanism of transport in these cases. The amounts of macromolecules transported in this way are extremely small, but sufficient to elicit their biological response.

Based on the relative slowness of this process and the very small amount of material that is transported, we assume that transcytosis probably does not play a role in the transport of most small molecule drugs across biological membranes. Although transcytosis is an important mechanism for the transport of a few large molecule drugs such as vaccines, it is a slow and relatively inefficient process and not significant for transport of most drugs across epithelia.

Summary of Transport Across Epithelial Tissues. Overall, a drug molecule or other substance can cross an epithelial membrane if it meets one of the following criteria:

- Is lipophilic enough to cross the lipid bilayer of epithelial cells passively
- Has a transporter that can transport it across epithelial cell membranes
- Has characteristics that allows it to use transcytosis mechanisms.

Passive transcellular diffusion is the primary mechanism for transport of drugs across epithelia. Thus, polar drugs that do not have adequate lipophilicity cannot cross epithelial tissues by this mechanism.

The only way polar molecules and very large molecules such as proteins can cross epithelia is by a carrier-mediated mechanism or by transcytosis. This is an exception rather than the rule.

As a result, epithelia are not permeable to most polar molecules or large molecules, and are only permeable to molecules with an adequate set of physicochemical properties (size, ionization state, partition coefficient).

The Endothelium

A specialized type of epithelial tissue, called the endothelium or endothelial membrane, makes up the walls of blood vessels, lymph vessels, and the internal surfaces of body cavities. Endothelial cells line the entire circulatory system, from the heart to the smallest capillary, with a single layer of endothelial cells forming the walls of most capillaries. Endothelial cells are more loosely packed than epithelial cells. Gaps between cells contain a loose network of proteins that act as filters, retaining very large molecules and letting smaller ones through.

Drug Transport Across the Capillary Endothelium

The capillary endothelium is the most important endothelial membrane for us to consider because of the role of the circulatory system in the distribution of drugs in the body. Once a drug crosses an epithelial membrane from the site of action into the body, it must enter the bloodstream across the capillary wall, and then leave the bloodstream at various sites in the body. Because of the looser junctions between endothelial cells, the paracellular pathway is very important for transport of drug molecules across the endothelium.

Paracellular Transport Across the Endothelium. The size of capillary endothelial junctions is in the range of 5 to 30 nm. Generally, molecules with molecular weights up to about 20,000 to 30,000 can diffuse paracellularly through the capillary endothelium; i.e., between the blood and the *extravascular* (outside the vascular system, or the blood and lymph vessels) space. The molecular size cut off is not exact: small molecules such as water (MW 18) move rapidly. The rate of transport decreases as the size of the molecule increases. Macromolecules of MW > 100,000 transfer very slowly, if at all. Proteins and blood cells, which are larger than the capillary endothelial junctions, are not capable of paracellular diffusion through them, except in diseases where these junctions become even leakier.

Paracellular transport is a passive diffusion process, so molecules can diffuse through cellular junctions if they are smaller that the junction diameter, and if there is a concentration gradient across the endothelial membrane. Thus, movement of individual drug molecules in and out of capillaries proceeds freely regardless of polarity or lipophilicity of the drug; this is the key difference between passive transcellular transport and passive paracellular transport.

The rate of paracellular diffusion across an endothelial membrane is given by an equation based on Fick's Law:

$$\text{Rate} = -\frac{D \cdot A \cdot (C_1 - C_2)}{h} \quad \text{(Eq. 5.6)}$$

As expected, the rate of passive paracellular diffusion of molecules depends on the concentration gradient, the area (A) and thickness (h) of the membrane, and the diffusion coefficient of the molecule through the tight junction. The rate of paracellular diffusion of uncharged molecules is found to be proportional to the diffusion coefficient, as predicted by Equation 5.6. The diffusion of positively charged molecules is observed to be somewhat slower than that predicted, presumably owing to repulsion by positive charges on membrane proteins in the endothelial junctions.

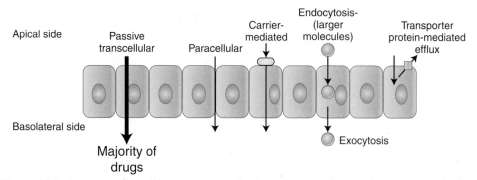

Figure 5.21. Summary of possible processes involved in transport of materials in and out of cells, and across an epithelial or endothelial barrier.

Transcellular Transport Across the Endothelium. Paracellular transport is an important mechanism for most drug molecules to cross the capillary endothelium. However, transcellular transport pathways are also available for molecules with adequate lipophilicity (transcellular passive diffusion), or with a transporter (carrier-mediated transport) or that are amenable to transcytosis. The principles underlying these mechanisms are exactly the same as we saw before.

Passive transcellular diffusion remains an important mechanism of transport for drugs that have adequate lipophilicity and are at least partially in the un-ionized state. Carrier-mediated pathways and receptor-mediated transcytosis are less prevalent, but occur more readily in endothelial membranes as compared to epithelial membranes. The transcytosis process for transport of materials through the capillary endothelium is illustrated in Figure 5.20.

Transport Across Specialized Endothelia. Our discussion on capillary endothelium so far focused on peripheral capillaries; i.e., those at the terminal end of the circulation in most of the body, excluding the brain and the heart. Even among peripheral capillaries, the ion- and size-selectivity of the paracellular pathway differs somewhat across the body, and is regulated by different physiological and pathological stimuli. In some special organs,

the capillary endothelium is quite different than that found in peripheral capillaries. For example, endothelial cells in liver capillaries are very loosely packed, and allow large molecules and even red blood cells to diffuse through cell junctions. In contrast, the endothelial junctions of brain capillaries are tighter than those of most epithelial membranes, allowing almost no movement of small molecules through these junctions.

Blood–Brain Barrier. The blood–brain barrier (BBB) is the specialized system of capillary endothelial cells that protects the brain from harmful substances in the bloodstream while supplying it with essential nutrients. Unlike peripheral capillaries that allow relatively free exchange of small molecules between blood and tissues, the BBB strictly limits transport into the brain through both physical (tight junction) and metabolic (enzyme) barriers. Capillaries bringing blood to the brain have tightly packed endothelial cells, with junctions similar to tight junctions in epithelial tissue. Cell-to-cell contacts between adjacent endothelial cells are essentially sealed, forming a continuous blood vessel. These tight paracellular junctions do not allow drugs and other small molecules to move between the blood and the brain; molecules may enter and leave the brain capillaries by transcellular pathways only.

The BBB has a number of highly selective carrier-mediated mechanisms to transport nutrients and other essential molecules into the brain. For example, receptor-mediated endocytosis occurs for endogenous macromolecules such as transferrin, insulin, and leptin.

The BBB is often the rate-limiting factor in determining permeation of drugs into the brain. The general rule is that the higher the lipophilicity of a substance, the greater its transcellular passive diffusion into the brain. Even if a drug molecule is lipophilic enough to diffuse transcellularly through the capillary endothelium, there are other processes that oppose uptake into the brain. One significant opposing process is carrier-mediated efflux, a major obstacle for many drugs with sites of action in the brain. Another is the presence of metabolizing enzymes in the capillary endothelium that break down the drug before it can enter the brain. Poor delivery into the brain remains a major challenge for many central nervous system (CNS) drugs.

Multiple Transport Pathways

It is important to understand that a solute may be able to cross membranes using several transport pathways simultaneously. Consider a solute that has good lipophilicity, fits through the endothelial paracellular junction, and can bind to a specific transporter in the capillary membrane. This solute can be transported across the capillary wall by passive transcellular diffusion, carrier-mediated transport, and paracellular diffusion.

The dominant mechanism of transport for this solute may vary from membrane to membrane. For example, passive transcellular diffusion may be dominant for intestinal absorption of this solute, paracellular transport may be controlling for its distribution in and out of peripheral capillaries, and active transport may be important for its entry into the brain.

The different pathways involved in transport of materials across a cell or tissue membrane are depicted in Figure 5.21.

Key Concepts

- The cell membrane is composed of a lipid bilayer with embedded membrane proteins.
- Membrane proteins are responsible for controlling transport, communication, and recognition between cells.
- Diffusion of drugs through hydrophilic cell membrane protein channels is insignificant.
- Most drugs cross cell membranes by passive diffusion across the lipid bilayer.
- The rate of passive diffusion is governed by Fick's law.
- Only un-ionized, lipophilic drug molecules cross the lipid bilayer by passive diffusion.
- Most proteins cannot diffuse passively across the cell membrane because they are too large and too polar.
- Ion trapping on either the donor or receiver sides can occur if their pHs are different.
- Carrier-mediated processes and efflux pumps play an important role in determining intracellular concentrations for some drugs and solutes.
- Epithelial tissue lines the internal cavities and external surfaces of the body.
- Tight junctions prevent paracellular transport of most drugs through the intercellular space between epithelial cells.
- Passive transcellular diffusion is the primary mechanism for transport of drugs across epithelia.

- Drugs can cross endothelial membranes (e.g., the capillary endothelium) by paracellular diffusion through cell junctions or by transcellular diffusion.

- Specialized endothelia (blood–brain barrier) can restrict paracellular transport, and behave more like an epithelium.

Review Questions

1. What are the typical constituents of a mammalian cell membrane?
2. What are the primary functions of the cell membrane?
3. Describe the composition and characteristics of the lipid bilayer.
4. Describe the types and functions of membrane proteins.
5. What does the term semipermeable mean? Describe the features of a cell membrane that regulate the transport of small molecules across it.
6. How do most ions and very small solutes enter and leave cells?
7. How do most small molecule drugs enter and leave cells? What parameters control the rate of this transport?
8. What role do transport proteins play in the transport of solutes in and out of cells? Why are only some solutes transported in this manner?
9. Explain the processes of endocytosis and exocytosis. What types of materials are transported predominantly by this mechanism?
10. Which of the transport mechanisms are saturable? Why?
11. Explain the difference between paracellular and transcellular transport across a functional membrane. What characteristics must a solute have to be transported paracellularly or transcellularly?
12. What are the types and functions of epithelial tissue?
13. Describe the three major types of cell junctions. What are their functions?
14. What role do tight junctions play in transport across epithelia? How do most drugs cross epithelial barriers?
15. How does the capillary endothelium differ from most other epithelia? What mechanisms are available for a drug to cross the capillary endothelium?
16. What is the blood–brain barrier? What types of compounds can cross the blood–brain barrier?

CASE STUDY 5.1

Why does my tooth still hurt?

A patient with an infected tooth goes to a dentist to have the tooth extracted. Before extraction, the dentist numbs the local nerve by injecting a solution of lidocaine (Xylocaine®), a common local anesthetic, into the space around the tooth. After the usual time for achieving anesthesia, the dentist checks the area around the tooth and finds that it is still not numb enough. She has to inject even more lidocaine before the area is numb enough for extraction. She later relates this incident to her pharmacist friend and wonders why the normal lidocaine dose did not work in this patient.

Background

For nerve cells (neurons) to conduct a stimulus like pain, sodium ions must first enter the neuron through Na^+ ion channel proteins in the neuronal cell membrane. Local anesthetics (LA) bind to a receptor on the Na^+ ion channel protein. This reduces transport of Na^+ into the nerve cell cytoplasm and blocks nerve conduction. To be effective, the LA must cross the cell membrane because the receptor is located on the cytoplasmic side of the Na^+ ion channel protein. A sufficient concentration of lidocaine needs to enter the neuron to block nerve conduction adequately.

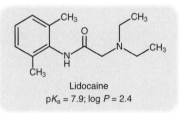

Lidocaine
$pK_a = 7.9$; log $P = 2.4$

Questions

1. Lidocaine solution is injected near a nerve around the tooth. Assume the extracellular fluid pH outside the neuron = 7.4. What % of the lidocaine molecules is ionized and un-ionized in this extracellular fluid?

2. Lidocaine can only cross the neuronal cell membrane by passive transcellular diffusion, and only the cationic form of lidocaine can bind to the ion channel receptor. If the pH of both intracellular and extracellular fluids is 7.4, explain how lidocaine can enter the cell and also bind to the receptor.

3. The binding of the cationic form to the receptor inside the neuron could potentially "tie up," some of it inside the neuron. How could this affect the further transport of lidocaine into the cell?

4. How does the numbness around the tooth caused by the local anesthetic eventually wear off? In other words, what makes the lidocaine eventually leave the cell?

5. The patient has an infected tooth. In many tooth infections, the extracellular tissue fluid pH is much lower, around 5. How will this impact the rate of transport of lidocaine into the cell? What might be the result on the time taken to achieve numbness of the gum?

6. If you were the dentist's pharmacist friend, how would you explain the lower efficacy of lidocaine in this patient?

7. You work for a drug company that would like to introduce a new and better lidocaine-like local anesthetic by optimizing the pK_a. In what direction would you change the pK_a of lidocaine (up or down) to achieve a faster rate of transport into the neuron (to give a quicker anesthetic effect)? In what direction would you change the pK_a to increase drug–receptor binding inside the cell (to give a longer duration of action)? Assume an extracellular and intracellular pH of 7.4, and no significant change in P or molecular size. Explain your rationale.

Additional Readings

Alberts B, Johnson A, Lewis J, Raff M, Roberts K, Walter P. Molecular Biology of the Cell, 5th ed. Garland Science, 2008.

Hillery A, Lloyd A, Swarbrick J (eds). Drug Delivery and Targeting: For Pharmacists and Pharmaceutical Scientists. CRC Press, 2001.

Shargel L, Wu-Pong S, Yu A. Applied Biopharmaceutics and Pharmacokinetics, 5th ed. McGraw-Hill/Appleton & Lange, 2004.

Washington N, Washington C, Wilson C. Physiological Pharmaceutics: Barriers to Drug Absorption, 2nd ed. CRC Press, 2000.

CHAPTER 6

Drug Absorption

Drugs are given to patients at a variety of locations in or on the body called sites of administration. The drug must travel from the site of administration and reach its site of action in a timely and predictable manner, where it can perform its function. There are many ways to administer a drug to a patient, and drugs are available in a variety of dosage forms. The choice of administration method and dosage form depends on, among other factors, the physicochemical properties of the drug, physiological limitations of the administration or absorption site, and the clinical situation.

In some situations, the site of action is localized and is readily accessible; in these cases the drug can be administered very close to, or right at, this site. Such an approach to drug administration is termed topical, nonsystemic, or local administration. An example is the application of a cream to the skin to treat a rash, or use of a local anesthetic during dental procedures.

In many conditions, the site of action is difficult to reach; an example is clinical depression where the site of action is the brain. Or, the drug may not penetrate deep enough into the tissue after topical administration to be completely effective, as in a fungal infection of the toenail. So, the drug has to be administered at some other convenient location, from where it is absorbed into the bloodstream which carries it to the site of action. In other cases, the site of action is not a single location but involves many tissues; an example is allergic reactions that involve the eyes, nose, lungs, and skin. The drug must reach all these sites to effectively treat the patient, so the best approach is to use the bloodstream to carry drug to all the target sites. Such an approach to drug administration is called systemic administration. The first step in the journey of a systemically administered drug is absorption into the bloodstream; only then can the drug reach the sites of action. In contrast, a drug administered topically needs merely to enter the desired tissue at the site of administration; absorption into the bloodstream is not necessary.

Table 6.1 summarizes the various routes of systemic and nonsystemic administration available for drug delivery. Some routes may be used for either systemic or nonsystemic dosing. For example, a drug can be applied to the skin for treating a local rash (nonsystemic application), whereas another drug can be applied to the skin to elicit a systemic effect (such as nicotine patches for smoking cessation). In the latter case, the drug is absorbed into the bloodstream and carried to the site of action.

TABLE 6.1. Classification of the Available Routes of Administration for Drugs	
Systemic	**Nonsystemic**
Oral	Oral
Parenteral	Parenteral
Intravenous	Intracardiac
Intramuscular	Intrathecal
Subcutaneous	Intralumbar
Intraarterial	
Rectal	Rectal
Sublingual/buccal	Buccal
Transdermal	Dermal
Pulmonary	Pulmonary
Nasal	Nasal
Vaginal	Vaginal
	Ophthalmic
	Otic
	Urethral

Systemic Administration

Systemically administered drugs may be absorbed directly from the site of administration into the bloodstream. For example, transdermal patches are applied to the skin (site of administration) and absorption of the drug occurs from the skin into the bloodstream. Therefore, for the transdermal route, the skin is both the site of administration as well as the site of absorption. For other systemically administered drugs, the drug must travel from the site of administration to a different region from where it is absorbed. For instance, orally administered drugs are administered in the mouth and swallowed; absorption usually occurs from the small intestines. Therefore, the site of absorption is the small intestines for oral administration. Regardless of where the site of absorption is located, the drug must be dissolved in body fluids at the site of absorption for it to be absorbed. We will discuss the dissolution process in more depth in Chapter 7.

Dissolved drug molecules have to cross the epithelial tissue at the absorption site, and then the capillary endothelium of blood vessels at the absorption site, to enter the bloodstream. Most drugs are small enough to cross the capillary endothelium readily by paracellular passive diffusion, regardless of their physicochemical properties. Thus, the slowest, or *rate-limiting*, step in absorption is usually the drug's ability to cross epithelial membranes at the absorption site, and this is what determines the overall rate of absorption.

Rate of Absorption

Absorption of *most* drugs across *most* epithelia occurs by passive transcellular diffusion. The absorption rate depends on physicochemical properties of the drug, permeability of the epithelial membrane at the site of absorption, surface area of the membrane exposed to drug at the absorption site, and concentration gradient of drug between the absorption site and the bloodstream. The equation for the rate of absorption is similar to Fick's law of diffusion:

$$\text{absorption rate} = \frac{P \cdot A \cdot D \cdot (C_a - C_p)}{h} \quad \text{(Eq. 6.1)}$$

The partition coefficient P and diffusion coefficient D depend on the structure and molecular size of the drug, respectively. The term A is the surface area of the membrane, and h is the thickness of the epithelial membrane at the absorption site; this membrane may be composed of one or more layers of epithelial cells. We ignore transport across the capillary endothelium in this analysis because it is much faster than transport across the epithelium. In other words, we assume that as soon as drug crosses the epithelial barrier, it can enter the capillaries readily. Equation 6.1 is the same as Equation 5.4 in the chapter Transport Across Biological Barriers; the only difference is that, in this context, C_a is the concentration of drug at the absorption site (donor side) and C_p is the concentration of drug in blood (receiver side). Remember also that for passive transcellular transport (the most common absorption mechanism for drugs), the concentration gradient of the *un-ionized* form drives transport.

Let us look more closely at the concentration gradient term $(C_a - C_p)$. Obviously, the higher the concentration of dissolved drug at the absorption site, the faster the rate of absorption will be. C_a is controlled by the dose of drug administered, the volume of fluid at the site of absorption, and the dissolution rate of drug in this fluid. On the receiver side (blood), if the site of absorption is well perfused (i.e., has good blood supply), blood flows through the absorption site so rapidly that drug is carried away in the circulation almost as soon as it enters the capillaries. Consequently, the concentration of drug in the capillaries is very small relative to the concentration at the absorption site. This maintains a positive concentration gradient for continued absorption until all administered drug is absorbed.

If we assume that C_p is approximately 0 for the reasons above, Equation 6.1 simplifies to

$$\text{absorption rate} = \frac{P \cdot A \cdot D}{h} C_a \quad \text{(Eq. 6.2)}$$

Combining D, A, P, and h to give a new constant k, we can write

$$\text{absorption rate} = k \cdot C_a \quad \text{(Eq. 6.3)}$$

The constant k is called the *permeation rate constant*. Note that the permeation rate constant is related to the permeability coefficient defined in the chapter Transport Across Biological Barriers (eq. 5.5). The permeation rate constant is the permeability coefficient of a particular membrane for a particular drug, multiplied by the area of membrane exposed to the drug.

Equation 6.3 shows that if the absorption site has good blood flow, absorption is directly proportional to the concentration of dissolved drug at the absorption site. Therefore, fast dissolution of drug from the dosage form and good perfusion of the absorption site facilitate rapid absorption of drug after administration. How much of the drug is in its un-ionized, absorbable form depends on the drug pK_a and the pH of fluids at the site of absorption. Note that a pH that favors ionization will increase dissolution rate but will hinder rate of permeation. This again underlines the concept that drugs must have an optimal balance between hydrophilicity and lipophilicity.

The actual rate of absorption may be less than that predicted by Equation 6.3. One factor is efflux pumps in many epithelial cells that pump a drug out of epithelial cells at the absorption site as they are being absorbed, and return them to the donor side. This protective mechanism contributes to the poor absorption of many drugs.

A few very low molecular weight drugs may be absorbed to some extent by paracellular passive diffusion, especially if the epithelial membrane is "leaky". In such cases, lipophilicity is not needed and the permeation rate constant will not depend on the partition coefficient. Drugs that resemble substrates of carrier proteins may be absorbed by an active transport process. For these drugs, the rate of absorption per unit surface area is described an equation similar to the Michaelis-Menten equation we discussed in Chapter 5:

$$\text{absorption rate} = \frac{V_{max} C_a}{K_m + C_a} \quad \text{(Eq. 6.4)}$$

In this context, C_a is the concentration of drug at the absorption site. Note that it is the concentration of drug, rather than the concentration gradient, that controls rate of absorption in active transport. When the concentration of drug at the administration site is low compared to the number of transporters available, C_a $<< K_m$, so eq. 6.4 simplifies to:

$$\text{absorption rate} = \frac{V_{max}}{K_m} C_a \qquad \text{(Eq. 6.5)}$$

If the concentration of drug at the administration site is high compared to the number of transporters available, C_a $>> K_m$, and eq. 6.4 approximates to:

$$\text{absorption rate} = V_{max} \qquad \text{(Eq. 6.6)}$$

The rate of absorption now becomes a constant, equal to the maximum rate at which the carrier can transport the drug. Any increase in concentration of drug has no effect on the rate of absorption, and we say that the transporter is saturated.

The Oral Route

Oral administration, in which a drug product (e.g. a tablet, capsule, suspension) is administered by mouth, is the most common and patient-preferred route of systemic administration. The dosage form moves down the gastrointestinal (GI) tract, and can be absorbed in any of several regions. Oral administration is an effective means of dosing if the drug is able to cross the epithelial membranes of the GI tract efficiently.

Structure of the Gastrointestinal Tract

The primary organs of the GI tract are the stomach, the small intestine (made up of the duodenum, jejunum, and ileum), and the colon (large intestine); these are shown diagrammatically in Figure 6.1. The GI tract ends in the rectum. The various parts differ in structure, length, secretions, and pH, all of which influence drug absorption. Although an oral product starts in the mouth and travels down the esophagus, the drug spends so little time here that

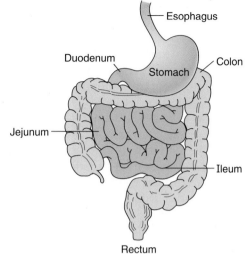

Figure 6.1. Diagram of the esophagus and gastrointestinal tract, showing the different parts.

the esophagus has no significant role in absorption of most oral medications.

The GI tract is lined with four concentric layers of tissue. Starting from the *intestinal lumen*, successive layers are the *mucosa, submucosa, muscular tissue,* and *serosa.* The mucosa consists of three layers: a single layer of epithelial cells in contact with intestinal contents, an underlying lamina propria containing blood vessels and lymphatic vessels, and a layer of muscle fibers. Absorption of drugs takes place across the epithelium into the blood capillaries of the lamina propria, from which the drug is carried in the bloodstream to the rest of the body. Epithelial cells of the GI mucosa are closely packed with very tight junctions. The diameter of these gaps has been estimated to be about 1.5 nm, too small for most drugs to cross paracellularly. The primary mode of transport of drugs across the GI epithelium is passive transcellular diffusion.

The lumenal sides of the GI epitheium contain various transporters whose primary function is the carrier-mediated absorption of nutrients from the GI lumen into the bloodstream. These transport pathways are especially important for polar molecules that cannot be absorbed by passive transcellular diffusion. There is growing evidence, however, that these transporters may also play a role in the absorption of some drugs. This is another reason why oral drug absorption cannot be predicted based solely on Equation 6.3.

The Stomach. An orally administered drug product arrives in the stomach very quickly after administration. The empty stomach, a pouch-like organ, contains approximately 100 mL of gastric fluid, with a maximum capacity of about 1 L. The primary functions of the stomach are to reduce ingested food into a liquid mixture called chyme, and to begin the process of digestion. The epithelial lining of the stomach also contains cells that secrete mucus, hydrochloric acid, and digestive enzymes, all of which make up gastric fluid (normal pH range 1–3).

For orally administered drugs, the stomach is a site for drug dissolution. The absorption of drug from the stomach into the bloodstream is either modest or negligible, regardless of whether a drug is a weak acid or weak base. One reason is the short time that dissolved drug spends in the stomach. Once a drug dissolves in gastric fluid, it moves quickly into the small intestines, leaving little time for significant absorption in the stomach. A second and equally important reason is that the surface area of the stomach is relatively small, making permeation slow.

Therefore, although some passive transcellular absorption of a drug *could* occur from the stomach given sufficient time, the stomach plays a negligible role in the absorption of most drugs under normal circumstances. The primary function of the stomach, then, is to grind up a solid dosage form and facilitate release and dissolution of drug for subsequent absorption from the small intestines. We will learn more about the dissolution process in the next chapter, Drug Delivery Systems.

The Small Intestine. The small intestine is a long and narrow tube about 6 to 7 m

(20 to 23 feet) in length. The first part is the duodenum, a short section following the stomach that receives stomach contents, and digestive secretions from the pancreas and liver. Next is the jejunum (roughly 40% of the small intestine), which is followed by the ileum (about 60% of the small intestine).

The intestinal epithelium, or gut wall, acts as a barrier between two distinct body compartments—the gut lumen and the systemic circulation. Maintenance of this barrier is required to prevent ingested pathogens and toxins from gaining ready access to internal organs and tissues. At the same time, the intestinal epithelium is designed for efficient absorption of nutrients, and is also the most important region for absorption of orally administered drugs.

The main reason for the absorptive capability of the small intestines is the extremely large surface area of epithelial tissue. Although the small intestine looks like a long tube, its absorptive surface area is tremendously enhanced by its unique internal structure, as shown in Figure 6.2. Another reason is the relatively long time (about 4 hours) intestinal contents spend in this region, as they travel from the duodenum to the end of the ileum.

The inner surface of the small intestine is not flat, but has circular folds (folds of Kerckring), which not only increase surface area about threefold, but help to mix intestinal contents by acting as baffles. Each fold has fingerlike protrusions called villi that increase surface area by another factor of 10. Villi are lined with epithelial cells called enterocytes (through which absorption takes place) and other cells that secrete mucus and digestive fluids. Enterocytes have brush-like projections called microvilli that extend into the intestinal lumen and increase absorptive surface area by another factor of 20. Because microvilli resemble a brush, the enterocyte surface is often called the *brush border*. Consequently, the actual absorptive surface area of the small intestinal epithelium is about 600 times that

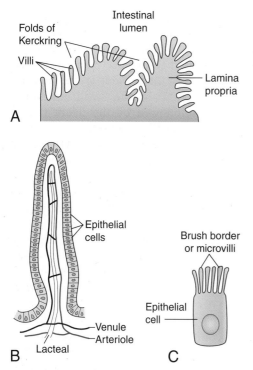

Figure 6.2. A. Layers of the small intestines and the folds of Kerckring. B. Schematic cross-section of a villus. C. Interpretation of the structure of the brush border of a single intestinal epithelial cell.

of a simple cylinder. This extraordinarily large surface area and the relatively long time (about 4 hours) that a drug spends in the small intestines explain the excellent absorptive ability of this region.

Villi are well perfused by blood and lymph, further facilitating absorption from the small intestines. Within each villus is a network of capillaries, and a lymph duct called the lacteal. Small intestinal capillaries combine to form the portal vein; most drugs are absorbed into blood in the capillaries and carried away by the portal vein. The main function of the lacteals is to absorb digested fat; lipophilic drugs are often absorbed with digested fats into the lymphatic circulation. The excellent perfusion of the small intestines by blood also contributes to its absorptive capability. Absorbed drug is carried away rapidly,

maintaining a positive concentration gradient for continued absorption.

Intestinal fluid is a complex mixture. Cells of the intestinal membrane secrete mucus and digestive enzymes into the intestinal lumen. In addition, digestive juices from the liver (bile) and pancreas (pancreatic juice) empty into the duodenum as needed after a meal. The pH of small intestinal contents varies slightly in different regions. The duodenal fluid is somewhat acidic (pH 5.5 to 6.5) due to the influence of entering gastric juices. In the jejunum and ileum, the pH is modified by alkaline pancreatic juice and bile, raising it to approximately 6.5 to 7.5.

The Large Intestine. The large intestine is the end of the GI tract, and consists of the cecum, the colon, the rectum and the anal canal. The large intestine is wider but shorter than the small intestine, measuring about 1.5 m (5 feet) in length. It is structurally somewhat similar to the small intestines but does not have villi on its inside surface, limiting the surface area available for absorption. The main functions of the colon are to absorb water and electrolytes from the remaining indigestible food matter, and to pass waste material from the body as feces. Undigested food may take as long as 30–40 hours to move through the large intestines. In spite of this long residence time, nutrients or drugs are not generally absorbed significantly from the large intestines. However, small amounts of some drugs that remain unabsorbed may be absorbed in this region; for example, theophylline is partially absorbed from the colon. In general, if a large amount of unabsorbed drug reaches the colon, it is excreted in the feces.

An important feature of the large intestine is the numerous species of bacteria that live in this region (colonic microflora) and perform a variety of functions. Bacteria help to ferment unused energy substrates, prevent growth of pathogenic bacteria, and produce vitamins such as biotin and vitamin *K* for absorption.

Bacteria may also metabolize some unab-sorbed drugs that reach the colon.

Oral Drug Absorption

As a result of the large surface area and long residence time, the small intestine is the main region for drug absorption. The drug must be dissolved in the intestinal fluids for it to permeate through the intestinal epithelium. Therefore, before absorption can occur, the drug needs to be either pre-dissolved in the drug product (e.g. an oral solution), or must dissolve in GI fluids from a solid dosage form after administration.

The rate of dissolution of weak acid and base drugs in the GI tract depends on their total solubility, which in turn depends on intrinsic solubility and extent of ionization. The latter, in turn, depends on drug pK_a, and the pH in the stomach or small intestine. In the stomach, a drug that exists predominantly in its ionized form will dissolve better (because of a higher solubility) than one that exists predominantly in its un-ionized form. Consequently, weak bases dissolve better in gastric fluid than weak acids. Weak acids will dissolve better when they move into the small intestines where the pH (and weak acid solubility) is higher. Remember that the intrinsic solubility also contributes to total solubility; drugs with a low intrinsic solubility will dissolve slowly even if they are mostly ionized. A drug must dissolve rapidly enough so that there is sufficient time it to permeate through the intestinal epithelium as it moves down the intestines towards the colon.

We often use the terms 'highly soluble' or 'poorly soluble' when referring to drugs. These are relative terms. In the context of drug absorption, the dose of the drug must also be considered. For example, consider a drug with an aqueous solubility of 0.05 mg/mL. If the therapeutic dose of this drug was 10 mg, the 250 mL of fluid in the stomach (swallowing a tablet with a glass of water) would be sufficient

to dissolve it completely. However, if the dose were 200 mg, dissolution could be incomplete and might pose a problem.

Most orally administered drugs are absorbed across the small intestinal epithelium by passive transcellular diffusion. A few may be absorbed by carrier-mediated processes. The absorption of several drugs is limited by efflux pumps in the intestinal epithelium.

Passive Transcellular Diffusion. As we learned in the chapter on Drug Transport, passive transcellular diffusion is the primary mechanism for transport of drugs across epithelia, including the intestinal epithelium. Only uncharged drugs and un-ionized forms of weak acids and weak bases can permeate across the intestinal epithelium by passive diffusion. The ionization of a drug will depend on its pK_a, and the pH of the intestinal fluid. The composition, volume, and pH of GI fluids vary down the length of the tract; Table 6.2 lists the pH ranges of the various GI fluids.

In the small intestines, a dissolved drug that exists predominantly in its un-ionized form will permeate faster than one that exists predominantly in its ionized form. Consequently, bases of pK_a 10 or higher and acids of pK_a less than 3 are poorly absorbed, because these are completely ionized at intestinal pH. In general, weak bases are absorbed better than weak acids. The ionization equilibrium of drugs

TABLE 6.2. Typical pH Values of the Various Regions of the Human GI Tract

GI Region	Normal pH
Mouth	6.5–7.0
Esophagus	5.0–6.0
Stomach	1.0–3.5
Duodenum	5.5–6.5
Jejunum	6.5–7.0
Ileum	7.0–7.5
Colon	6.0–7.0
Rectum	7.0–7.5

is rapid. This means that as the un-ionized form of the drug is absorbed and leaves the intestinal lumen, equilibrium reestablishes to produce more un-ionized drug. Thus, if a drug has a high enough partition coefficient and is at least partially un-ionized in the small intestines, it can be absorbed.

The dissolution and absorption of nonelectrolyte drugs will not be influenced by pH in the GI tract. If such drugs have adequate intrinsic water solubility they will dissolve sufficiently in the stomach and small intestines. If they also have adequate lipophilicity, they will permeate the small intestinal epithelium rapidly by passive transcellular diffusion.

The Biopharmaceutics Classification System (BCS) is a scientific framework for classifying orally administered drugs based on aqueous solubility and intestinal permeability. The BCS takes into account two major factors that control the rate and extent of drug absorption from solid oral drug products: aqueous solubility and intestinal permeability. According to the BCS, drug substances can be classified into the following categories:

- Class I: High solubility–high permeability (e.g., propranolol, verapamil, metoprolol)
- Class II: Low solubility–high permeability (e.g., naproxen, ketoprofen, carbamazepine)
- Class III: High solubility–low permeability (e.g., cimetidine, ranitidine, atenolol)
- Class IV: Low solubility–low permeability (e.g., furosemide, hydrochlorothiazide, taxol)

Figure 6.3 shows a graphical view of the BCS. The intestinal permeability of drugs is measured by appropriate laboratory techniques. Classification of a drug as high solubility or low solubility in the BCS depends on the oral dose of the drug. A drug is considered to have "high" solubility if the highest oral dose is soluble in the 250 ml of water between the pH

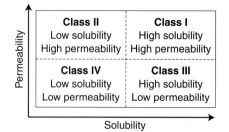

Figure 6.3. A graphical representation of the Biopharmaceutics Classification System (BCS). A drug is classified as having "high solubility" if the highest dose is soluble in the average fluid volume present in the GI tract (250 ml) between the typical GI pH values of 1.0–7.5. The intestinal permeability is measured by appropriate laboratory techniques.

values of 1.0–7.5. This medium is chosen to represent the average fluid pH and volume in the GI tract. If the dose is not completely soluble in 250 mL, the drug is considered to have "poor" solubility. The important concept here is that, for two drugs with the same aqueous solubility, the drug with a lower dose drug will be absorbed to a greater extent than the one with a higher dose.

The BCS allows the roles of dissolution and permeability in drug absorption to be separated. If absorption is poor as a result of inadequate aqueous solubility, the drug is said to have dissolution-limited absorption. On the other hand, if low lipophilicity compromises absorption, the drug is considered to exhibit permeability-limited absorption. Appropriate strategies can then be developed to improve either dissolution or permeation, depending on which one is the problem.

Carrier-Mediated Absorption. A wide variety of transporters are found in the intestinal epithelium, and are involved in the absorption of essential nutrients (such as amino acids, small peptides, vitamins, minerals, and sugars) as well as drugs. Each transporter exhibits its own substrate specificity, and some have broader specificities than others. These transporters may also help to absorb drugs that are structurally similar to the natural substrates. For example, the amino acid transporter in the small intestines helps in the absorption of many oral cephalosporins. Peptide-like drugs (such as β-lactam antibiotics and angiotensin-converting enzyme (ACE) inhibitors) are known to be absorbed via organic ion transporters. Many antiviral and anticancer drugs (e.g. zidovudine, cladribine, acyclovir, cytosine arabinoside, and dideoxycytidine) are nucleoside analogs; carrier-mediated absorption through sodium-dependent nucleoside transporters may play a role in their absorption. Recall that lipophilicity is not necessary for carrier-mediated processes. However, ionization may be important because the transporter may preferentially bind to either the ionized or un-ionized form of the drug.

Carrier-mediated transport can be saturated at high substrate concentrations. Therefore, drugs that need a transporter for absorption may have to compete with the transporter's natural substrates (nutrients), resulting in lower absorption. Genetic differences in the expression of transporters can also cause variability of absorption among individuals.

Intestinal Drug Efflux. The role of multidrug resistance (MDR) transporters as efflux pumps is becoming increasingly apparent in explaining poor oral absorption of a variety of drugs which we would expect to be well-absorbed by passive transcellular diffusion. Hydrophobic drugs appear to be more susceptible to these efflux systems than hydrophilic drugs. Epithelial cells of the small intestines express the multidrug transporter, which transports drug unidirectionally, from the enterocyte back into the intestinal lumen. In other words, the drug enters the intestinal epithelial cell by passive diffusion, but rather than moving on into the bloodstream, is effluxed back into the intestinal lumen. For example, the HIV-1 protease inhibitors ritonavir, saquinavir and indinavir are poorly absorbed after oral administration because of P-glycoprotein (P-gp)–mediated efflux. Recall that carrier-mediated transport, which is governed by Michaelis–Menten kinetics, can become saturated when a large concentration of the substrate is present. This is illustrated in the dose-dependent absorption of celiprolol, a cardiovascular drug. It is absorbed in much greater proportion after an oral dose of 400 mg than after a dose of 100 mg. The efflux pumps become saturated at higher doses and a greater proportion of the 400 mg dose can escape efflux and reach the systemic circulation.

Substances that inhibit efflux pumps also have an effect on drug absorption. For instance, grapefruit juice contains various flavonoids that have inhibitory effects on P-gp–mediated transport; one glass of grapefruit juice can inhibit P-gp for up to 24 hours. Therefore, when cyclosporine, a P-gp substrate, is co-administered with grapefruit juice, a large increase in cyclosporine absorption is observed. This type of interaction also provides a potential application to increase absorption of drugs like cyclosporine that are P-gp efflux substrates. The use of P-gp inhibitors to increase intracellular concentrations of chemotherapeutic agents in tumor cells is also being evaluated in patients with multidrug-resistant tumors.

Transcytosis. Transcytosis, or a related process–receptor-mediated transcytosis–, is uncommon for the absorption of most small molecule drugs from the GI tract. Even for large molecules and particles, the process is inefficient, in that only a small proportion of the material in the intestinal lumen can be absorbed in this way. For some macromolecular drugs, even this small degree of absorption may be sufficient to obtain a pharmacological effect. It is believed that many orally administered vaccines are absorbed by transcytosis, and can be effective because only a small degree of absorption is necessary.

TABLE 6.3. Drug or Patient Characteristics That Make Oral Administration Unsuitable

Drug Properties

- Instability in GI fluids and consequent rapid degradation
- Irritation of the gastric or intestinal epithelium
- Poor lipophilicity for passive transcellular diffusion
- Large molecular size resulting in a slow absorption rate

Patient Characteristics

- Unable or unwilling to swallow medications
- Needs immediate response; not provided by relatively slow oral absorption
- Suffering from GI distress (nausea, vomiting, diarrhea)
- Suffering from GI disease that may be exacerbated by oral administration, or that compromises drug absorption
- Taking another medication that is incompatible with drug

Nonoral Routes for Systemic Administration

Most patients prefer to take drugs orally than by other routes. However, it is not always possible to administer a drug orally when drug properties or patient characteristics are unfavorable or inappropriate. These are listed in Table 6.3. Some drugs may never be developed as oral products. Other drugs may be available in both oral and nonoral products; the appropriate dosage form and route will depend on the specific clinical situation.

The Parenteral Route

When oral administration is not feasible, one option is to administer the drug parenterally. Although parenteral means "other than enteral," the term is reserved for routes in which a drug (usually in a liquid) is injected into the body through a hollow needle that punctures the skin. Parenteral administration avoids the epithelial barriers that can be difficult for some drugs to cross. The drug may

be injected directly into the bloodstream by intravenous (IV; in a vein) or intra-arterial (in an artery) administration. Alternatively, the drug may be injected into a tissue from which it can reach the bloodstream, such as in subcutaneous (SC; under the skin), intramuscular (IM; in a muscle), or intraperitoneal (IP; in the abdomen) administration.

Absorption is not an issue for IV and intra-arterial administration because the drug is placed directly in the bloodstream. These routes ensure that the entire dose of drug enters the bloodstream, representing the fastest systemic ways of getting drug to the site of action. Polar, nonpolar and large molecule drugs can all be administered effectively by these routes. IV administration is more common because veins are easily accessible for administration.

In contrast, SC, IM, or IP administration requires drug to travel through the tissue at the administration site before it can enter the blood in nearest capillaries. Fortunately, this entails crossing the more permeable endothelial capillary wall rather than epithelial barriers with tight junctions. Therefore, drugs administered by SC, IM, or IP injections usually enter the bloodstream much more readily and completely than those administered orally, although there still is a lag time before the drug reaches the bloodstream.

SC, IM, or IP routes can be used to administer both lipophilic and hydrophilic drugs. Hydrophilic drugs will enter capillaries by paracellular transport through the large gaps in the capillary endothelium; lipophilic drugs can use both paracellular and transcellular diffusion mechanisms. Even small proteins can cross the capillary endothelium and enter the bloodstream after SC, IM, or IP administration. SC and IM injections are easier and more convenient to administer than IP injections.

The Rectal Route

Most drugs given orally can also be administered rectally. Rectal dosing involves administration through the anus into the rectum (lower portion of the large intestines). The drug is administered either by a suppository or by a retention enema. Drugs are absorbed from the rectum in the same way as from other parts of the GI tract—by crossing the epithelial membrane lining the rectum, primarily by passive transcellular diffusion.

Although the rectal region has a fairly good blood supply, it has a much lower surface area than the small intestines because of the absence of villi. Thus, absorption is much slower compared with the oral route, and is often more variable. This method of systemic drug delivery is reserved for situations in which oral administration is difficult, such as in children or the elderly. It may also be used in patients who are vomiting or unable to take medications orally. An example is the rectal administration of diazepam to children having an epileptic seizure and in whom intravenous access is difficult.

The Buccal or Sublingual Route

These routes involve placing the medication in the mouth, without swallowing, enabling absorption through buccal (cheek) or sublingual (below the tongue) mucosal membranes. The oral mucosa is very well perfused and allows rapid absorption of lipophilic drugs by passive transcellular diffusion. These routes are generally used for drugs that are destroyed by the low pH in the stomach, decomposed by enzymes of the GI tract, or extensively metabolized by first-pass metabolism (discussed in the chapter on Drug Metabolism). Sublingual administration is used for nitroglycerin, a drug used to treat angina.

The Transdermal Route

Although many drugs are applied to the skin for local action, systemic absorption of drugs through the skin is also possible. In transdermal delivery, the intention is to deliver drugs systemically through the skin into the bloodstream.

The skin is a formidable barrier that protects the body against entry of undesirable substances. It has three main layers: epidermis, dermis, and subcutaneous fat. The outermost part of the epidermis is the stratum corneum, consisting of several layers of dead cells. This is the main barrier to drug absorption. If a drug can cross the stratum corneum, it can travel easily through the rest of the epidermis into the dermis. The dermis is well perfused with blood; once a drug arrives in the dermis, it can enter the bloodstream. Therefore, if physicochemical properties of a drug are suitable for transport through the stratum corneum, it will be absorbed systemically.

The dead cells of the stratum corneum are very tightly packed with junctions that do not allow paracellular transport. Thus, passive transcellular diffusion is the only means of transdermal drug absorption; only lipophilic drugs with small molecular size can penetrate the stratum corneum and be absorbed. The surface area for absorption is the area of the skin the drug is applied to, and is very small compared with extensive absorptive surface area available after oral administration. Therefore, absorption through the skin is usually a slow process, and transdermal administration is reserved for long-term therapy.

Scientists have been able to design effective sustained-release transdermal delivery systems so that once-daily or once-weekly therapies are possible. For example, once-weekly administration of estrogen in transdermal patches is used for hormone replacement therapy.

The Pulmonary Route

In this route (also called the inhalation or respiratory route) a drug is inhaled through the mouth into the lungs where absorption takes place. The drug, suspended in air, travels from the mouth, down the trachea into the bronchial tree that forms the lungs. The bronchial tree consists of the primary bronchi, which divide successively into smaller branches: bronchioles, terminal bronchioles, respiratory bronchioles, and finally, clusters of tiny air sacs called alveoli. The alveolar epithelial membrane is very thin with a large surface area and an extensive blood supply. Once drug reaches the alveoli, it can be rapidly absorbed into the bloodstream by passive transcellular diffusion through the alveolar epithelium. There is also some evidence that macromolecular drugs, such as insulin, are absorbed in the alveolar epithelium by vesicular transport and receptor-mediated endocytosis.

The majority of the pulmonary absorptive surface is in the terminal bronchioles and alveoli, so substances must reach this region to be effectively absorbed. If a drug can travel down the bronchial tree and reach the alveoli, its absorption will be rapid and complete. Inhaled gases and vapors (general anesthetics, for example) have no difficulty reaching this region, and are rapidly and completely absorbed after inhalation. However, drugs inhaled as solid particles or liquid droplets have a more difficult time reaching the lower bronchial tree. Drug particles or droplets have to be small enough to be able to fit through the increasingly smaller passages of the bronchial tree. Only particles less than 5 µm in diameter are small enough to reach the lower bronchial tree. Thus, although the lung is a great site for systemic absorption, getting a sufficient dose of the drug to the absorptive regions is a challenge.

The Nasal Route

Nasal delivery involves depositing drug in the nose, usually as drops or a liquid spray. The nasal mucosa is very permeable and has a good blood supply, so drugs can be absorbed rapidly. Although nasal delivery seems like a convenient route for systemic administration, it has

several limitations. The anatomical and physiological features of the nose are not ideal for drug administration for several reasons. It is often difficult to get a large enough dose into a small volume of liquid to spray into the nose. The nasal mucosa has a relatively small surface area (150 cm^2) for absorption, and the drug does not remain in contact with the nasal mucosa long enough for complete absorption. Many drugs also irritate the nasal lining and can damage it with long-term use. Therefore, the nasal route is not commonly used for systemic administration when alternative routes, especially oral, are available.

The nasal route is a good option when oral absorption is problematic. An example is nasal delivery of vitamin B12 to patients with Crohn's disease and irritable bowel syndrome. The nasal route is also very attractive for macromolecular drugs that are not orally absorbed. Peptide hormone analogs such as antidiuretic hormone and calcitonin are given as nasal sprays. These drugs are destroyed in the GI tract if given orally.

Systemic Absorption of Macromolecular Drugs

Proteins and other macromolecular drugs present a difficult delivery problem because of their large molecular size, high polarity, and their extreme sensitivity to the surrounding environment. Such drugs cannot cross epithelial tissues effectively and in sufficient concentrations to be effective, so parenteral administration is still the most common route of delivery. Because parenteral administration is invasive and inconvenient, researchers continue to investigate nonparenteral delivery strategies.

Alternative routes have had limited success. Oral administration of proteins and large peptides is being studied, but no completely effective system has yet been developed. The hydrochloric acid and digestive enzymes in the stomach rapidly degrade proteins and peptides. Even if the molecules could somehow be protected, it is difficult for large molecules to cross the intestinal epithelium in sufficient quantities for therapeutic benefit. No acceptable transdermal delivery systems have been found because inherent physicochemical properties prohibit these large polar molecules from crossing the stratum corneum without the addition of potentially irritating additives called penetration enhancers.

The pulmonary route has shown success with macromolecular drugs delivered either as solutions or fine powders. The properties and composition of lung fluid are similar to those of blood, so pulmonary delivery is very similar to injection into the bloodstream. The lungs can absorb many macromolecules and some small particles, presumably by transcytosis in the alveoli. Once absorbed in the deep lung, the drug passes readily into the bloodstream. The body's protective mechanisms, however, pose a problem in getting drug to the deep lung. Large molecules and particles may be removed by metabolism, and by phagocytosis by white blood cells. Nevertheless, if the drug is delivered efficiently to the lower pulmonary regions, a sufficient quantity can be absorbed into the bloodstream to exert a therapeutic effect. For example, the pulmonary delivery of insulin has been successful, and that of other protein drugs is showing success in clinical trials.

Local Administration

Systemic administration is appropriate when we need to use the bloodstream to get drug to the site of action. However, the bloodstream also carries the drug to all other organs and tissues in the body, which often leads to unwanted side effects.

Sometimes, it is possible to administer the drug at or close to the site of action so that absorption into the bloodstream is unnecessary; this approach to drug administration is called nonsystemic or local. To exert its action, the drug has to merely stay at the site of application, or travel only a short distance through the tissue. High local concentrations are achieved at the intended site, usually much higher than those possible by a systemic route. Therefore, a much lower dose can be used for local delivery compared with administration of the same drug systemically.

Because absorption in the bloodstream is not necessary, local delivery avoids many systemic side effects. This does not mean, however, that all the drugs remain at the site of application. Some of the administered drug may enter the bloodstream (by the processes discussed above under Systemic Administration) and travel to the rest of the body. As a result, some systemic side effects may occur with locally applied medications, particularly with inappropriate use.

Many of the systemic routes discussed earlier can also be employed to treat localized conditions. Although the oral route is most commonly used for systemic administration, orally administered drugs also treat ailments of the GI tract locally. Examples are antacids to neutralize stomach acid and antibiotics for the treatment of GI infections. In these situations, the site of action is the GI tract, and the drug does not need to be absorbed into the circulation.

Local parenteral delivery involves injecting the drug near the site of action, as in intracardiac (in the heart), intrathecal (in the cerebrospinal fluid), or intralumbar (in the lumbar space) application. These routes are only used in specialized situations, when other routes of administration cannot achieve adequate concentrations of drug in the tissues.

Examples of buccal delivery for local treatment are sprays applied to gums, mouth, and throat for local infections or pain, and lozenges for dissolution in the mouth to soothe the mouth and throat regions.

Rectal suppositories and enemas are used to relive constipation and for clearing out the lower intestines before surgical procedures. Ointments and creams are applied rectally for the relief of hemorrhoids and itching.

Dermal delivery involves application of medications to the skin for local treatment. Medications can be applied to skin for protection (e.g., sunscreens), to fight infection (e.g., antibacterials and antibiotics), or to modify properties of the skin (e.g., anti-acne products, anti-aging products, or chemical peels). Many of the latter are considered cosmetics rather than drug products, but the distinction is often blurred.

Pulmonary delivery of drugs is more common for local treatment than for systemic application. It is widely used to treat pulmonary conditions such as asthma, emphysema, and lung infections. Nasal delivery is also more common for treatment of local conditions. Nasal allergies and nasal congestion are frequently treated with drops or sprays applied in the nostrils.

The ophthalmic route is reserved for local application to the eye only and is generally not used for systemic administration. The eye is a very delicate organ and is easily irritated and damaged by introduction of foreign substances. Therefore, medications are applied to the eye only when necessary to treat ophthalmic diseases. Eye infections and inflammatory conditions can be treated by eye drops or ointments. Ophthalmic products are also used to treat glaucoma, with the drug traveling through the cornea into the aqueous humor.

Vaginal and urethral application is also reserved for treating local conditions, vaginal application being more common. Solution, creams, or tablets can be applied to the vagina for contraception or to treat infections. Small tablets can also be used for treating urethral infections.

Key Concepts

- Drugs can be administered either systemically or locally.
- Absorption rate is influenced by drug physicochemical properties and the physiological conditions at the site of absorption.
- Absorption rate depends on the dissolution rate of drug as it arrives at the absorption site, and the permeability of drug through the membranes at the absorption site.
- Most drugs are absorbed by passive transcellular diffusion. Only the un-ionized form of the drug diffuses through epithelial barriers at absorption sites.
- Carrier-mediated absorption enhances the absorption of some drugs, whereas opposing efflux pumps limit the absorption of others.
- Local administration does not require drug absorption into the bloodstream; however, absorption may occur.

Review Questions

1. Differentiate between systemic and local (nonsystemic) drug administration, and list the routes used for each.
2. Explain the term permeability as it applies to a drug crossing a membrane. What makes some membranes more permeable to a drug than others?

3. What is the primary mechanism for drug absorption across epithelial membranes? What parameters control the rate of absorption of a drug?
4. Discuss the role of transporters in increasing or decreasing drug absorption.
5. Describe the role of the esophagus, stomach, small intestines, and colon in oral drug absorption. Why are most drugs absorbed from the small intestines?
6. How does the pH of GI fluids influence the release and absorption of weak acid and weak base drugs?
7. When is it appropriate to use nonoral routes for systemic delivery? List the key features of each route.

CASE STUDY 6.1

Things go better with Coca Cola

Drug Absorption

KM is a 30 year old female who was recently prescribed one 200-mg tablet of ketoconazole (Nizoral™) daily for treatment of a persistent vaginal yeast infection. Ketoconazole is an antifungal drug.

KM's physician told her to take the ketoconazole tablet with Coca Cola rather than with water because the Coca Cola "makes the drug work better". KM does not like Coca Cola, so she called her brother who is a pharmacy student, and asked him what other liquid she can use instead of Coca Cola.

Background

Ketoconazole is a weak dibasic compound with pK_a values of 2.9 and 6.5. It is practically insoluble in aqueous fluids unless *both* weak base groups are ionized.

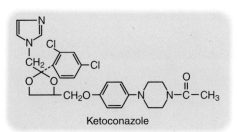

Ketoconazole

Questions

1. Calculate the % of ketoconazole that is uncharged, singly charged, and doubly charged at pH 6 and pH 2.
2. Qualitatively describe how pH of the solution will influence the aqueous solubility of ketoconazole. Will ketoconazole be more soluble in the stomach or in the small intestines?
3. Explain how ketoconazole can be absorbed from the small intestines if it is not very soluble at pH 6, the usual pH of intestinal fluids.
4. Some elderly persons have achlorhydria, or insufficient production of gastric acid. Gastric pH in these individuals may be as high as 5–6. Ketoconazole has been show to be poorly absorbed in these patients. Explain.
5. The pH values of some carbonated beverages are given below. Drinking water has a pH of 6.5–7.0. Explain why KM's physician recommended that she take ketoconazole with Coca Cola. Which of the others may also work? How does the drink "make the drug work better"?

Beverage	pH
Coca-Cola	2.5
Pepsi	2.5
7-Up	3.3
Canada Dry Ginger Ale	2.7
Diet Coke	3.2
Diet Pepsi	3.2
Diet 7-Up	3.4

6. KM tells her grandson that she does not like Coca Cola or most carbonated beverages. What other beverages can he suggest?
7. Even if KM does not have achlorhydria, what other types of drug products can raise gastric pH, and should be avoided by KM while she is taking ketoconazole?

Additional Readings

Banker GS, Rhodes CT (eds). Modern Pharmaceutics, 4th ed. Marcel Dekker, 2002.

Dipiro JT, Talbert RL, Yee GC, Matzke GR, Wells BG, Posey LM (eds). Pharmacotherapy: a Pathophysiologic Approach, 5th ed. McGraw-Hill/Appleton & Lange, 2002.

Gennaro AR (ed). Remington—The Science and Practice of Pharmacy, 20th ed. Lippincott Williams & Wilkins, 2000.

Shargel L, Yu ABC. Applied Biopharmaceutics and Pharmacokinetics, 4th ed. McGraw-Hill/Appleton & Lange, 1999.

CHAPTER 7

Drug Delivery Systems

The development and effective therapeutic use of a new pharmaceutical product involve more than just the discovery of a compound with intrinsic pharmacological activity. That is where drug delivery comes in. Once appropriate routes of administration, whether systemic or local, have been identified, scientists must design drug products that enable the drug to reach the site of action at the appropriate time, and maintain an effective concentration for the desired duration. This is not a trivial issue; the development of an appropriate delivery system is often as complex as the discovery of the drug molecule itself.

The three important considerations in the design of a delivery system are release of drug for absorption, stability, and elegance. Release is necessary because a drug must dissolve in order to be absorbed and to bind to the target. Stability is important to ensure that a product retains its characteristics for a sufficient duration, and provides reproducible performance over its shelf life. Elegance is critical to make sure the product's appearance, smell, taste, and method of administration are acceptable to patients.

Dosage Forms

As pure compounds, drugs are usually solid substances (amorphous or crystalline) or, in rare cases, liquids. Drugs are combined with several inert materials called excipients, and these mixtures are processed into distinct units called dosage forms. Each excipient plays an important role in the overall performance of the dosage form. An excipient may facilitate drug release, improve drug stability, protect the product from microbial contamination, provide elegance, or make the product easy to manufacture on a large scale.

Examples of dosage forms are tablets, capsules, suspensions, solutions, and ointments. Dosage forms can be administered to patients via several different routes of administration (e.g., oral, injectable, rectal), as discussed in Chapter 6. Many dosage forms have to be used with a specialized administration device, such as an inhaler, a nasal spray, or a transdermal patch. The complete system of dosage form and administration device is called the drug delivery system, or drug product.

The physicochemical properties of a drug (solubility, pK_a, lipophilicity, particle size, chemical stability) are important when determining which route, dosage form, and excipients will be best suited for a particular application. Also important are the requirements of the individual patient. Many drugs are available in several different doses and dosage forms, for administration by several routes. Each clinical situation requires an analysis of which product is best suited for the patient. The science of the design, evaluation, and manufacture of drug delivery systems is called *pharmaceutics*.

Need for Dosage Forms

In the past, pure drug substances were often given directly to patients in preweighed quantities; this type of dosing is almost never used today. Dosage forms provide control and accuracy of dosing, allow a convenient means of administration, protect the drug, and prevent contamination. They also make it possible for the drug to be delivered at a rate appropriate to the needs of the patient or the disease.

The design of a good drug product takes into account the properties of the drug, the requirements of the disease that it treats, and the needs and preferences of patients. An optimized drug product delivers the drug in a manner that produces maximum effectiveness, safety, and reliability. The characteristics of an ideal drug delivery system are as follows:

- Releases drug at the appropriate location in the body
- Releases drug at a controlled, predictable rate unique to each situation
- Is not affected by physiological variability such as gastric pH, diet, and patient health.
- Is convenient and easy for the patient to take
- Has a long shelf life when stored under various environmental conditions
- Is easy to manufacture on a large scale
- Is cost-effective
- Is elegant (taste, smell, appearance, texture).

Although it is difficult to achieve all objectives for every drug, these considerations are important in designing drug products.

Types of Dosage Forms

Dosage forms are broadly classified according to their gross physical nature as

- Solutions
- Dispersions
- Semisolids
- Solids

The drug in the dosage form is often referred to as the active ingredient and is present along with several excipients.

In a solution, the drug is completely dissolved in a medium, usually aqueous. Excipients added to drug solutions may be cosolvents, buffers, preservatives, stabilizing agents, flavors, and colors. Solutions are commonly administered orally, by injection, or can be applied to the nose, ear, or eye. Nonaqueous solutions, although not common, are also available. Examples include drugs dissolved in oils for administration by injection, or dissolved in other lipids for dermal application.

Dispersions are products with two phases, one phase dispersed in a medium of another phase. Examples are suspensions (solid drug dispersed in a liquid) and emulsions (a liquid dispersed in another immiscible liquid). To keep the active ingredient uniformly suspended throughout the liquid, a suspending or thickening agent is usually added. Other excipients are similar to those found in solutions. Dispersions are often given orally or by injection, or can be applied to the nose, ear, eye, or skin. Specialized dispersions of drug in a nonaqueous medium also exist, e.g., metered-dose inhalers, which contain drug dispersed in a liquid propellant mixture.

Semisolids such as ointments, creams, and gels are dosage forms generally meant for application to the skin. They may also be applied to the eye as ophthalmic ointments, and rectally or vaginally as suppositories. In addition to the active ingredient, semisolid dosage forms may contain oils or lipids, water, buffers, polymers for thickening, and preservatives for stability.

Solids are the most common types of dosage forms; examples are tablets, capsules, and powders. Solid dosage forms vary greatly in shape, size, weight, and many other properties. They are usually given orally, but powders may be formulated for application to the skin or for inhalation. Some powders are designed to be added to a liquid and made into a solution or suspension just prior to administration.

Drug Release and Dissolution

Regardless of the type of dosage form, drug must be in solution at the absorption or administration site before it can cross membranes or enter cells. The first medium most drugs encounter in the body is usually aqueous; this is why it is important for drugs to have adequate water solubility.

In solution dosage forms, the drug is already dissolved in the product, and is available for absorption immediately after administration to a patient. However, in other types of dosage forms (tablets, capsules, suspensions, and so forth), the drug is present as a solid. Before the drug can be absorbed or reach its target, it must be released from the dosage form; in other words, it must dissolve in the fluids at the site of absorption. Undissolved drug cannot be absorbed. Even if the drug product is intended for local action and does not require systemic absorption, dissolution is necessary for the drug molecules to reach the site of action and interact with the target. If the drug does not dissolve completely, the amount of drug available for absorption or action will be less than the dose administered.

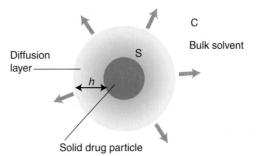

Figure 7.1. Schematic diagram of the dissolution process. The concentration of drug at the solid surface is equal to the solubility S of the drug in the dissolution medium, C is the concentration of drug in the bulk solvent, and h is the thickness of the diffusion layer.

Dissolution Rate

Dissolution is a process by which a compound goes from the solid state into solution in a solvent. Let us first consider dissolution of a sample of pure drug. The dissolution process can be characterized mathematically using the diffusion layer model, depicted schematically in Figure 7.1. The model assumes that, as a drug particle dissolves, a thin layer of liquid (called a diffusion layer or stagnant layer) of thickness h is formed adjacent to the surface of the particle. This layer remains stagnant or unmixed, while the bulk liquid in the solution is completely mixed. At the solid/liquid interface, the drug dissolves rapidly forming a saturated solution. The overall rate of dissolution is governed entirely by the diffusion of dissolved drug molecules through the stagnant layer from solid surface to the bulk liquid.

Let us follow what happens in the stagnant layer when a drug particle dissolves in water at a particular pH, etc.

- Initially, (*time* = 0) the concentration of dissolved drug immediately around the particle is S, the saturated solubility in the medium. There is no drug yet dissolved in the bulk, so the drug concentration at the other end of the stagnant layer is zero. Thus, there is a concentration gradient in the stagnant layer, with a high drug concentration (S) at the surface of the particle and a low concentration (zero) in the bulk solvent. Drug molecules diffuse through the stagnant layer into the bulk solvent, and more drug dissolves from the particle to maintain a saturated solution at the particle's surface.

- Partway through the dissolution process (*time* = *t*), the concentration at the particle surface is still S, while the concentration in the bulk has now increased to some concentration C. As long as $C < S$, there will be a concentration gradient in the stagnant layer, and dissolution will continue. The rate of dissolution will be slower, however, because the concentration gradient in the stagnant layer is smaller.
- Dissolution will eventually stop (*time* = ∞) when either of the following two conditions is reached. If there is sufficient solvent to allow the particle to dissolve completely, then there will be no solid drug left to maintain a saturated solution at the particle surface, and no concentration gradient. The concentration in the entire stagnant layer will be the concentration in the bulk (C). If, on the other hand, there is insufficient solvent to dissolve the drug, dissolution will stop when the concentration in the bulk (C) becomes equal to S. Even if the particle is not completely dissolved, no further dissolution will occur because there is no concentration gradient.

Mathematically, the dissolution rate of a drug is the rate of increase in its bulk concentration as a function of time. It is described by the modified Noyes–Whitney equation, derived from Fick's first law of diffusion

$$\text{Dissolution rate} = \frac{dC}{dt} = \frac{D \cdot A(S-C)}{h}$$

(Eq. 7.1)

In this equation, A is the surface area of solid drug exposed to the dissolution medium, S is the drug solubility in the dissolution medium, C is the concentration of the drug in the bulk dissolution medium, D is the diffusion coefficient of the drug, and h is the thickness of the diffusion layer. Thus, ($S - C$) is the concentration gradient that drives the dissolution process. A plot of this concentration gradient at different times is shown in Figure 7.2. Dissolution will be fast initially (time = 0) when the concentration gradient is the highest. Dissolution will become slower as ($S - C$) becomes smaller (time = t); and dissolution will eventually stop ($S - C = 0$ at time = ∞). This condition is reached either when a saturated solution is formed in the bulk ($C = S$) or when the entire solid dissolves. Although we denote the time as ∞, the time taken could vary from hours to days, depending on the conditions.

Equation 7.1 tells us that dissolution will be fast for a drug with high solubility, diffusion coefficient, and surface area, and in a medium with a small diffusion layer thickness.

Equation 7.1 is often written as

$$\text{Dissolution rate} = k \cdot A(S-C) \qquad \text{(Eq. 7.2)}$$

The constant k is called the *intrinsic dissolution rate constant* of the drug in the medium. It is directly proportional to diffusion coefficient (D) of the drug (which in turn depends on drug molecular weight), and is inversely proportional to thickness (h) of the diffusion layer. Diffusion layer thickness can be reduced by stirring the medium or by decreasing its viscosity.

Dissolution of Drug from Dosage Forms

Equation 7.1 allows us to identify all the factors that control the dissolution rate of a drug. If the solid drug were dissolving in a beaker of solvent, we could

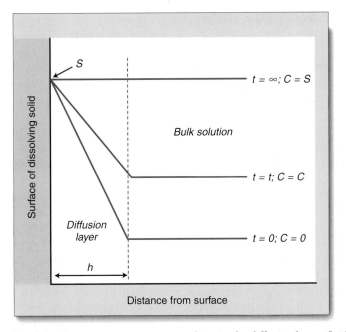

Figure 7.2. A plot of the changing concentration gradient in the diffusion layer of a dissolving particle at time $= 0$, time $= t$, and time $= \infty$. The solubility of the solid is S and the thickness of the diffusion layer is h. The concentration (C) in the bulk solvent increases as dissolution progresses, reducing the concentration gradient and dissolution rate. Dissolution progresses as long as $C < S$, and stops when C becomes equal to S.

easily determine how to change each parameter (S, A, D, or h) to increase or decrease dissolution rate. However, for a drug in a dosage form dissolving in the body, there are several constraints on which parameters can be modified and to what degree.

Drug Solubility

It is intuitively obvious that the solubility, S, of a drug is an important parameter in determining dissolution rate. Drugs with a high solubility in the medium will dissolve faster than those with a low solubility. In Chapter 4, we learned that intrinsic water solubility depends on the solid state structure of the drug, and that total solubility of weak acids or weak bases further depends on pH of the medium. Consequently, dissolution rate is influenced by these factors as well.

Solid State Structure. If a drug exhibits polymorphism, the metastable or *high-energy* polymorph (with a lower melting point) has a higher intrinsic solubility and faster dissolution rate compared with the stable polymorph (with the higher melting point). The crystal lattice of the metastable polymorph is more readily broken, allowing the drug to dissolve. It would seem logical to select the metastable polymorph if a fast dissolution rate is needed.

Unfortunately, metastable polymorphs revert to the stable, less soluble polymorph with time. This process is usually difficult to control and nonreproducible. Thus, although metastable polymorphs are attractive for their faster dissolution, they are rarely used in drug products. Pharmaceutical companies usually identify and select the most stable polymorph for development. In general, the stable polymorph has the highest melting point, the lowest solubility, and the maximum stability.

pH of the Medium. Since the ionized form of a drug has a higher aqueous solubility than the un-ionized form, drugs dissolve faster if they are able to ionize in the dissolution medium. A higher total drug concentration is achieved at the particle surface, increasing the concentration gradient for dissolution. For drug dissolution at various sites of administration and absorption, the local physiological pH has a tremendous influence on dissolution rate, and consequently could have a big influence on absorption rate.

For example, stomach fluids have pH values between 1 and 3.5, whereas the small intestinal fluid pH is in the range 5.5 to 7.5. A weak acid drug will have a lower solubility and dissolution rate in the stomach and a higher solubility and dissolution rate in the small intestines. The opposite is true for weak base drugs.

Salts of weak acids and bases often have faster dissolution rates than the parent acid or base, as we learned in Chapter 4. The faster dissolution rate is a reflection of higher water solubility of the salt because of a local pH effect; the salt effectively acts as its own buffer and facilitates ionization and dissolution. The type of salt, i.e., the counter-ion, also influences dissolution; each type of salt of a particular acid or base drug has a different solubility product and therefore a different dissolution rate. Selection of the appropriate salt for fast dissolution is an important step in new drug development.

Role of Solubility in Absorption Rate. In Chapter 6, we saw that oral drugs are classified according to the BCS to predict whether solubility or permeability is more important for absorption. Solubility is used to estimate the ability of the drug to dissolve in gastrointestinal fluids.

The dissolution process is critical for BCS Class II (low solubility–high permeability) and Class IV drugs (low solubility–low permeability). These low solubility drugs will have slow dissolution rates that could lead to incomplete absorption. Differences between dissolution rates among dosage forms may translate into significant differences in absorption and efficacy. Much of the product development effort for such drugs is spent trying to speed up dissolution rate.

On the other hand, faster dissolution may not necessarily translate to better absorption for BCS Class III drugs (high solubility–low permeability). For such drugs, it is the membrane permeability rather than dissolution rate that limits absorption. It is possible that a solid dosage form of such drugs will have the same rate of absorption as a solution product. Improvement of dissolution rate may not be a high priority during the development of these drugs.

Concentration Gradient

Although a high drug solubility will give a high dissolution rate, it is actually the concentration gradient $(S - C)$ that is the driving force for dissolution. A high solubility (S) will help to give a large concentration gradient. So will a low value for C. This is why the rate is highest when dissolution begins, and slows down as we approach equilibrium $(S = C)$. If we could somehow keep C at a low value, we could keep the dissolution rate high. This is what occurs during the dissolution and absorption process in the body. As the drug dissolves, some or all of it is absorbed into the bloodstream and removed from the absorption site. This maintains the concentration gradient, and allows dissolution to continue.

Particle Size

In addition to solubility, the size of drug particles plays a role in dissolution rate. If a large particle of drug is ground up to give many small particles, the total surface area exposed to the solvent (A in Eqn. 7.1) increases, and dissolution rate increases proportionately. Thus, a common approach to increasing dissolution rate is to reduce the average size of the solid particles to only a few microns in diameter, a process known as *micronization*.

Diffusion Coefficient

The diffusion coefficient of a drug in a medium depends on the molecular weight of the drug and the characteristics of the medium. A drug with a high molecular weight has a lower diffusion coefficient (D) and will dissolve slower than one with a small molecular weight, everything else being the same. However, we cannot change the molecular weight of the drug without changing its structure and, therefore, its other properties. Thus, this is not a parameter that can be readily modified to change dissolution rate.

Diffusion coefficient also depends on the viscosity of the medium; a high viscosity results in a low diffusion coefficient. Thus, the viscosity of the physiological fluid in which the drug is dissolving will affect dissolution rate. This, too, is not generally a parameter that can be readily changed.

Diffusion Layer Thickness

A thick diffusion layer (i.e., a large h) means that a dissolving drug molecule has to diffuse across a longer path to get from the solid particle to the bulk. This slows the overall rate of dissolution. While the other parameters discussed earlier were characteristics of the drug, diffusion layer thickness is a property of the medium. Diffusion layer thickness can be reduced by increasing temperature, decreasing the viscosity of the medium, or by agitating the medium. In general, the dissolution medium in the body is the physiological fluid at the site of administration and cannot be readily modified.

Approaches to Drug Delivery

Immediate-Release Products

The goal for most drug delivery systems is rapid dissolution of drug after administration; such products are called immediate-release systems. The objective with these is to get drug to the site of action or into the bloodstream as quickly as possible. The product is designed to give the fastest dissolution rate possible, with the assumption that this will give the fastest absorption and effect. As discussed, rapid dissolution can be achieved by increasing surface area A of drug particles (reducing particle size) and by using appropriate excipients to enhance solubility of drug in diffusion layer.

Figure 7.3 illustrates the drug release and dissolution process of an oral tablet. Immediate-release tablets are designed to undergo rapid disintegration to smaller granules and subsequent deaggregation to fine particles. A larger surface area is exposed to the dissolution medium, resulting in a faster dissolution rate than if the tablet were to dissolve intact. Excipients that facilitate disintegration (*disintegrants*) and deaggregation (*surfactants*) are usually included in immediate-release solid dosage forms.

When an immediate-release product is administered, the drug concentration in blood rises rapidly, peaks soon after administration, and then declines. If the peak concentration is too high, the drug may exhibit undesirable side effects. If the decline in blood concentration is also rapid, the product will have to be dosed frequently to maintain therapeutic blood levels. Such a large fluctuation in blood concentration may not be suitable for some drugs, or may require dosing frequencies that are impractical.

Controlled-Release Products

In contrast to immediate-release products designed to release drug as fast as possible, a controlled-release product releases

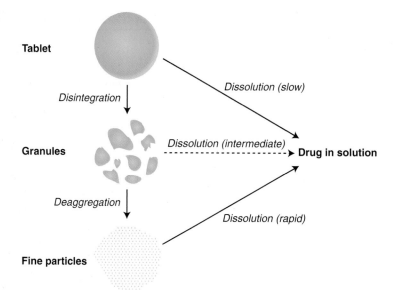

Figure 7.3. The processes involved in dissolution of a drug from a tablet in the presence of fluids. Although dissolution can occur from the whole tablet, granules, and fine particles, the large surface area of the granules and even larger surface area of the fine particles give faster dissolution rates.

drug in the body in a manner precisely controlled to suit the clinical situation. Its goal is to achieve a constant, effective drug concentration at the site of action for the necessary duration. Controlled release requires predictability and reproducibility of drug dissolution from the dosage form.

The term *controlled release* refers to a variety of methods that modify release of drug from a dosage form. This term includes preparations labeled as "extended release," "delayed release," "modified release," or "sustained release." Unlike immediate-release products from which the entire dose of drug is released rapidly after administration, controlled-release products gradually release specific amounts of drug over a longer time period. Major benefits include less frequent dosing, less fluctuation of drug concentration in the blood, fewer side effects, and better patient compliance.

The most common application of controlled release is sustained release, in which dissolution rate is deliberately reduced to achieve continuous release

and absorption of drug over a long time. For an oral sustained release product, the drug is slowly released and absorbed as it travels down the GI tract, rather than being released rapidly in the stomach. Clearly, this means that the drug properties and physiological conditions should allow absorption along the entire length of the small intestines. The absorption rate of sustained release systems is programmed to match the rate of elimination of drug from the bloodstream, so that a relatively constant concentration is maintained in the blood.

We can examine Equation 7.1 again to understand how the various parameters can be manipulated to give slow dissolution.

- The solubility can be reduced by choosing a low solubility form of the drug (e.g., weak acid/base instead of the salt).
- The pH in the diffusion layer can be modified to reduce S, by adding acidic or basic excipients.
- Surface area can be reduced by not allowing the product to disintegrate or deaggregate.

- Diffusion layer thickness can be increased by adding viscosity-increasing excipients; this will also decrease diffusion coefficient D of the drug.
- Drug particles can be coated with a slow dissolving excipient, so the medium cannot reach the drug rapidly.

All of these approaches are used in the design of the sustained release drug products on the market today.

Sustained-release products contain a much larger amount of drug than a single dose of an immediate-release product, because they are supposed to maintain therapeutic concentrations for a prolonged period. This poses one of the biggest problems in using such products—the danger that inappropriate manufacture or use may result in a large amount of drug being released and absorbed rapidly, causing toxicity.

Not all drugs can or should be formulated in sustained-release systems. The physicochemical or ADME properties of the drug may make sustained-release delivery unfeasible. Moreover, constant blood levels may not be pharmacodynamically or therapeutically desirable for some drugs or disease states.

Targeted Drug Delivery

The therapeutic potential of many of today's highly potent drugs, such as many chemotherapeutics, is limited by serious side effects. In the traditional systemic delivery systems discussed so far, the drug becomes distributed throughout the body via the bloodstream. Only a small fraction of drug reaches site of action, while the rest goes to unintended organs and tissues, causing side effects. Targeted or site-specific drug delivery is an approach to concentrate drug in the tissues of interest, while minimizing drug concentration in the other tissues. By controlling the precise level and/or location of drug in the body, side effects are reduced, lower doses can be used, and new therapies are possible.

One way of minimizing side effects is to design very selective drugs that bind to only the desired receptor subtype. The objective is to improve fit, affinity, and binding to the specific receptor that ultimately will trigger the pharmacological activity. Unfortunately, the target receptor may be distributed in several organs of the body. Also, it is difficult to achieve the desired level of specificity necessary to avoid all side effects. Therefore, a more common approach of drug targeting is by designing delivery systems that localize the drug primarily at the site of action. Although there are only a few successful commercial examples of such products, drug targeting continues to be very active area of research.

Successful drug targeting, however, is very complex. It involves modifying various aspects of absorption and distribution, as well as sometimes drug metabolism and excretion. There are a number of important parameters to be considered such as the biological and cellular membranes at the site of action, type and distribution of drug receptors, type and distribution of enzymes that metabolize the drug, and local blood flow.

The three major approaches to drug targeting can be classified as physical, biological, and chemical.

The physical approach to targeting uses a controlled release approach to achieve a sustained, relatively constant blood and/or tissue concentration of a drug. Targeting is achieved by localizing the delivery system at or around the target organ so that some differential distribution of drug is achieved. Physical targeting has been used for pilocarpine delivery to the eye from a polymeric device or the contraceptive sustained release of progesterone from a vaginal polymeric insert. This approach is successful if the site is readily accessible, like with local or nonsystemic delivery. Other examples are drug-embedded implants that are surgically placed at or near the intended site, but these have limited value because of their invasiveness.

Biological targeting systems are based on attaching the drug to an antibody that is specific for a particular protein on the cell membrane of targeted cells. The antibody–drug conjugate is then taken up only by these cells, and broken down to release drug preferentially in or near the cell. Tumors can be targeted in this manner. There are, however, a number of problems related to the actual distribution of an antibody–drug conjugate in the body. The antibody specificity is often altered by conjugation with the drug, the amount of drug that can be carried by antibodies is small; and the antibody–drug conjugate may break down too fast or too slow. In most cases, this critical process, producing pharmacologically active local concentrations of the drug, is the major problem.

Chemically targeted systems involve adding a targeting group to the drug's chemical structure. Recall that a drug molecule's structure can be divided into a pharmacophore, and carrier and vulnerable groups, as discussed in Chapter 2. To enable drug targeting in the current context, the carrier group, now called the targetor, must be enhanced to give it additional properties. The targetor now is responsible for optimizing molecular properties controlling distribution and elimination as with conventional drugs, as well as determining site targeting, site specificity, and site retention. Often, the targetor makes the compound inactive in its parent form, but allows drug release only after being broken down by enzymes at the site of action.

A detailed discussion of targeted delivery is outside the scope of our discussion.

Drug Stability

A good drug product should maintain its performance (effectiveness, safety, and reliability) for a sufficiently long time to allow use by the patient. Unfortunately, the performance of most drug products changes with time. The shelf life is the period (in days, months, or years) after manufacture during which a product is expected to perform as intended, within specified limits, when stored under the recommended conditions. The expiration date specifies the exact date after which a particular batch of product cannot be guaranteed to be safe and effective. Each batch will have the same shelf life, but different expiration dates, depending on the date of manufacture. Ideally, we would like drug products to have a long shelf life; in other words, we would like them to be very stable or to have good stability.

The term "stability," with respect to a drug dosage form refers to the chemical and physical integrity of the dosage unit and, the ability of the dosage unit to maintain protection against microbiological contamination. Thus, the types of instability that can determine the shelf life and expiration date of a product are

- Chemical degradation of the drug or excipients
- Microbiological contamination
- Physical changes.

The shelf life of a particular drug product may be limited for chemical, microbiological or physical instability reasons.

Chemical Stability

Chemical stability characterizes the change in concentration or amount of the active drug in the product with time. The drug may degrade over time as a result of chemical reactions such as hydrolysis, oxidation, or photolysis. Chemical instability decreases in the amount of drug in the dosage form and reduces the dose provided to the patient. Moreover, the degradation products formed can be undesirable or toxic. Thus, chemical instability results in a gradual decline in the effectiveness and/or safety of a drug product. Although we focus mainly on the chemical stability of the drug itself, degradation of any of the excipients in the product may also compromise product performance. Usually, manufacturers select excipients that do not pose significant stability problems.

Common Degradation Reactions

Hydrolysis, the decomposition of a chemical compound by reaction with water, is the most significant reaction for chemical instability of drugs. This is because many drugs have functional groups (ester, amide, lactone, lactam) that are prone to hydrolytic attack, and because water is present to some extent in most drug products and in the environment. Hydrolysis rates depend on the pH of the product, the temperature and humidity at which the product is stored, and excipients in the product. Oxidation, particularly oxidation catalyzed by light (*photooxidation*), is the second most common degradation reaction of drugs, because of the ubiquitous presence of oxygen in the environment. Oxidation is often catalyzed by heavy metal ions.

Degradation reactions are generally fastest in solutions and slowest in solid dosage forms. Therefore, solid dosage forms of a drug are usually more stable than its liquid dosage forms. Excipients are frequently added to drug products to improve chemical stability. Appropriate buffers and cosolvents can reduce hydrolysis rates, and chelating agents and antioxidants reduce oxidation rates. Many solid dosage forms may be coated with a protective film to slow the entry of moisture and oxygen into the product.

The package in which the product is provided also plays a role in drug product stability. Hydrolysis and oxidation rates can be reduced by using airtight, sealed containers. The use of desiccants (such as silica) in the container helps to reduce moisture content and, therefore, hydrolysis rates. Opaque containers protect products from light and reduce photooxidation.

Chemical Shelf Life

Almost all drugs chemically degrade to some extent with time, resulting in a decrease in the concentration of the active ingredient in the product. Small changes in concentration are not clinically significant, so the accepted limit of chemical decomposition for most drug products is $\pm 10\%$, i.e., drug products should contain 90% to 110% of the active ingredient claimed on the label. The chemical shelf life is the time period after manufacture for which the drug concentration remains within these limits. When the active ingredient concentration goes outside these limits, the product is considered to have *expired*.

Microbiological Stability

The microbiological stability of a drug product is a measure of its resistance to microbial (bacterial and fungal) contamination during storage and use. Contamination may occur due to exposure of the product to the environment (e.g., atmosphere) or due to inadvertent addition of an organism during use. Even if only a few microbes are introduced into the product, they may grow and multiply, seriously compromising the safety of the product.

Microbial growth is especially likely in products with high moisture content such as aqueous solutions, dispersions, and water-based semisolids. Most such products contain an antimicrobial preservative to minimize microbial growth. Most solid dosage forms contain relatively small amounts of water and do not require an antimicrobial preservative.

Certain pharmaceutical products, such as injectable and ophthalmic products, are also required to be *sterile* (free from contaminating microorganisms) throughout their shelf life. When these products are designed for single use (such as a prefilled syringe for injection), an antimicrobial preservative may not be necessary. However, sterile multidose products need to be preserved to maintain sterility during use.

Physical Stability

Many physical characteristics of dosage forms may also change with time. Examples of physical characteristics are dissolution rate, uniformity, appearance and color, taste, odor, texture, etc. These changes also influence effectiveness, safety, and reliability of the product. The effect of a changing dissolution rate on drug absorption and effectiveness is obvious. However, a patient's perception of the effectiveness and safety of a drug product is also influenced if a product's color, taste, odor, or other aspect of appearance changes with time. Thus, even if a drug product has good chemical and microbiological stability, physical changes may result in a shorter overall shelf life.

Delivery of Macromolecular Drugs

Advances in biotechnology have made possible the development of biopharmaceutical drug products based on very large molecules such as proteins, peptides, and nucleic acids. Although they offer a new approach to therapy, macromolecules pose many challenges in designing safe, stable, and effective drug products that are convenient to administer. We discussed the challenges in absorption of macromolecular drugs in Chapter 2. Consequently, most macromolecular drugs are administered as injectable products. Unfortunately, injectable delivery has poor patient acceptance because of inconvenience, discomfort, and the potential for infection at the injection site. An example is the administration of insulin injections to patients with diabetes, in which patient compliance and long-term complications are serious problems. With the introduction of many new chronically administered macromolecular drugs such as interferons and growth factors, there is a need for the development of alternative, noninvasive, and more convenient methods of administration.

As far as shelf life goes, chemical and physical instability problems are often more serious for macromolecules. Conformational changes in protein structure can often inactivate a product or make it immunogenic, even though the molecule has not chemically degraded. We will discuss more details of biopharmaceutical products in Chapter 18. Special excipients and packaging approaches are necessary for optimum stability of macromolecular drugs. A detailed discussion is outside the scope of this book.

Key Concepts

- Design of a good drug delivery system is important in optimal drug therapy.
- Excipients are added to drug products to enhance release, stability, elegance, or manufacturability.
- Drug dissolution is a necessary first step before absorption or efficacy.
- Dissolution rate is described by the Noyes–Whitney equation, and can be controlled by modifying key parameters.

- Immediate-release products are designed to dissolve fast for rapid absorption.
- Sustained-release products dissolve slowly to maintain steady blood levels.
- Targeted drug delivery is an area of research to enhance efficacy and reduce side effects.
- The chemical, microbiological, and physical stability of a drug product together determine its shelf life.

Review Questions

1. What are the advantages of using a delivery system to administer drugs? What are the characteristics of an ideal delivery system?
2. Discuss the mathematical expression describing the dissolution of a solid drug particle. What parameters can be changed to increase or decrease dissolution rate, and how?
3. What are the differences between immediate-release and sustained-release products? Under what conditions is a sustained-release product a better therapeutic option than an immediate-release product of the same drug?
4. Describe the meaning of targeted or site-specific delivery. What are the approaches to achieving site-specific delivery?
5. What is meant by the shelf life and expiration date of a drug product? Discuss the various aspects of stability of a drug product.
6. What are the unique delivery challenges of macromolecular drugs?

CASE STUDY 7.1

Is this patient becoming an addict?

Drug Delivery

DT is a 32-year-old female who had Roux-en-Y gastric bypass surgery 2 years ago to help with weight loss. She lost 115 lb, has been in good health, and does not take any medications except a daily vitamin. She recently had a skiing accident, broke her foot and had to have surgery. The doctor prescribed Tylenol with codeine, but it did not control DT's pain. Her physician then prescribed Oxycontin® 10 mg tablets, an opioid analgesic product. DT only gets some relief with Oxycontin®, but needs to take it every 6 hours, rather than every 12 hours as indicated. DT contacted her doctor and asked for a higher dose and more refills. The doctor is concerned that DT is either diverting the product or becoming addicted to it, and is considering not giving her any more refills.

Background

Oxycontin® tablets are a sustained release dosage form containing oxycodone hydrochloride, a schedule II controlled substance with an abuse potential similar to morphine. Oxycodone, like morphine and other opioids used in analgesia, is addictive, can be abused, and is sometimes illegally diverted by patients. Oxycodone has a pKa of 8.5; and an aqueous solubility of 100 mg/mL between pH 1.0 and 6.5. In normal adults, oxycodone is well absorbed orally with about 80% of the dose reaching the systemic circulation.

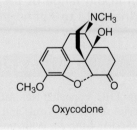

Oxycodone

The Roux-en-Y procedure (RYGB) is a common gastric bypass surgical procedure. Stomach size is reduced by converting it into a small pouch to limit food intake. The pouch is connected to the lower part of the small intestines (ileum), so that a majority of the small intestines is by-passed during food intake. The connection between pouch and intestine is narrow, to slow emptying from the pouch and maintain a longer feeling of fullness after a small meal. Since ingested material bypasses the lower stomach and a majority of the small intestine (duodenum and jejunum), food is incompletely digested and absorbed, further contributing to weight loss.

Questions

1. Is oxycodone a weak acid or weak base? Why do you think the manufacturer used oxycodone hydrochloride in the tablets as opposed to oxycodone?

   Questions 2 to 6 are general questions about the impact of the RYGB procedure on drug absorption.

   Questions 7 to 9 deal specifically with oxycodone and DT's case.

2. What is the role of the normal stomach (dissolution absorption, or both) in oral drug delivery? Explain. What might be the consequence if the stomach is reduced to a small pouch?

3. The pouch contains fewer parietal cells and produces much less hydrochloric acid than the normal stomach. The gastric pH in RYGB patients is often in the range of pH 4 to 5 rather than pH 1 to 3 of normal gastric juice. How might this affect the dissolution of weak acid and weak base drugs? Explain.

4. What is the role of the small intestines in oral drug therapy? How might the absorption of orally administered drugs be different in patients who have had the Roux-en-Y procedure? Explain.

5. Which BCS classes of drugs might be most affected by the RYGB procedure?

6. RGBY patients are advised to take vitamin supplements. Why?

7. Explain why DT is not getting sufficient relief with Oxycontin. Based on the physicochemical properties of oxycodone and the type of dosage form, do you expect dissolution, absorption or both to be the problem?

8. What options for oxycodone administration would you suggest to provide pain relief for DT? Consider higher dose (20, 40, 100 mg Oxycontin sustained release tablets are available), immediate-release oxycodone tablets (Roxicodone), different route of delivery.

9. The general recommendation for RYGB patients is to only use immediate-release products for oral dosing, and to further crush all solid medications before use. Why do you think crushing is recommended? Would you recommend that DT crush her Oxycontin tablets?

Additional Readings

Allen LV, Ansel HC, Popovich NG, Allen LV. Pharmaceutical Dosage Forms and Drug Delivery Systems, 9th ed. Williams & Wilkins, 2010.

Aulton ME (ed). Pharmaceutics: The Science of Dosage Form Design, 2nd ed. Churchill Livingstone, 2001.

Banker GS, Rhodes CT (eds). Modern Pharmaceutics (Drugs and the Pharmaceutical Sciences vol 12), 4th ed. Marcel Dekker, 2002.

Hillery AM, Llyod AW, Swarbrick, J. Drug Delivery and Targeting. CRC Press, 2001.

PART III

Drug Disposition

The whole is simpler than the sum of its parts
—Willard Gibbs

Chapter 8 Drug Distribution

Chapter 9 Drug Excretion

Chapter 10 Drug Metabolism

Chapter 11 Pharmacokinetic Concepts

Drug Distribution

A drug administered systemically relies on the circulatory system to take it to the site of action and to other tissues in the body. After absorption into blood, most drugs must leave the bloodstream and enter the site of action to exert their effect. For a drug administered topically (nonsystemically), entry into or exit from the blood is not necessary. Topical drugs merely need to travel a short distance from the site of administration (i.e., the skin surface for dermal administration) to the site of action (i.e., dermis). However, it is possible for topical drugs to enter the systemic circulation and cause side effects. We must understand the mechanisms of drug transport into and out of the bloodstream so that it can be enhanced when needed, and minimized when not needed. In general, drug distribution is the reversible transfer of drug from one location in the body to another.

To simplify the distribution process, the body is considered to be composed of two distinctive fluids: vascular fluid and extravascular fluid. Vascular volume (i.e., blood) includes the fluid in the heart and vascular system of the body. Extravascular volume is everything outside the vascular space and includes many fluids such as cellular, interstitial, and lymphatic fluids. For our discussion in this chapter, distribution is the reversible transfer of drug between the vascular space and the extravascular space. Drug can enter the vascular space by intravenous (IV) administration, or after absorption of drug administered by another route.

A drug's pattern of distribution depends on its physicochemical properties, on the efficiency of blood circulation, and on the characteristics of the extravascular tissue. Distribution is uneven throughout the body because of differences in regional pH and blood perfusion, tissue binding, and permeability of cell membranes. The dynamic nature of drug distribution also means that drug concentrations in blood and tissues are constantly changing as drug is absorbed, distributed, metabolized, and excreted.

The Circulatory System

The circulatory system is the major conduit for transporting nutrients, gases, waste products, hormones, drugs, etc. through the body. It is composed of the cardiovascular system, which distributes blood, and the lymphatic system, which distributes lymph.

The Cardiovascular System

The blood, heart, and blood vessels form the cardiovascular system. It may be divided into three distinct sections: pulmonary circulation for oxygenation of blood, coronary circulation for nourishment of the heart, and systemic circulation for nourishment of all other tissues. The latter is most relevant to our discussion of drug distribution.

Blood

Blood is composed of plasma, red blood cells, white blood cells, and platelets, as described in Figure 8.1. The average 70-kg adult has 5 L of blood (0.07 L/kg), approximately 55% of which is a fluid called plasma, and 45% is cells and platelets. Plasma is a pale yellowish fluid with a volume of 0.04 L/kg, or 3 L in a 70-kg individual. It contains water, plasma proteins (albumin, globulin, immunoglobulin, prothrombin and fibrinogen) and many other dissolved substances such as amino acids, sugars fatty acids, and ions. As we will see later, plasma proteins play an important role in the distribution behavior of drugs.

The Heart and Cardiac Output

The primary function of the heart is to generate and sustain the necessary arterial blood pressure to provide blood flow to all organs. The heart does this by contracting its muscular walls around a closed chamber (the left ventricle) to create sufficient pressure to propel blood from the left ventricle, through the aortic valve and into the aorta.

The heart pumps blood through a closed system of vessels that carries blood to the rest of the body. The volume of blood pumped by the heart per minute is called cardiac output, the product of heart rate (HR) and stroke volume (SV).

$$\text{Cardiac output} = HR \times SV \quad \text{(Eq. 8.1)}$$

In healthy adults, SV at rest in the standing position averages between 60 and 80 mL of blood per ventricular contraction. Therefore, cardiac output at a resting HR of 80 beats per minute varies between 4.8 and 6.4 L/min. This means all the blood is pumped through the average adult heart very rapidly, about once every minute.

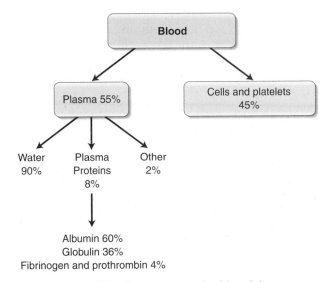

Figure 8.1. Typical composition of blood in an average, healthy adult.

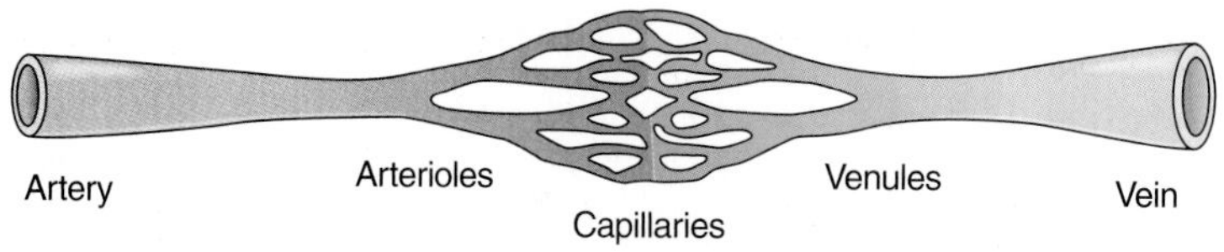

Figure 8.2. The branching arrangement of arteries, capillaries, and veins that make up the blood vessels of the circulatory system.

Blood Vessels

The human cardiovascular system is closed, meaning that the blood does not leave the network of blood vessels, and the volume of blood remains fairly constant. A branching system of arteries and veins (Fig. 8.2) takes blood to all parts of the body and back to the heart. Arteries carry blood away from the heart and progressively become finely divided into arterioles. Blood then flows into capillaries, the smallest vessels, where most of the exchange of materials between vascular and extravascular fluids occurs. The vessels get larger again, forming venules that join and enlarge to form veins to carry blood back to the heart. The distinction between arteries and veins is based on direction of blood flow, not oxygen content.

Arteries and arterioles have elastic fibers and smooth muscle cells that enable these vessels to withstand high pressures and to change their diameter, altering their resistance and, thus, blood flow. Veins, on the other hand, are less elastic and often contain unidirectional valves to prevent backflow of blood. Capillaries are very small tubes, 7 to 9 μm in diameter, whose walls are composed of a single flat layer of endothelial cells, resting on a basement membrane. In Chapter 5, we learned that endothelial cells are more loosely packed than epithelial cells. Gaps between endothelial cells contain a loose network of proteins that act as filters, retaining very large molecules and letting smaller ones through. Thus, blood cells, platelets, and plasma proteins are retained in the capillaries, while water and small molecules (and most drugs) can pass freely between the vascular and extravascular space.

Capillary Exchange

The *microcirculation* generally includes the arterioles, capillaries, and venules. Exchange of gases, nutrients, metabolites, and drugs between the blood and tissues occurs almost exclusively in the microcirculation. Blood does not come into direct contact with the cells it nourishes, but fluid readily exchanges between vascular and extravascular spaces across the capillary wall. When blood enters the arteriole end of a capillary, it is still under some pressure produced by contraction of the heart. This slight pressure difference between arterial blood and tissue fluid allows some water and dissolved solutes to be "squeezed out" paracellularly, through the endothelial cell junctions, into the interstitium (the space between cells in a tissue) of the surrounding tissue. This process, known as filtration, is an additional mechanism by which solutes can leave the vascular space along with fluids. Although filtration is not significant for drug distribution in most tissues, it becomes important in the kidney, as we will see later.

Although blood cells and most plasma proteins are too large to leave capillaries through endothelial junctions, small amounts of plasma proteins may be forced out with water due to the hydrostatic pressure at the arterial end. The resulting interstitial fluid (ISF, also called tissue fluid) bathes cells in the body. Typical volume of ISF in a healthy adult is 0.13 L/kg or 9 L in a 70-kg individual. Plasma and ISF are the two main types of *extracellular fluids* (ECF) in our body. The composition of ISF is similar to that of plasma, but with a much lower concentration of proteins compared to plasma.

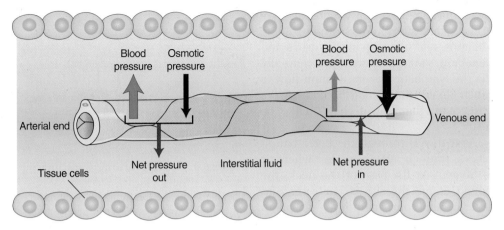

Figure 8.3. The exchange of fluids between circulating blood in capillaries and interstitial fluid (ISF). At the arterial end, there is a net movement of fluid out of capillaries. At the venous end, the balance of pressure sends fluid back into capillaries.

Because of this difference in composition, ISF has a lower osmotic pressure compared to plasma. An osmotic pressure gradient is set up across the capillary wall, allowing much of the interstitial water to re-enter the capillary. The exchange of fluids between blood and the interstitium is illustrated in Figure 8.3. Overall, the average pressure in the capillaries and ISF is similar, and there is only a small net flow of water out of the vasculature, except in some special tissues or in some disease states.

Near the venous end of capillaries, blood pressure is reduced and filtration pressure decreases. Waste products and other substances secreted by cells diffuse from the ISF into capillaries and are carried away in venous blood. ISF and plasma are together called extracellular fluid. The total volume of ECF in a healthy adult is approximately 0.17 L/kg, or 12 L in a 70-kg individual.

The Lymphatic System

There is a small net movement of fluid from vascular to extravascular compartments in most capillary beds in the body. In other words, the volume of fluid leaving the capillaries is greater than the volume reentering capillaries. This would cause fluid accumulation in the interstitium if it were not for the lymphatic system of vessels that removes excess fluid from the interstitium and returns it to the vascular space.

Lymphatic Vessels

The lymphatic system is made up of lymph vessels and lymph nodes. Lymph vessels divide to form microscopic dead-end lymph capillaries that extend into most tissues, paralleling blood capillaries. Lymph capillaries differ from blood capillaries in important ways. A blood capillary has an arterial and a venous end, whereas a lymph capillary has no arterial end. Instead, each lymph capillary originates as a closed tube; thus, lymphatic vessels only carry fluid away from tissues. The endothelium of lymph capillaries is much more permeable than that of blood capillaries; larger paracellular junctions allow movement of larger molecules (e.g., proteins) in and out of lymph capillaries.

Lymph

ISF that enters a lymphatic capillary is referred to as lymph. It is similar in composition to plasma, and also contains particles such as viruses, pathogens, and cell debris. Certain lipophilic compounds,

including long-chain fatty acids, triglyc-
erides, cholesterol esters, lipid-soluble
vitamins, and other lipophilic drugs and
xenobiotics are transported preferentially
via the lymphatic system. Lymph flow is
much slower than blood because of the
absence of a pumping mechanism like the
heart.

As it travels through the body, lymph
passes through lymph nodes where it
is filtered. At the base of the neck, the
lymph enters the subclavian veins and
once again becomes part of the plasma in
the bloodstream. About 2 to 4 L of lymph
is returned to the vascular circulation per
day.

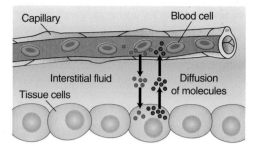

Figure 8.4. Dynamics of drug distribution
processes. Drug molecules can move out of
a capillary into the ISF, from the ISF into the
intracellular fluid of tissue cells, and from the
intracellular fluid back into the ISF and return
to the capillary. The extent to which each of
these steps can occur depends on the physicochemical properties of the drug.

Functions of the Lymphatic System

The main functions of the lymphatic system are to

• Collect and return ISF, including
  plasma proteins, to the vascular space
  and thus help maintain fluid balance
• Defend the body against disease by
  producing lymphocytes
• Absorb lipids from the intestine and
  transport them to the blood.

The last function of the lymphatic system allows lipophilic drugs to be absorbed
along with dietary fats into the lymphatic
circulation, and eventually into the blood.
For this reason, many oral lipophilic
drugs are absorbed more completely when
given with food, particularly with meals
containing fat. A detailed description of
lymphatic transport is outside the scope
of our discussion.

Drug Distribution Processes

Although blood and lymph are essentially
confined to the vessels that carry them,
there is a constant exchange of fluid and
dissolved materials between vascular and
extravascular fluids. The overall distribution of a drug between blood and extravas-

cular space can be viewed as a series of
processes as illustrated in Figure 8.4:

• Movement of drug out of the bloodstream into ISF
• Movement of drug from ISF into tissue
  cells
• Movement of drug from cells into ISF
• Movement of drug from ISF back into
  blood.

Let us examine each of these distribution steps in some detail, assuming a drug
has been administered, absorbed, and is
in the circulation.

Drug Distribution Out
of Capillaries

The movement of a drug or other solute
in (and out) of capillaries occurs mainly
by diffusion; paracellular and transcellular. Therefore, the diffusion coefficient of
the drug (D), the concentration gradient
across the capillary endothelium (C_{plasma} −
C_{tissue}), and the thickness of the endothelium (h) are important factors that control
distribution rate, as discussed in Chapter 5.
In addition, filtration may play a role in
distribution in some specialized tissues,
as we will see.

Other factors that determine the rate of distribution out of the capillary are as follows:

- Type of capillary in the tissue
- Physicochemical properties of drug
- Blood flow to the tissue
- Binding of drug to plasma and tissue proteins.

Type of Capillary

The capillary endothelium plays a central and active role in regulating the exchange of macromolecules, fluid, and solutes (including drugs) between the blood and the ISF. Capillaries may be of three major types, based on endothelial structure: continuous, fenestrated, and discontinuous, as shown in Figure 8.5. Distribution behavior of a solute or drug out of the capillary will depend on the type of endothelium.

Continuous Capillaries. Continuous capillaries are the most common capillaries in the body and carry blood to many tissues such as the skin, nervous system, and muscle. Their endothelial cells form a continuous layer lining the capillary wall. Recall from Chapter 5 that these endothelial cells are generally loosely packed with cell junctions in the range of 5 to 30 nm. Thus, small molecules, regardless of lipophilicity or ionization state, can readily move paracellularly across the continuous capillary endothelium.

An important exception is the system of continuous capillaries that bring blood to the central nervous system. These capillaries have an endothelium with very tight junctions, forming the **blood–brain barrier** (BBB). Consequently, capillaries in the brain have the lowest paracellular permeability, making it difficult for drug molecules to enter the brain, as outlined in Chapter 5.

There are additional features of the BBB that hinder transport of solutes from the vascular space into the cerebrospinal fluid (CSF). The *glial membrane*, closely

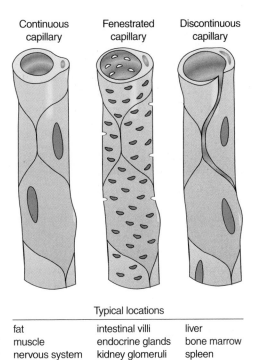

| Continuous capillary | Fenestrated capillary | Discontinuous capillary |

Typical locations

fat	intestinal villi	liver
muscle	endocrine glands	bone marrow
nervous system	kidney glomeruli	spleen

Figure 8.5. A comparison of continuous, fenestrated, and discontinuous capillaries. Continuous capillaries are lined by a layer of flat endothelial cells that form a continuous lining. Fenestrated capillaries have endothelial cells pierced by pores or channels. Discontinuous capillaries have very large cell junctions that allow extensive mixing between plasma and ISF.

attached to the capillary wall, is made up of cells called *astrocytes*; long projections from astrocytes completely cover the capillary endothelium (Fig. 8.6). A solute in blood must cross both the capillary endothelium and surrounding *astrocyte sheath* before entering the brain.

Paracellular transport through the BBB is impossible even for small solutes. This means that transcellular transport (either by passive diffusion or by a carrier-mediated process) and transcytosis are the only mechanisms for distribution of solutes into the brain. Even transcellular diffusion is slowed down considerably by the astrocyte sheath. Lipophilic compounds are able to enter the brain by passive transcellular diffusion, but polar drugs have a very difficult time entering

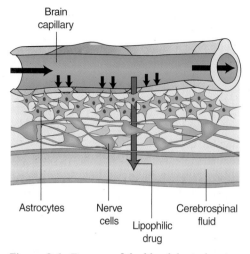

Brain capillary

Astrocytes   Nerve cells   Lipophilic drug   Cerebrospinal fluid

Figure 8.6. Features of the blood–brain barrier that make transport of drugs into the brain difficult. Small lipophilic molecules can enter the cerebrospinal fluid by passive transcellular diffusion.

brain tissue unless transported by a specific carrier-mediated process. In addition, distribution of lipophilic drugs to the brain may be counteracted by the presence of efflux pumps in the lumenal membrane of the brain endothelium. These efflux pumps actively drive drugs such as chemotherapeutics from the brain back to the blood and may thereby prevent significant distribution of antitumor agents in the brain. Metabolizing enzymes in the capillary endothelium may also break down a drug before it can distribute into the brain.

Thus, distribution is a formidable challenge when the site of action of a drug is in the brain. It is partly for these reasons that most classic chemotherapeutic drugs used to treat cancer outside the central nervous system are relatively ineffective in treatment of brain tumors.

Fenestrated Capillaries. The endothelial cells of fenestrated capillaries are pierced by pores or fenestrations (80 to 100 nm in diameter) that extend through the full thickness of the cell and provide channels across the capillary wall. Fenestrated capillaries are found in the kidney, where they allow a higher rate of exchange between intra- and extravascular fluids. Without them, the kidney could not perform its primary function of clearing low-molecular-weight waste products from the circulation. In addition, blood in these capillaries is under higher hydrostatic pressure than in the rest of the body, making filtration a dominant mechanism for distribution of drugs from blood into the kidney. Consequently, fenestrated capillaries filter water and dissolved solutes at rates 100 to 400 times faster than continuous capillaries. Blood cells and platelets are larger in size than fenestrae, and are not filtered out of the bloodstream in glomerular capillaries.

Many proteins present in blood are smaller than the size of fenestrae, yet very little protein is filtered out of renal capillaries. This is believed to be a consequence of the negative charge on most proteins slowing their movement through negatively charged protein pores in the basement membrane of capillaries. Drug molecules bound to plasma proteins will also remain in blood and will not be filtered out in the kidney. This becomes important in slowing the excretion rate of protein-bound drugs. We will discuss the kidney and excretion in more detail in Chapter 9.

Discontinuous Capillaries. Discontinuous capillaries (sinusoidal capillaries or sinusoids) are found in the liver, spleen, and bone marrow. They are special capillaries with very large endothelial junctions (30 to 40 μm in diameter), allowing passage of larger molecules (such as proteins), lipid particles, and cellular debris across the capillary wall. Another characteristic of the liver sinusoidal endothelium is its endocytotic capacity, enabling it to transport a wide variety of substances by transcytosis. The liver is the primary site of metabolism of xenobiotics, and needs this intimate contact between blood and liver enzymes. We will discuss the liver in more detail in Chapter 10.

Physicochemical Properties

Most small molecules diffuse easily out of capillary endothelial junctions as a result of the pressure gradient, coupled with a favorable concentration gradient. Generally, molecules with molecular weights <10,000 (plasma proteins have MWs >60,000) can move through paracellular gaps of the continuous capillaries, except in the brain. Lipophilic, un-ionized molecules can concurrently diffuse through capillary endothelial cells transcellularly. Macromolecular drugs with molecular weights >10,000 are too large to enter ISF in significant amounts, and tend to be retained in blood. For this reason, drugs bound to plasma proteins are also retained in the blood; only "free" or unbound drug molecules are able to leave capillaries.

Lipophilic solutes move rapidly through capillary endothelium by passive transcellular diffusion. The primary reason for this fast transport is the very large surface area of the capillary network in most tissues and the small thickness of the endothelial membrane. Although most lipophilic solutes also diffuse paracellularly through the capillary endothelium, passive transcellular diffusion is believed to be at least as fast, or faster. Differences in distribution rates between various lipophilic solutes can be directly related to differences in their partition coefficients. If there is a pH difference between blood and ISF in a tissue, ion trapping may either favor or hinder distribution of acidic or basic drugs, as discussed in Chapter 5.

Hydrophilic compounds, with poor lipophilicity, cannot diffuse efficiently through capillary endothelial cells and therefore can use the paracellular pathway if their size is smaller than the endothelial junction. Distribution rates for hydrophilic solutes can be directly linked to their diffusion coefficient (i.e., molecular size). Hydrophilic solutes generally have slower overall distribution rates than lipophilic compounds.

Macromolecular compounds such as proteins are too polar for transcellular diffusion and too large for paracellular diffusion through endothelial junctions. However, even these substances may distribute out of capillaries to a small extent by filtration as a result of arterial hydrostatic pressure, and by transcytosis (vesicular transport). In the liver, macromolecules are able to distribute out of the vascular space, because the capillary endothelium is discontinuous.

Blood Flow

The amount of blood flowing through a particular tissue in a given time is referred to as perfusion of that tissue. Perfusion depends on how extensive the network of capillaries is in that tissue, and the rate of blood flow in the capillaries. Well-perfused tissues (brain, kidney, liver, heart) need and have an extensive microcirculation. Other tissues do not need extensive blood flow, have a sparse capillary network, and are consequently poorly perfused (skin, muscle at rest, fat). Perfusion may decrease in some disease states (e.g., hypertension, congestive heart failure), or increase in certain situations (e.g., in skin and muscles during vigorous activity).

For drugs that can diffuse rapidly across the capillary endothelium, rate of distribution will depend on how quickly drug molecules arrive at the tissue, i.e., distribution will depend on perfusion. This type of behavior is called *perfusion-controlled distribution*, and is exhibited by low-molecular-weight lipophilic drugs. Distribution of perfusion-controlled drugs may be dramatically affected if the rate of blood flow to the tissue is altered.

Conversely, if a drug diffuses slowly across the capillary endothelium, changes in blood flow will not significantly affect distribution to that tissue. This behavior is termed *permeability-controlled distribution*. Conditions that change blood flow do not significantly alter distribution of such drugs; distribution is slow no matter the blood flow. Examples are the distribution of polar drugs across the BBB or other endothelia with tight junctions. However, conditions that change capillary permeability (e.g., inflammation) may alter the distribution rate of permeability-controlled drugs. It is important to note that these statements only address the *rate* at which drug distributes, not the total amount of drug that will eventually end up in a particular tissue. That depends on the physicochemical properties of the drug, which we will discuss later.

Drug Binding to Plasma Proteins

Many drugs bind reversibly to plasma proteins to form drug–protein complexes. Plasma proteins are relatively nonspecific in their binding behavior. Albumin, which makes up more than half of all plasma proteins, is the most important contributor to protein binding. Lipoproteins and globulins also play a significant but smaller role. The other relevant protein is α_1-acid glycoprotein (AAG), which is present in much lower concentrations than the other proteins, but can bind strongly to weak base drugs.

Plasma protein binding of drugs is relatively nonspecific, and binding does not occur at a unique active site on the protein. Physicochemical properties of the drug and protein are important in determining which drug will bind to which protein, and the extent of that binding. Generally, the higher the lipophilicity of a drug, the greater is its affinity for plasma proteins. The extent of binding also depends upon the total number of binding sites available (i.e., concentration of protein), the association constant between drug and protein, and the concentration of the drug. Plasma protein binding varies widely among drugs, ranging from almost no binding to greater than 99% bound. Overall, binding of drugs to plasma proteins is the norm rather than the exception.

Therefore, most drugs in plasma are present partly as free (unbound) drug and partly as protein-bound drug. Protein–drug complexes are too large to leave capillaries paracellularly (except in the liver), and too polar to leave it transcellularly. Thus, protein binding keeps the drug in the bloodstream and decreases its distribution into ISF. The overall distribution of a protein-bound drug between vascular and ISF is illustrated in Figure 8.7.

As free drug leaves capillaries, some of the complex will dissociate to release free drug and maintain equilibrium in blood.

The binding equilibrium between drug and plasma proteins can be written as follows:

$$D + P \rightleftharpoons D-P \qquad \text{(Eq. 8.2)}$$

where D denotes the free drug, P the protein, and $D-P$ the protein–drug complex or bound drug.

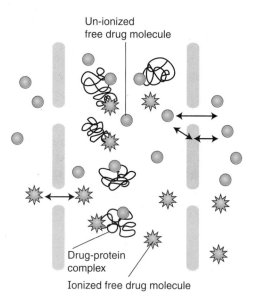

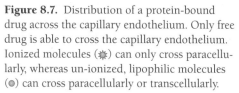

Figure 8.7. Distribution of a protein-bound drug across the capillary endothelium. Only free drug is able to cross the capillary endothelium. Ionized molecules (✳) can only cross paracellularly, whereas un-ionized, lipophilic molecules (●) can cross paracellularly or transcellularly.

| TABLE 8.1. Extent of Plasma Protein Binding of Select Drugs ||
Drug	% Bound
Gentamicin	3
Digoxin	25
Lidocaine	51
Phenytoin	89
Propranolol	93
Furosemide	96
Diazepam	99
Warfarin	99

The total plasma concentration of drug $[C_{p(total)}]$ is given by the sum of free $[C_{p(free)}]$ and bound $[C_{p(bound)}]$ drug concentrations:

$$C_{p(total)} = C_{p(free)} + C_{p(bound)} \quad \text{(Eq. 8.3)}$$

The ratio of free drug concentration to total drug concentration in plasma is called the free fraction, or fraction unbound (f_u), and is given by

$$f_u = \frac{C_{p(free)}}{C_{p(total)}} = \frac{C_{p(free)}}{C_{p(free)} + C_{p(bound)}}$$

$$\text{(Eq. 8.4)}$$

The free fraction is a unitless quantity. The extent of protein binding may also be expressed as percentage rather than a fraction. Table 8.1 lists the extent of protein binding of selected drugs.

Drug Distribution into Intracellular Fluid

It is only the free drug that can leave the vascular space and enter ISF. Once a drug has been distributed from the plasma into the ISF, and the process has reached equilibrium, there will be no net transport in or out of capillaries, and drug concentration in the ISF will be equal to the *free* drug concentration in plasma.

The free drug may continue to distribute from the ISF into the cells of the tissue. Lipophilic solutes, and the un-ionized form of weak acids and bases, can diffuse through cell membranes of tissue cells, into the intracellular fluid (ICF). For such solutes, the intracellular drug concentration will be equal to extracellular drug concentration at equilibrium, as we saw in the Chapter 5. In addition, solutes that have transport proteins in cell membranes will be able to enter cells by carrier-mediated processes. This may lead to higher drug concentrations in the ICF, allowing a drug to concentrate in the cell.

A drug that can enter tissue cells is thus distributed into a larger volume than a drug that remains in plasma, or a drug that can only distribute to the ISF from plasma. ESF and ICF together represent the entire fluid volume in the body; this is collectively called total body water and is approximately 40 L in a healthy adult. Figure 8.8 shows the relative volumes of body fluid into which a drug can distribute.

Just as drugs bind to plasma proteins, they may bind to tissue proteins, or other tissue components, as well. This binding will influence the concentration of free drug in tissue cells. The overall distribution of a protein-bound drug into plasma, ISF, and ICF is illustrated in Figure 8.9.

Drug Distribution from Tissues to Plasma

Distribution can occur in both directions, out of and into the bloodstream. As drugs distribute out of plasma, and are simultaneously removed from plasma by metabolism and excretion, plasma concentration becomes lower than tissue concentration. Now the drug will begin to distribute in the opposite direction, from tissues back into plasma. Transport out of tissues back into blood is important for eventual removal of drugs and metabolites from the body. The most common transport mechanisms are paracellular and transcellular diffusion; carrier-mediated transport may be possible for select solutes.

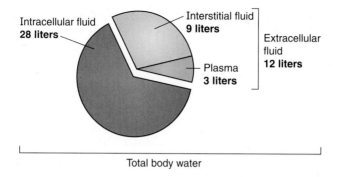

Figure 8.8. Relative volumes of body fluids into which a drug distributes. In a healthy 70-kg adult, the volume of blood in the body is 5 L, of which plasma constitutes 3 L. The volume of blood cells (2 L) is included in the volume of intracellular fluid. Plasma and ISF together constitute extracellular fluid. The extracellular and intracellular fluids together make up *total body water*.

Drug (or metabolite) concentration in the tissue must be higher than in blood for drug (or metabolite) to be transported back into blood. Drugs extensively bound to tissue components will tend to remain in tissues because free drug concentration in tissues is low and not enough to create a large concentration gradient. Lipophilic drugs, because of their high partition coefficient, can also accumulate in organs or sites with adipose (fat) deposits.

Volume of Distribution

A quantitative analysis of distribution is necessary to understand pharmacokinetics of a drug. We have just learned that each drug will distribute differently into tissues depending on its physicochemical properties. A drug can, therefore, be characterized by the volume of fluids into which it distributes. Because the exact volume of body fluids cannot be easily measured, we

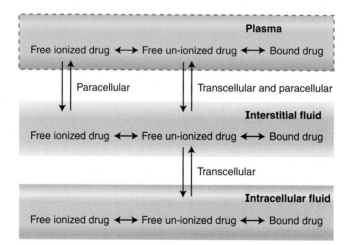

Figure 8.9. Illustration of the distribution of a protein-bound drug. Only free drug is able to cross the capillary endothelial membrane or cell membranes. Ionized molecules can only cross paracellularly across the capillary endothelium, whereas un-ionized, lipophilic molecules can cross both paracellularly and transcellularly. Furthermore, only un-ionized, lipophilic molecules can cross the cell membrane by passive transcellular diffusion to enter intracellular fluid. Exceptions to this are molecules with carrier-mediated transport pathways.

simplify the analysis by assuming that the body is a tank of fluid into which the drug is placed. If the total amount of drug (dose) put into the tank (body) is known, and the concentration of drug in the tank is measured, the volume of fluid in the tank can be calculated. For some drugs, the volume of fluid into which they can enter is small (plasma); for others it is large (plasma + ISF + ICF). This volume is called the apparent volume of distribution, V_d, of the drug. The term *apparent* signifies this is not a real volume (because the body is not a uniform tank), but a calculated number that helps us to model the distribution process and to compare different drugs.

Measuring V_d

The apparent volume of distribution of a drug may be determined by administering a known dose by intravenous bolus injection and measuring plasma drug concentration immediately after injection. After an IV injection, the drug mixes with blood, equilibrates swiftly in plasma, and is transported throughout the body. At an average cardiac output of 4.8 to 6.4 L/min, it is reasonable to assume that distribution to well-perfused tissues is complete within a couple of minutes after IV administration. For most drugs, these tissues are the major sites of distribution. If a blood sample is removed and analyzed immediately, drug concentration in plasma will depend on amount of drug administered (dose) and extent of drug distribution out of the vascular space. (If the blood sample were to be taken later, plasma concentration will be diminished as a result of elimination processes.)

The V_d can be calculated using the equation

$$V_d = \frac{X}{C_p} \qquad \text{(Eq. 8.5)}$$

where X is the IV dose of drug (in mg) and C_p is initial drug concentration in plasma. In general, we assume that C_p is the total concentration of drug (free and bound).

The volume of distribution depends on the drug's physicochemical properties, which control its ability to enter extravascular fluids and tissues. This is best understood by examining three general cases illustrating the distribution behavior of specific types of compounds.

V_d of a Macromolecular Drug

Assume that X milligrams of a protein drug (e.g., heparin) is injected IV, and the initial plasma concentration (C_p) measured. Macromolecules such as heparin cannot distribute out of capillaries and remain confined to the vascular volume; thus the plasma concentration of drug will be high. The V_d (calculated using Equation 8.5) will be approximately equal to the volume of plasma in the individual, usually around 0.04 L/kg, or 3 L in a 70-kg individual. Drugs such as heparin have their site of action in the vascular space, and so it is fine for them to be retained in the bloodstream.

Other macromolecular drugs may have sites of action outside the vascular space and will be need to distribute out of plasma via transporters in the capillary endothelium, or by transcytosis. The V_d of such macromolecular drugs will therefore be larger than 3 L.

V_d of a Polar Small Molecule Drug

Assume that X milligrams of a polar, small molecule compound (e.g., mannitol) is injected IV. Being a small molecule, mannitol can distribute into ISF, thus decreasing plasma concentration. It is not lipophilic enough to enter ICF and is thus is confined to ECF (plasma + ISF). The total volume of fluid into which mannitol distributes is thus greater than that for heparin.

Mannitol does not bind to proteins in plasma or tissues, so we can assume that the mannitol is uniformly distributed in ECF. The initial plasma concentration of mannitol, C_p, will be the same as the mannitol concentration in ECF (C_{ECF}). Thus, it is not necessary (nor convenient) to measure concentration of a drug in all tissue fluids; C_p is sufficient to calculate volume of distribution. The V_d of mannitol can be calculated as before

$$V_d = \frac{X}{C_{ECF}} \approx \frac{X}{C_p} \qquad \text{(Eq. 8.6)}$$

Because mannitol can distribute into ECF but not into ICF, the V_d calculated will be approximately 0.17 L/kg, or 12 L in a 70-kg individual.

V_d of a Lipophilic Small Molecule Drug

Consider a lipophilic drug that can diffuse into cells in various tissues; many drugs fall into this category. Assume the drug does not bind to plasma proteins. Thus, this drug can distribute from plasma into ECF and ICF; i.e., into total body water. The total volume of fluid into which such a drug distributes is thus greater than that for heparin or mannitol.

If X milligrams of this drug is given IV, initial drug concentrations in plasma, ISF, and ICF can be assumed to be equal (assuming no ion trapping). Although this is not strictly true, it is a reasonable assumption for most purposes. Thus, the volume of distribution of such a drug will be given by

$$V_d = \frac{X}{C_{TBW}} \approx \frac{X}{C_p} \qquad \text{(Eq. 8.7)}$$

The V_d calculated in this case will be close to the volume of total body water (approximately 0.57 L/kg, or about 40 L in an average 70-kg individual). Examples of drugs that distribute in total body water are phenytoin, methotrexate, diazepam, and lidocaine.

Physical Significance of V_d

In examining these three types of drugs, it is clear that as the drug is able to distribute into a larger volume of body fluid, its initial plasma concentration will be lower and the V_d calculated will be larger. Conversely, the V_d of a drug is an indication of its permeability into various fluids and tissues. A word of caution is necessary here. Although some general patterns of distribution may be deduced based on the numerical value of V_d, it is incorrect to equate a given value of V_d too closely with a certain anatomical region of the body. Many factors such as drug binding to proteins and to other physiological components can complicate interpretation of V_d. Table 8.2 lists apparent volumes of distribution of selected drugs.

Protein Binding and V_d

V_d is usually determined using the total concentration of drug in plasma. However, we know that only free drug (not bound to plasma proteins) can distribute out of plasma. Drugs extensively bound to plasma proteins have a low f_u, are less extensively distributed to tissues, and *generally* have lower apparent volumes of distribution. Examples of this type of behavior are seen for warfarin, valproic acid, and the penicillins. Drugs with less extensive plasma protein binding have a higher f_u, diffuse to a greater extent out of the vascular space, and

TABLE 8.2. Examples of Apparent Volumes of Distribution of Select Drugs in a 70-kg Individual	
Drug	V_d *(L)*
Furosemide	8
Gentamicin	18
Phenytoin	45
Lidocaine	77
Propranolol	270
Digoxin	440
Nortriptyline	1,300

generally have higher apparent volumes of distribution. Because protein binding, lipophilicity, and ionization influence V_d, the situation is more complex than these statements imply.

Although plasma protein-bound drugs cannot cross the capillary endothelium, it is important to remember that protein binding is a dynamic equilibrium (Eqn 8.2) between bound and free drug. As free drug leaves vascular space, the protein binding equilibrium will readjust to replenish the free drug. This released free drug can also leave vascular space. In this way, a drug with a very low f_u can exhibit a higher than expected volume of distribution. Several drugs, such as amiodarone, digoxin, and tricyclic antidepressants, although highly bound to plasma proteins, are bound with greater affinity to tissue proteins, resulting in a large V_d.

Because only free drug can be excreted by the kidney, the bloodstream acts as a reservoir for protein-bound drugs, prolonging the half life of drug in the body. For many drugs, only free drug can be metabolized, again prolonging half life. As free drug is removed from the body by metabolism and excretion, the protein-bound drug is released to maintain the equilibrium shown in Eqn 8.2.

Protein binding has to be taken into account when determining dose and frequency of administration of a drug. Plasma protein concentrations are usually similar in most healthy adults, so dose and dosing frequency can be standardized. However, plasma protein concentrations may change significantly in some disease states. In such situations, the dose must to be adjusted to avoid either overdosing or underdosing.

Complications also arise when a patient is taking several drugs that bind to the same plasma protein; one drug may displace another significantly enough to require a dosing adjustment. In some cases, such drugs should not be given together. The extent of the problem will depend on the degree of protein binding. For example, if drug X is 98% bound to albumin and 2% of bound X is displaced by another drug, then the free concentration of X almost doubles. On the other hand, if drug Y is 70% bound and 2% of bound Y is displaced by another drug the free Y concentration will not change significantly.

Binding and Accumulation in Tissues

Many drugs can bind to tissue proteins and other components as well as to plasma proteins. The large V_d of some drugs can be directly attributed to tissue binding. Indeed, tissue binding often plays a more important role in drug distribution than does plasma protein binding. Many lipophilic drugs such as amphetamine and meperidine are extensively bound in tissues and thus have an apparent volume of distribution larger than total body water. Conversely, when the V_d of a drug is calculated to be much larger than TBW, it indicates that there is extensive tissue binding of the drug—i.e., very little of the dose is in the vascular space, while most is in the tissues.

Tissue binding may be slow, so the distribution pattern becomes apparent only after several doses rather than after a single dose. For such drugs, V_d is measured after multiple dosing which allows the drug to equilibrate in all fluids; this condition is termed *steady state*. Measuring V_d at steady state rather than after a single dose gives a more physiologically relevant value.

Some drugs have such a strong affinity for a tissue component that they concentrate in that tissue, depleting drug from plasma. The main result is accumulation and "storage" of the drug in the body for prolonged periods because only free drug in plasma can be metabolized and excreted. One example is accumulation of lipophilic drugs in adipose (fat) tissue—such drugs have apparent volumes of distribution much greater than TBW. Another common example is the binding and accumulation of tetracycline antibiotics in bones and teeth, due to chelation between the drug and calcium in these tissues.

Key Concepts

- Distribution occurs via the circulatory system, which transports drug throughout the body.
- Distribution is a dynamic process, and concentrations of drug in plasma and tissues are constantly changing as drug is absorbed and eliminated from the body.
- Distribution patterns depend on physicochemical properties of drug, nature of the capillary endothelium in the tissue, perfusion and blood flow of the tissue, and drug–protein binding.
- Only free, unbound drug is able to distribute across membranes.
- The apparent volume of distribution characterizes the extent to which a drug leaves vascular space and distributes into tissues.
- A large volume of distribution results in longer retention of drug in the body.

Review Questions

1. Why is the capillary endothelium more permeable to drugs than epithelial tissue?
2. What physicochemical properties allow a drug to easily leave the vascular space? What types of drugs cannot leave the vascular space?
3. What are the different types of fluid compartments in the body? What physicochemical properties of a drug allow it to enter each of these types of fluids?
4. What are the primary transport mechanisms for drug distribution in and out of capillaries?
5. Why does the blood–brain barrier prevent entry of drugs into the brain? What physicochemical properties are necessary for a drug to distribute into the brain?
6. Discuss how the capillary endothelia in the kidney and liver are specialized for their respective functions.
7. How can the apparent volume of distribution of a drug be measured? What assumptions are made in this calculation?
8. How can the numerical value of the apparent volume of distribution be interpreted? What does it tell us about the drug?
9. Why does plasma and tissue protein binding of drugs influence drug distribution?
10. When is the apparent volume of distribution after multiple dosing a better measure of distribution than after a single dose?

Practice Problems

1. After a 50 mg IV bolus dose of theophylline, amphetamine, and tolbutamide to healthy individuals, the plasma concentrations were measured immediately and found to be as follows:

Drug	Plasma Concentrations (mg/L)
Theophylline	1.2
Amphetamine	0.15
Tolbutamide	6.0

Assume no plasma protein binding in answering the following questions:

a. Calculate the V_d for each of these drugs. Explain why the initial plasma concentrations are so different even if the same 50 mg dose of each was administered for all the drugs.

b. Based on the values of V_d calculated, explain which fluids (plasma, ISF, ICF) each of the drugs distributes into.

c. What IV dose of theophylline will be needed to reach an initial plasma concentration of 3.6 mg/L?

d. The V_d of theophylline is much lower in patients with cardiovascular disease. To achieve an initial plasma concentration of 1.2 mg/L in these individuals, will the IV dose of theophylline need to be greater or lower than 50 mg? Explain.

2. Tetracycline (TET) ($V_d = 1.3$ L/kg; 55% plasma protein bound) and doxycycline (DOX) ($V_d = 0.6$ L/kg; 90% plasma protein bound) are two broad spectrum antibiotics.

a. Calculate the V_d of both drugs in a 70-kg individual. What do these numbers suggest about the fluid compartments into which these drugs distribute? Do the numbers point to extensive tissue binding?

b. What is the free fraction (f_u) of both drugs in plasma?

c. Although TET and DOX distribute into the same fluids and tissues, the measured V_d of DOX is lower than that of TET. Suggest a reason for this.

d. A severely ill patient experiencing nausea and vomiting is to receive an IV bolus dose of TET. The patient weighs 110 pounds. What IV bolus dose (in milligrams) of TET would yield an initial plasma concentration of 5 μg/mL?

e. Calculate the concentration of free TET if the total plasma concentration of TET in a patient is 5 μg/mL.

CASE STUDY 8.1

Where is that Beta-Blocker?

The beta-blockers are a class of drugs used in treating cardiovascular disorders, such as hypertension, cardiac arrhythmias, or ischemic heart diseases. The distribution behavior of three beta-blockers in healthy adults is summarized below:

Drug (Brand Name)	% Protein Binding	V_d (L/kg)	pK_a	P_{app} (pH 7.4)
Propranolol (Inderal®)	90	4	9.5	12
Metoprolol (Lopressor®, Toprol®)	12	10	9.7	1.0
Atenolol (Tenormin®)	6	5	9.5	0.02

Propranolol

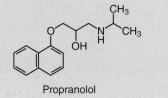

Propranolol

Atenolol

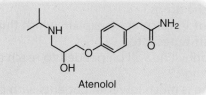

Atenolol

Metoprolol

Metoprolol

Questions

1. Are these drugs weak acids or weak bases?
2. Calculate the partition coefficient P of each drug based on the P_{app} at pH 7.4 and the pK_a. Rank the drugs in order of lipophilicity.
3. Which of these drugs is most likely to cross the blood–brain barrier? Why?
4. Explain how lipophilicity of a drug influences distribution behavior and the value of V_d. Explain how plasma protein binding influences distribution behavior and V_d.
5. Atenolol and propranolol have similar V_d values, even though their lipophilicity and plasma protein binding are very different. Discuss the reasons for this.
6. Calculate the initial plasma concentration of propranolol when a 5 mg IV bolus dose is given to a 70-kg adult. What is the concentration of free and bound propranolol?

7. Some patients taking propranolol complain of central nervous side effects (such as sleep disturbances, psychosis, depression, and hallucinations) during therapy. Would either metoprolol or atenolol be better at avoiding these side effects?
8. All three beta-blockers are bound mainly to AAG in the plasma, rather than to albumin. Explain why AAG plays a more important role than albumin in protein binding of these drugs.
9. Concentrations of AAG are significantly higher in the plasma of elderly patients. Discuss how this might alter plasma concentration (total and free) and V_d of propranolol and atenolol in the elderly. For which drug would this difference be more significant?

Additional Readings

Dipiro JT, Spruill WJ, Wade WE, Blouin RA, Pruemer JM. Concepts in Clinical Pharmacokinetics, 5th ed. American Society of Health Systems Pharmacists, 2010.

Ritschel WA, Kearns GL. Handbook of Basic Pharmacokinetics, 7th ed. American Pharmaceutical Association, 2009.

Rowland M, Tozer TN. Clinical Pharmacokinetics and Pharmacodynamics: Concepts and Applications, 4th ed. Lippincott Williams & Wilkins, 2010.

Shargel L, Yu A. Applied Biopharmaceutics and Pharmacokinetics, 5th ed. McGraw-Hill/Appleton & Lange, 2004.

CHAPTER 9

Drug Excretion

After a drug has been administered and is distributed, the body immediately begins to get rid of the drug by several processes. Drug elimination is the removal of drug from the body by these processes. More specifically, we define elimination as the removal of drug from *plasma*, resulting in a decrease of plasma concentration with time. A drug may be removed from the plasma physically and put into an aqueous fluid such as urine (excretion), or may be chemically transformed into metabolites (biotransformation or metabolism). As drug is eliminated from plasma, distribution equilibria pull drug out of tissues and return it back into plasma. Elimination continues, and drug is progressively removed from the bloodstream and tissues (including the site of action), until no more drug remains in the body. The consequence of elimination is a progressive decrease and eventual loss of the pharmacological action of the drug.

Excretion is a process by which a drug is eliminated from the body without any chemical change. We say that drugs are excreted *unchanged*, *intact*, or as the *parent drug*. This is to distinguish excretion from metabolism, where the drug is chemically changed into different compounds called *metabolites*. The body excretes drugs and other substances by taking them out of plasma and putting them in a waste fluid such as urine. Excreted drugs can also appear in other fluids such as saliva, bile, sweat, breast milk, and exhaled air. Generally, the contribution of these alternative excretion fluids is small compared to urine, except for excretion of volatile anesthetics in exhaled air.

The physicochemical properties of a drug (lipophilicity, ionization, protein binding) determine if it is more likely to be excreted in urine, or to be metabolized. Many drugs are eliminated by both these pathways. In general, polar compounds are more likely to be eliminated by excretion, while lipophilic compounds must be metabolized. We will discuss drug metabolism in the Chapter 10. Table 9.1 lists examples of drugs eliminated primarily by excretion and those eliminated primarily by metabolism.

Excretion by the Kidneys

The kidney is the main organ of excretion of the body's waste products, and of drugs and drug metabolites. Although the kidneys perform many important functions, those most relevant to drug excretion are as follows:

- Cleansing of blood
- Regulation and maintenance of fluid and chemical balance

TABLE 9.1. Examples of Drugs Excreted Primarily in the Unchanged Form and Primarily as Metabolites	
Excreted Mostly Unchanged	*Excreted Mostly as Metabolites*
Digoxin	Phenacetin
Streptomycin	Morphine
Amphetamine	Chloramphenicol
Ampicillin	Isoniazid
Guanethidine	
Penicillin	
Tetracycline	

- Production of urine to remove waste materials.

Urine is the most important fluid for excretion of waste materials (resulting from various cellular processes), as well as drugs and metabolites, from the body.

The kidneys are constantly adjusting urine composition to reflect the body's needs, by either removing or adding water and chemicals to the blood. The kidney removes wastes from blood, and also removes common components of blood present at greater-than-normal concentrations. For example, when excess water, sodium ions, calcium ions, and so forth are present in blood, the excess quickly passes out in urine. On the other hand, the kidney steps up reclamation of these same substances when they are present in blood at less-than-normal amounts. Thus the kidney continuously regulates the composition of blood within narrow limits.

Structure of the Kidneys

Although a thorough description of kidney structure will not be given here, we will briefly review the main components important for excretion. The basic structural and functional unit of the kidney is the nephron; each kidney contains about one million nephrons arranged in several renal pyramids. The kidneys' extraordinary excretory and regulatory functions are achieved through processes of glomerular filtration, tubular reabsorption, and tubular secretion, all of which occur in the nephron.

Blood enters the kidney via the renal artery, which branches several times into smaller vessels, and eventually leads into each nephron through an *afferent arteriole*. Each nephron can be divided into two sections: the renal corpuscle and renal tubule, shown diagrammatically in Figure 9.1. The renal corpuscle (Fig. 9.2) is the initial filtering unit, made up of a network of capillaries known as the glomerulus, that receives blood from the

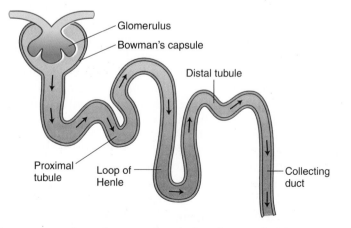

Figure 9.1. Schematic view of a nephron, composed of renal corpuscle (glomerulus and Bowman's capsule), tubules (proximal tubule, loop of Henle, and distal tubule), and collecting duct.

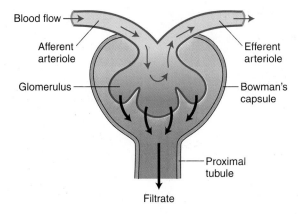

Figure 9.2. The renal corpuscle showing the glomerulus and surrounding Bowman's capsule. Blood enters the renal corpuscle and flows through the glomerular capillaries where it is filtered. The filtrate is collected in the Bowman's capsule.

afferent renal arteriole. This is the "gateway" through which blood first passes to be cleansed by the nephron. The glomerulus is nestled inside the Bowman's capsule, a cup-shaped structure that receives fluid after filtration of blood flowing through the glomerulus. Glomerular filtration is the term used for the renal process in which plasma is filtered across the glomerulus and into the Bowman's capsule (or Bowman's space).

The filtered fluid flows into the renal tubule which may be divided into four functional parts: the *proximal tubule, loop of Henle, distal tubule*, and *collecting duct*. The tubule is surrounded by a network of peritubular capillaries, formed by the efferent arteriole from the glomerulus. The renal corpuscle is important for filtration, whereas the tubule and peritubular capillaries are responsible for secretion of ions and reabsorption of water and other substances, as we will see later. Secretion and reabsorption processes change the composition of the filtrate as it flows along the tubule into the collecting duct. The collecting ducts of all the nephrons join and drain into the *ureter*, which carries the resulting fluid, now called urine, to the bladder for storage.

Cleansed blood from the peritubular capillaries leaves the nephron via an *efferent arteriole*. These efferent arterioles have a smaller diameter than the afferent arterioles, creating hydrostatic pressure in the glomerulus. It is this pressure that causes plasma to be filtered (squeezed out) into the Bowman's space. The efferent arterioles from all nephrons eventually merge and cleansed blood then leaves the kidney via the renal vein. Figure 9.3 is a diagram showing the parts of a nephron and its blood supply.

Urine Formation

Urine is made by the kidneys to excrete water-soluble materials that are either waste products or present in excess in the body. The composition of urine varies considerably, adjusting to the needs of the body. In general, urine is about 95% water, the rest being dissolved compounds and ions. It is produced as a result of three precisely regulated processes in the nephron: glomerular filtration, tubular reabsorption, and tubular secretion.

Glomerular Filtration

This process is often called *ultrafiltration*, reflecting the fact that the glomerular filtration barrier involves a very fine molecular sieve that allows filtration of small molecules but restricts passage of macromolecules.

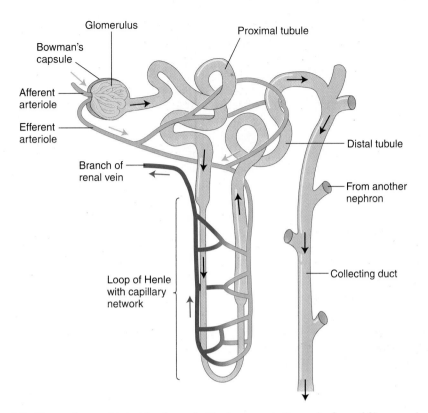

Figure 9.3. The nephron with its blood supply. Black arrows indicate the flow of filtrate and purple arrows indicate the flow of blood.

Glomerular Filtration Barrier. The wall of the glomerular capillaries consists of three layers: fenestrated endothelium, basement membrane, and podocytes (specialized epithelial cells that wrap around the capillary). Together, these three layers form the renal filtration barrier, regulating the transport of substances from blood into the Bowman's space. The first layer of the filtration barrier is the capillary endothelium, with large fenestrations that allow free passage of all molecules with diameters up to 100 nm, thus excluding blood cells, platelets, and large plasma proteins.

The second layer, the glomerular basement membrane, represents the major barrier to the filtration of macromolecules. It is made of fibrous proteins that intertwine to form a meshwork with smaller openings through which selective filtration occurs. The crossed fibers act as a size barrier and restrict the filtration of large molecules. This layer also contains anionic proteins that further inhibit filtration of negatively charged ions.

The third layer of podocytes forms narrow elongated, slits about 25 to 60 nm wide, lined with negatively charged proteins. These narrow slits combined with the negative charges provide the final barrier to movement of plasma proteins (which are negatively charged) through the glomerular membrane.

Filtration is greatly assisted by a high hydrostatic pressure within the glomerulus, compared to other capillaries in the body. The higher pressure is primarily due to the smaller diameter of the efferent arteriole compared to the afferent arteriole. As a result, a large volume of fluid (along with dissolved small molecules) is forced out of the glomerulus and into the Bowman's space during filtration. Blood cells, platelets, and plasma proteins are too large to be filtered and remain in the bloodstream. At this point, the filtered fluid in the Bowman's capsule is called the glomerular filtrate. Simply, it is plasma minus plasma proteins.

The "effective pore size" of the glomerular filter is a complex concept and depends on a range of factors such as the size, shape, and charge of filtered substances, as well as on the characteristics of the glomerulus itself. There is no barrier to filtration for molecules up to a molecular weight of about 5,000, but above that charge and shape become progressively more important determinants of filtration. All solutes up to a molecular weight of approximately 5,000 are present in the glomerular filtrate at the same concentration found in plasma. Even low-molecular-weight proteins up to a molecular weight of 25,000 are filtered to some extent. However, many of these are either reabsorbed as they travel down the tubules, or broken down into amino acids, so very little intact protein is excreted in the urine. Larger molecular weight plasma proteins such as albumin (MW ~69,000) and globulins (MW ~160,000) are not filtered. Damage to the glomerular filtration barrier may result in these proteins, and blood cells, appearing in the urine.

Glomerular Filtration Rate. Blood enters the kidney through the renal artery and reaches each nephron via the afferent arteriole. The kidneys constantly receive about 20% of the cardiac output, a very substantial portion of the total blood flow. An average adult male with a cardiac output of 5.5 L/min has a total renal blood flow of 1.1 L/min. Since blood is composed of about 55% plasma, the total renal plasma flow is 600 mL/min.

Obviously, not all the plasma entering the nephron ends up as glomerular filtrate. Only about 20% of plasma flowing through the two kidneys is converted into filtrate. We know that normal renal plasma flow is 600 mL/min, giving a plasma glomerular filtration rate (GFR) of approximately 120 mL/min in an adult with normal renal

function. The GFR is, therefore, defined as the volume of plasma filtered by the kidneys per minute. Note that this is *not* how much blood passes through the kidney each minute, but instead, how much filtrate is removed from the blood each minute. One hundred and twenty milliliters per minute is still a very large volume, and the body would become dehydrated if all this fluid were excreted as urine. Fortunately, the body has mechanisms to recover much of the water from the glomerular filtrate and return it to the bloodstream.

Tubular Reabsorption

The glomerular filtrate travels from the Bowman's capsule along the renal tubule; we now refer to it simply as *filtrate*. The renal tubule is lined with a single layer of epithelial cells in close contact with the peritubular capillary network. Reabsorption is the transport of substances out of the filtrate back into the peritubular blood. Many essential nutrients (e.g., amino acids, glucose) and ions (Na^+, K^+, Cl^-, HCO_3^-) are *actively* transported from the filtrate into the peritubular capillaries by specific carriers in the tubular epithelium. This is a mechanism by which the body reclaims substances it does not want to excrete. Various hormones are released as needed to regulate reabsorption to maintain homeostasis. In a healthy individual, glucose is entirely reabsorbed back into the blood from the proximal tubules, while sodium ions and other ions are only partially reabsorbed, as needed.

The reabsorption of select solutes and ions from filtrate into the blood sets up an osmotic gradient that simultaneously drives reabsorption of water from the filtrate into blood. The enormous length of the tubules allows plenty of opportunity to reabsorb water. Thus, as filtrate moves from Bowman's capsule to the collecting duct, a lot of water is reabsorbed, select solutes are actively reabsorbed, and the filtrate becomes progressively more concentrated in the remaining solutes, eventually turning into a concentrated fluid we call urine.

Urine is thus an aqueous fluid with a high concentration of urea, unwanted excess salts, and other substances. The rate of urine formation varies between 15 mL/hr and 1,500 mL/hr, but is usually around 60 to 120 mL/hr or between 1 to 2 mL/min; this volume goes to the bladder for storage. Since we started out with 120 mL/min of glomerular filtrate, it is apparent that over 98% of water in the filtrate is reabsorbed in the kidneys and returned to blood.

Tubular Secretion

Although urine formation is a result primarily of the filtration and reabsorption mechanisms described earlier, an auxiliary mechanism called tubular secretion is also involved. Just as certain solutes can be reabsorbed from the tubular filtrate back into blood, the reverse process can also occur. Cells of the tubular epithelium remove certain molecules and ions (such as H^+ and K^+) from peritubular blood and *secrete* these into the filtrate within the tubules. The filtrate is more concentrated in these solutes than is plasma (as a result of extensive water reabsorption), so an active transport process has to be in place to move substances from plasma into filtrate against the concentration gradient. Thus, secretion is an active, energy-requiring process that uses carrier proteins in tubular epithelium to transport substances into the filtrate.

Tubular secretion of H^+ is important for maintaining control of the pH of blood. When pH of blood starts to drop, more H^+ is secreted into urine. If blood should become too alkaline, secretion of H^+ is reduced. Thus, pH of urine can vary between a value as low as 4.5 or as high as 8.5 to maintain a blood pH within its normal limits of 7.3 to 7.4. Normally, urine is more acidic than blood.

The processes of glomerular filtration, tubular reabsorption, and tubular secretion are shown diagrammatically in Figure 9.4. Reabsorption and secretion modify the

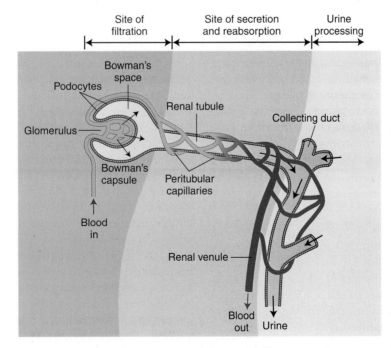

Figure 9.4. Schematic diagram of the processes of glomerular filtration, reabsorption, and secretion in a nephron.

composition and volume of glomerular filtrate as it travels down the nephron to the collecting tubule. Once these processes are complete, the modified, concentrated filtrate, now called urine, is transported to the bladder for storage until it can be removed from the body.

Renal Excretion of Drugs

The kidneys are involved to some extent in the excretion of almost every drug or drug metabolite from the body. The processes of filtration, reabsorption, and secretion discussed earlier determine which and how much drug or metabolite is excreted in urine.

Glomerular Filtration of Drugs

We learned that all solutes in plasma, except large proteins and macromolecules, are filtered in the glomerulus and enter the filtrate. Therefore, most plasma protein–drug complexes will not be filtered and will remain in the bloodstream. In other words, only free drug is able to leave the bloodstream and enter the Bowman's space. Because filtration is driven primarily by hydrostatic pressure in the glomerulus, the concentration of a drug (or metabolite) in the filtrate will be equal to its *unbound*, or *free* concentration in plasma. Since we usually measure plasma concentrations of drug as total drug rather than free drug, the following equations are helpful:

$$C_{\text{filtrate}} = C_{\text{(free)plasma}} = f_u \times C_{\text{(total)plasma}}$$

$$(\text{Eq. 9.1})$$

The GFR of fluid through normal kidneys is about 120 mL/min. We can also define a GFR for each drug, a term that describes the rate at which the particular drug is filtered. GFR of a drug depends on its extent of protein binding, and is given by the equation

$$\text{GFR}_{\text{drug}} = f_u \cdot \text{GFR}_{\text{plasma}} \quad (\text{Eq. 9.2})$$

where f_u is the fraction of unbound drug in plasma. Highly protein-bound drugs (i.e., those with a low f_u) have a low GFR and are retained in plasma. Conversely, a drug that is not protein bound will have the same GFR as plasma, 120 mL/min.

Tubular Reabsorption of Drugs

Although the tubular epithelium contains specific transporters for reabsorption of essential ions and molecules, no special transporters exist for reabsorption of drugs. Thus, the only mechanism available for drug reabsorption from filtrate to blood is passive transcellular diffusion through the epithelial membrane of the tubules. As filtrate containing drug travels through the tubules, water reabsorption causes it to become more concentrated in drug, resulting in a higher concentration of drug in tubular filtrate compared with peritubular blood. A concentration gradient is set up between filtrate and peritubular plasma, allowing drug molecules to diffuse from filtrate back into plasma *if* their physiochemical properties (such as partition coefficient and pK_a) are appropriate. Passive drug reabsorption can occur along the entire renal tubule.

Influence of Filtrate pH. We know that only uncharged, lipophilic molecules can diffuse passively through epithelial membranes, including the tubular epithelium. Thus, drug reabsorption depends on extent of ionization of drug in the tubular filtrate—and, therefore, on filtrate pH—and on the partition coefficient of (unionized) drug. A filtrate pH that favors drug ionization will reduce its rate and extent of reabsorption, and vice versa. Because the pH of the two fluids (plasma and tubular filtrate) across the tubular epithelial membrane can be (and usually is) different, an *ion-trapping* situation is set up. In alkaline urine, acidic drugs are more ionized, less reabsorbed, and more readily excreted, whereas basic drugs are more un-ionized, more reabsorbed, and less readily excreted. The reverse is true in acidic urine.

Ion trapping can be exploited to slow down or speed up excretion of drugs by appropriately altering urine pH. In a drug overdose situation, it may be possible to increase excretion of a drug by suitable adjustment of urine pH. Acidifiers such as ammonium chloride and aspirin lower urine pH, whereas alkalinizers such as calcium carbonate, sodium bicarbonate, and sodium glutamate increase urine pH. Acidic foods (citrus fruits, cranberry juice) and basic foods (milk products) can also change urine pH to some extent. An example of altering urine pH in clinical situations is in the case of pentobarbital overdose; renal excretion of pentobarbital (a weak acid) can be increased by alkalinizing urine with sodium bicarbonate injections.

Tubular Secretion of Drugs

Secretion involves transporting drugs from peritubular blood to filtrate against a concentration gradient (from plasma to a more concentrated filtrate) and thus requires active transport. Scientists have identified a variety of tubular proteins (primarily located in the epithelium of the proximal tubule) responsible for transport of organic cations and organic anions, and a few specific agents such as prostaglandins. Organic anion transporters (OATs) and organic cationic transporters (OCTs) play a key role in tubular secretion of many drugs. These transporters have rather broad substrate specificities; OATs will bind to and transport many ionized organic acids, and OCTs will do the same for ionized organic bases.

Although transporters bind to only the free drug, most protein–drug complexes in blood dissociate rapidly enough to make additional free drug available when some of it has been removed from plasma by secretion. Tubular transporters are so active with some drugs that drug can be completely stripped off plasma proteins

in one pass of blood through the kidney. Therefore, plasma protein binding of a drug has relatively little influence on its rate of tubular secretion.

Because the transporters bind to and secrete only the ionized form of drug, the pH of plasma and its relationship to pK_a of drug are important. A drug that is highly ionized at pH 7.4 will be secreted to a somewhat greater extent than a drug only slightly ionized at this pH.

There are two important consequences arising from these active secretion mechanisms.

- Competitive drug interactions: Many drugs share the same secretion transporters, so competition for transporters can occur, leading to desirable or undesirable drug interactions. For example, penicillin and probenecid are both substrates for the organic anion transporter, so probenecid is used clinically to compete with penicillin and reduce its renal excretion. Cimetidine and procainamide are basic drugs that compete with each other for the organic cation transporter and thus reduce each other's renal excretion.
- Saturable kinetics: The active secretion processes are saturable, so renal excretion can reach a plateau at high doses of a drug. This will lead to a lower excretion rate than expected and, consequently, a higher than anticipated plasma concentration.

Rate of Renal Excretion of Drugs

The rate at which a drug is excreted in urine is the net result of glomerular filtration, reabsorption, and secretion. These processes depend not only on physicochemical properties of drug but also on the rate of blood flow in the nephron, both in the glomerulus and in tubular capillaries. A more rapid blood flow to the nephron increases the rate of all these processes and usually results in an overall higher drug excretion rate. Plasma GFR is a direct measure of perfusion of the kidneys; the greater the blood flow to the kidneys, the higher the GFR.

Secretion and reabsorption of drugs proceed simultaneously in the tubules; secretion increases concentration of drug in the filtrate, whereas reabsorption decreases it. Secretion is favored by ionization of drug in the pH 7.4 plasma; reabsorption is favored by lack of ionization of drug in the (usually) more acidic filtrate.

Thus, the overall rate of drug excretion in urine is governed by a complex relationship between physicochemical properties of drug (pK_a, partition coefficient, and protein binding), pH of plasma and urine, and plasma GFR. In general, the kidneys readily excrete drugs that are water soluble and ionized in the filtrate, but cannot efficiently excrete drugs that are lipophilic and predominantly un-ionized in the filtrate.

Renal Clearance

Clearance (CL) is a term that indicates the rate at which a drug is removed from plasma. A drug is removed from plasma by two main elimination processes: excretion of unchanged drug and metabolism of drug to metabolites. The faster the body can eliminate drug, the higher the clearance of that drug. Total body clearance is the sum of clearances from all elimination pathways.

One would expect that the units of clearance would be amount/time (e.g., mg/hr), so we know how much drug is removed in a given time, and can compare it to the dose administered. However, this number would not be constant, and would change depending on the plasma concentration (and thus with time and dose given). A less intuitive but more useful way to define clearance is in units of volume per time (e.g., mL/min or L/hr). Clearance, therefore, is defined as the hypothetical volume of plasma from which drug is removed, totally and irreversibly, per unit time. The concept of clearance is illustrated in Figure 9.5.

Renal clearance (CL_r) is a component of total body clearance, and represents the efficiency of removal of unchanged drug in urine by renal excretion. It is the volume of plasma that contained the amount of drug appearing in urine per unit time. The rate at which plasma is cleared of drug by the kidneys cannot be directly measured, so an indirect method is used. Renal clearance of a drug can be expressed as:

$$CL_r = \frac{\text{excretion rate in urine}}{\text{plasma concentration}} \quad \text{(Eq. 9.3)}$$

The concentrations of drug in urine and plasma (C_u and C_p, respectively) and volume of urine formation per unit time

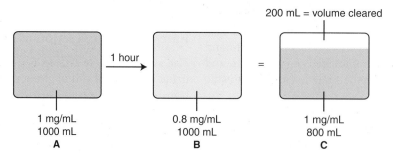

Figure 9.5. A clarification of the concept of clearance. The box (A) represents 1,000 mL of plasma containing 1 mg/mL of a drug. After 1 hour, the plasma concentration of drug drops to 0.8 mg/mL in 1,000 mL due to elimination (B). In other words, after 1 hour, only 800 mL of plasma contains the original concentration of drug (1 mg/mL), whereas 200 mL of plasma is completely free of drug, as shown in (C). Thus, the clearance of drug in this example is 200 mL/hr.

(V_u) are measured. From this, CL_r can be calculated using the following equation:

$$CL_r = \frac{C_u \times V_u}{C_p} \qquad \text{(Eq. 9.4)}$$

Here, $(C_u \times V_u)$ represents the excretion rate of drug in urine.

Physicochemical Properties and Renal Clearance

The susceptibility of a compound or drug to be eliminated by the kidneys depends on its physicochemical properties. In particular, renal excretion depends on plasma protein binding (influences glomerular filtration), ionization in plasma (influences secretion), ionization in the filtrate (influences reabsorption), and lipophilicity (influences reabsorption). This relationship is best understood by examining renal clearance in some special cases.

Renal Clearance of Inulin. Consider a substance such as *inulin*, a carbohydrate from plants (do not confuse with the hormone *insulin*, which is a protein). Inulin does not bind to plasma proteins and so is completely filtered in the glomerulus, which means that

$$C_{inulin(filtrate)} = f_u \times C_{inulin(plasma)}$$
$$= C_{inulin(plasma)} \qquad \text{(Eq. 9.5)}$$

In other words, inulin concentration in the glomerular filtrate is the same as its total concentration in plasma. Inulin is not reabsorbed in the tubules (it does not have a high enough partition coefficient) and is not secreted (it is not ionized in plasma). Therefore, glomerular filtration is the only mechanism that contributes to renal excretion of inulin. In other words, plasma is cleared of inulin at the same rate that plasma is filtered in the glomerulus. There is no secretion to increase inulin clearance and no reabsorption to decrease clearance. Therefore

$$CL_{r(inulin)} = GFR_{inulin} = f_u \times GFR_{plasma}$$
$$= 120 \text{ mL/min} \qquad \text{(Eq. 9.6)}$$

The renal clearance of inulin is the same as plasma GFR, or approximately 120 mL/min in an adult with normal kidney function. As the filtrate travels down the tubules it becomes concentrated as a result of the reabsorption of water; the final inulin concentration in urine will therefore be significantly higher than in plasma.

If rate of urine formation, V_u, is about 1 to 2 mL/min (the normal range for adults) and inulin CL_r is 120 mL/min, then the ratio of concentrations of inulin in urine and plasma can be calculated by rearranging Eqn 9.4 as follows:

$$\frac{C_u}{C_p} = \frac{CL_r}{V_u} = \frac{120 \text{ mL/min}}{2 \text{ mL/min}} = 60 \qquad \text{(Eq. 9.7)}$$

In other words, the concentration of inulin will be about 60 times higher in urine than in plasma.

Conversely, inulin CL_r can be calculated by measuring inulin concentrations in urine and plasma. In fact, renal clearance of *creatinine*, an endogenous substance with properties similar to those of inulin, is often measured to determine an individual's plasma GFR and provide an indication of kidney function.

Creatinine Clearance. Creatinine is a waste substance in the blood, produced by normal breakdown of muscle during physical activity. Creatinine is not protein-bound, not reabsorbed, and is minimally secreted in the tubules; thus it is cleared almost exclusively by glomerular filtration like inulin. Healthy kidneys excrete sufficient creatinine in urine to maintain a stable plasma creatinine concentration. Under normal conditions, creatinine excretion is approximately equal to creatinine production, to keep plasma creatinine concentration fairly constant. When plasma GFR is reduced in renal impairment, creatinine builds up in plasma. The accumulation of creatinine will depend on the degree of loss of glomerular filtration.

Creatinine clearance (CL_{Cr}) is defined as the ratio of urinary excretion of creatinine to plasma creatinine. In the clinic, creatinine clearance (CL_{Cr}) is determined by collecting urine for 24 hours and taking a blood sample at the midpoint of this time interval. The creatinine concentration is measured in both samples, and CL_{Cr} of the patient is calculated by using Eqn 9.4 as follows:

$$CL_r = \frac{C_u \times V_u}{C_p} \qquad \text{(Eq. 9.8)}$$

A small fraction of creatinine is secreted, and there is some non-renal elimination as well. As a result, CL_{Cr} slightly overestimates the actual plasma GFR, but is nevertheless a clinically useful measure of kidney function. A CL_{Cr} significantly lower than 100 mL/min indicates a problem with a patient's filtration process and kidney function.

Renal Clearance of _p_-Aminohippuric Acid. Consider a slightly more complex case: a compound not significantly plasma protein bound, very efficiently secreted by the tubules, but not reabsorbed because of complete ionization in the filtrate. An example is _para-aminohippuric acid_ (PAH), a weak acid completely ionized in the filtrate. PAH will be filtered in the glomerulus just like creatinine or inulin. However, as filtrate travels down the tubules, the concentration of PAH will increase not only because of water reabsorption but also because of PAH secretion from peritubular blood. In fact, PAH is secreted so efficiently by tubular epithelial transporters that plasma in the tubular capillaries is completely cleared of PAH as it flows through.

Thus, the kidneys remove _all_ PAH from plasma in a single pass; blood leaving the kidneys in the renal vein contains virtually no PAH. The CL_r of PAH is, therefore, equal to the rate of plasma flow through the kidneys because that entire volume of plasma has been cleared of drug. The rate of normal renal plasma flow is about 600 mL/min in adults, which represents the highest renal clearance for any substance. Renal clearance of PAH in a patient can give valuable information about kidney function; a PAH clearance much less than 600 mL/min may indicate problems with blood flow to the kidneys. Note that PAH is a very special compound, and its rapid CL_r is a very special case. Any drug that is cleared this rapidly will have an unacceptably short retention in the body and will not be therapeutically useful.

Renal Clearance of Glucose. Now consider the other extreme—a substance that is not cleared by the kidneys at all. An example is glucose, a compound that is completely reabsorbed in the tubules (glucose, being an essential nutrient, is reabsorbed by a carrier-mediated process). Glucose is not protein bound, and so is filtered efficiently. However, after glomerular filtration, glucose is completely reabsorbed into plasma as the filtrate travels through the tubules. Thus, urine contains no glucose in a healthy individual, and CL_r of glucose is zero.

Renal Clearance of Drugs

The three cases discussed earlier illustrate special situations of renal excretion and establish minimum and maximum values for renal clearance. CL_r can range from zero at one extreme to approximately 600 mL/min as the maximum CL_r. The CL_r of most drugs lies somewhere in this range. The CL_r of a drug cleared by filtration only, with no secretion or reabsorption, will be given by

$$CL_r = f_u \times GFR_{plasma} \qquad \text{(Eq. 9.9)}$$

In other words, its renal clearance will be equal to its GFR.

In the case of a drug for which secretion exceeds reabsorption, CL_r will be higher than its GFR.

$$CL_r > f_u \times GFR_{plasma} \quad (Eq. 9.10)$$

In the case of a drug for which reabsorption exceeds secretion, CL_r will be lower than its GFR.

$$CL_r < f_u \times GFR_{plasma} \quad (Eq. 9.11)$$

Rate Versus Extent of Renal Clearance

As we have seen, renal clearance of a drug is the *rate* at which the kidneys excrete it in the urine. The higher the CL_r, the faster the drug is cleared in urine, and the lower the CL_r, the slower the drug is cleared in urine. As drug is being eliminated in urine, it may also be simultaneously metabolized (hepatic clearance) or eliminated by other mechanisms. For example, 60% of a drug may be cleared renally and 40% hepatically. This refers to the *extent* of clearance, or the percentage of the administered dose cleared by each of these two elimination pathways. In general, more drug is cleared by the faster pathway.

A drug with a low CL_r may still be 100% cleared by the kidneys. This means that although renal clearance is slow, it is the only mechanism by which drug is eliminated by the body, and metabolism or other pathways are not significant. In the next chapters we will discuss the factors that determine the relative contribution of various elimination pathways to the overall clearance of a drug.

Excretion by the Liver

Although the primary role of the liver in drug elimination is via metabolism, the liver also secretes a fluid called bile that may play a role in drug excretion. Bile is an aqueous solution of bile acids, bile salts, cholesterol, and inorganic salts. It is sent to the gallbladder for storage, from where it empties into the small intestines as needed to aid in digestion of food. The extent of bile production depends on the type of food present, with food high in proteins resulting in greatest bile secretion. Typically, the liver secretes 0.25 to 1.0 L of bile per day, which is further concentrated up to 10-fold in the gallbladder before reaching the intestine.

Biliary Excretion of Drugs

Blood supply to the liver comes via the hepatic artery from the systemic circulation and via the portal vein from the intestines. The liver removes drugs and other substances from the portal and arterial blood for metabolism. While in the liver, these drugs can also be secreted into bile in much the same manner as the kidney secretes drugs into urine. This is believed to be an active transport process involving anion and cation transporters in hepatocytes (liver cells). Drugs secreted into bile are emptied along with bile into the duodenum, from where they can be removed from the body in the feces; this elimination pathway is called biliary excretion.

Since bile is an aqueous solution, it is suitable for dissolving hydrophilic drugs. In addition, the presence of micelle-forming bile acids allows some solubilization of lipid-soluble drugs in bile. Thus, all types of species (anions, cations, and un-ionized molecules), polar and lipophilic, can be secreted into bile. The main criterion for significant biliary secretion seems to be a molecular weight greater than about 500. Lower molecular weight compounds are reabsorbed from the bile before being transported into the small intestines, and are generally excreted only in negligible amounts in bile. Drug metabolites, many of which have higher molecular weights than the parent drug, can also be secreted into bile.

When the bile concentration of the drug is the same as its plasma concentration, biliary clearance is equal to the bile flow and, therefore, is small. A drug has a high biliary clearance when its bile concentration is much higher than its plasma concentration. This occurs for drugs or metabolites that can be actively transported across the biliary epithelium against a concentration gradient.

Biliary secretion can be saturated at high plasma drug concentration. Also, substances with similar physicochemical properties may compete with each other for secretory transporters.

Enterohepatic Recirculation

Once bile and its constituents reach the intestines, many organic biliary constituents, including bile salts, cholesterol, and phospholipids, are reabsorbed from the intestines back into the blood with high efficiency. These components then return via the portal blood back to the liver. In fact, the human bile salt pool circulates 6 to 10 times per day.

Drugs excreted in the bile may recirculate in the same manner. If the drug has appropriate physicochemical properties (partition coefficient, pK_a), it can be partially reabsorbed from the intestines back into the bloodstream just like an orally administered drug; this process is known as enterohepatic recirculation. Such drugs continue to be secreted into bile and reabsorbed to some extent into blood, until some other process eventually eliminates them from the body. Enterohepatic recirculation, therefore, increases the persistence of drugs in the body, and reduces overall clearance in bile.

Biliary excretion represents an important elimination mechanism for some drugs such as morphine, warfarin, indomethacin, cardiac glycosides, and several antimicrobial agents (clindamycin, rifampicin, erythromycin, metronidazole,

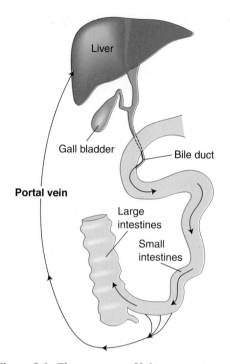

Figure 9.6. The processes of biliary excretion and enterohepatic recirculation of drugs and metabolites.

ampicillin, ceftriaxone, and doxycycline). Figure 9.6 illustrates the processes of biliary excretion and enterohepatic recycling of drugs and metabolites.

Overall, the extent of enterohepatic recirculation of drugs depends on a complex interaction of range of factors associated with gastrointestinal (GI) absorption, hepatic uptake, drug metabolism, and biliary secretion. Each of these processes depends on age, disease, drug properties, genetics, physiology, and coadministered drugs. A change in any one of these parameters may interrupt or enhance enterohepatic recirculation.

Therefore, drugs or metabolites excreted in the bile can be either irreversibly excreted into feces, or reabsorbed via enterohepatic recirculation. Although we know that biliary excretion is a significant pathway for the excretion of some drugs, measuring and predicting it quantitatively is a complex problem.

Excretion by Other Organs

Just as drugs are excreted into fluids such as urine in the kidney, and bile in the liver, they can be excreted into other fluids as well.

Excretion in Saliva

Several drugs are secreted into saliva made by salivary glands in the mouth. The mechanism for transport of drugs from blood into saliva is passive transcellular diffusion of free (unbound) drug. Salivary secretion is not a significant route of drug excretion because saliva is usually swallowed and enters the GI tract. The drug, therefore, can be reabsorbed from the small intestines, resulting in a process of salivary recycling. Drugs that appear in saliva include phenytoin, lithium, digoxin, and salicylates. One application of salivary drug excretion is for routine and noninvasive monitoring of drug levels in patients by measuring concentrations in saliva.

Excretion in Breast Milk

Many drugs pass into the milk of lactating mothers. The primary mechanism of transport is passive diffusion, with some contribution from ion trapping because breast milk has a lower pH (approximately 6.8) compared with blood (7.4). Thus, weak base drugs tend to be more concentrated in breast milk than in plasma. An illustrative example is erythromycin, which shows concentrations approximately eight times higher in breast milk than blood. Other examples include heroin, methadone, tetracycline, and diazepam. Some cases of active transport into breast milk have been seen as well. The appearance of high concentrations of drugs in breast milk can have serious consequences for the infant, and nursing mothers are cautioned against the use of drugs during breast feeding.

Excretion in Sweat

Sweat is a watery fluid produced primarily by glands distributed widely across the skin surface of humans. The primary purpose of sweat production is heat regulation; consequently, the amount of sweat produced is highly dependent on environmental conditions. Several drugs such as amphetamine, cocaine, morphine, and ethanol have been found in sweat. Because the volume of sweat produced is small, excretion in sweat is a possible but not significant mode of drug excretion. However, sweat is being examined as a convenient fluid for detecting illegal drug use.

Excretion in Expired Air

The lung is a major organ of excretion for gaseous and volatile substances, and is a significant route of excretion for volatile drugs such as anesthetics and ethanol. In fact, the Breathalyzer test is based on a measurement of pulmonary excretion of ethanol in expired air. Most organs that excrete drugs eliminate polar compounds more readily than lipophilic compounds. The exception to this premise is the lungs, in which volatility of drug or metabolite is more important than its polarity. Other examples of drugs that appear in expired air are sulfanilamide and sulfapyridine.

Key Concepts

- Drug excretion is the removal of unchanged (unmetabolized) drug from plasma.
- The kidney is the main organ for drug excretion, and transfers drug from plasma into urine for elimination.
- Renal excretion of drugs (and metabolites) depends on kidney function, physicochemical

properties of the compound, its plasma protein binding, and urine pH.

- Glomerular filtration is the first step in renal excretion. The GFR of a drug depends on its extent of plasma protein binding.
- Lipophilic, un-ionized compounds can be reabsorbed passively from the tubules, decreasing their renal excretion.
- Drugs ionized in plasma are actively secreted into urine, increasing their renal excretion. This process has the potential for saturation and competition.

- Renal clearance, CL_r, is the efficiency of removal of unchanged drug in urine by the kidneys.
- CL_r values can range between a minimum of zero to a maximum of 650 mL/min. The CL_r of most drugs lies in this range.
- Drugs and drug metabolites are also excreted by the liver in bile, and irreversibly removed in the feces. Biliary excretion may be reduced by enterohepatic recycling.
- Some drugs may also be excreted to a small extent in sweat, expired air, saliva, and breast milk.

Review Questions

1. What physicochemical properties favor (1) glomerular filtration, (2) secretion, and (3) reabsorption of drugs in the kidney?
2. Why is secretion the only process that can be saturated or competitively inhibited? What are the consequences of inhibition or saturation?
3. Why can some drugs be excreted in the urine without the need for metabolism? What types of drugs need to be metabolized before they can be eliminated?
4. Why does plasma protein binding decrease renal drug clearance?
5. How can urinary pH be altered to increase the excretion of (1) a weak acid and (2) a weak base?
6. Why is creatinine clearance a convenient indicator of kidney function?
7. What are the nonrenal pathways of drug excretion?
8. What types of drugs are successfully eliminated in the feces after biliary secretion?
9. What types of drugs undergo enterohepatic recycling?

Practice Problems

Consider three different drugs with properties as shown below.

Drug A	Weak acid, $pK_a = 4.4$	50% protein bound
Drug B	Weak base, $pK_a = 6.4$	20% protein bound
Drug C	Nonelectrolyte	30% protein bound

Assume that the tubular filtrate pH is 5.4 and the plasma pH is 7.4.

1. If the total plasma concentration of each drug is 25 μg/mL, what is the concentration of each drug in the glomerular filtrate?

2. What fraction of each drug will be ionized in the tubular filtrate? Based on this, which drug will have the greatest probability to be reabsorbed (assume all drugs have similar partition coefficients)?

3. If you want to increase reabsorption of these drugs to keep them in the body for longer, will you need to acidify or alkalinize the urine in each case?

4. What fraction of each drug will be ionized in plasma? Based on this, which drug will have the greatest probability for tubular secretion?

5. Will acidifying or alkalinizing the urine change the extent of secretion of these drugs?

6. What do you expect the GFR of each drug to be in an adult with normal kidney function?

7. Based on what you have deduced about reabsorption and secretion of each drug, determine if the renal clearance of each of these drugs will be equal to, greater than or less than its GFR calculated in #6.

CASE STUDY 9.1

Take With A Pinch of Baking Soda

Renal Excretion of Methotrexate

Methotrexate (MTX; molecular weight 454) is a drug used in the treatment of certain neoplastic diseases, severe psoriasis, and adult rheumatoid arthritis. It is a dicarboxylic acid with pK_a values of 4.8 and 5.5 for the two carboxylic groups. Here are some other important pharmacokinetic parameters for MTX:

Parameter	Value
Volume of distribution, V_d	0.6 L/kg
% Plasma protein bound	50%
Renal clearance, CL_r	2 mL/min/kg

MTX is generally well absorbed after oral administration of low doses. At high doses, absorption becomes saturated.

Renal excretion is the primary elimination pathway for MTX. The drug undergoes glomerular filtration, and tubular secretion and reabsorption. Because urinary excretion is the major elimination pathway for MTX from the body, high MTX concentrations are reached in the tubular filtrate. Impaired renal function can cause MTX toxicity.

After IV administration, 80% of the administered dose is excreted unchanged in the urine, 10% of the administered dose is excreted in the bile, presumably by biliary excretion, and the remainder of the dose is metabolized. It is believed that some MTX undergoes enterohepatic recirculation.

Questions

1. What is the volume of distribution of MTX in a patient weighting 70 kg? What does this number tell you about the fluids into which MTX distributes?

2. a. What is the ionization state (mostly ionized or un-ionized) of MTX molecules at physiological pH (7.4)? First, calculate the % ionized for the WA group of pK_a 4.8. Then calculate the % ionized for the WA group of pK_a 5.5. Then

put these two numbers together to figure out what % of molecules are un-ionized and what % have one or two charges.

b. Given the ionization state of MTX at pH 7.4, how can it be transported into and across tissue cells?

c. Oral absorption of MTX becomes saturated at high doses. What does this mean? What does this tell you about the primary mechanism of oral absorption?

3. a. Using the numbers given in the table, calculate the GFR of MTX in an individual with normal kidney function.

b. Using the numbers given in the table, calculate the CL_r of MTX in a 70 kg individual with normal kidney function.

c. Compare the GFR of MTX with the CL_r of MTX calculated in 3a and 3b. Based on this comparison, does secretion or reabsorption predominate in the urinary excretion of MTX?

4. MTX has poor intrinsic solubility and may precipitate in the urine, particularly at high doses. Precipitation can cause renal failure, will also delay further MTX elimination, and is a potentially life-threatening complication. To avoid precipitation of MTX in the urine, clinicians often hydrate patients aggressively, and administer sodium bicarbonate.

a. Explain how aggressive hydration can reduce the chances of MTX precipitation in the urine.

b. Explain how sodium bicarbonate can reduce the chances of MTX precipitation in the urine.

c. Will changing urine pH by sodium bicarbonate have any effect on the extent of glomerular filtration, tubular secretion, or tubular reabsorption of MTX? How might this alter the CL_r of MTX?

5. KR, a lymphoma patient taking MTX, had unexpected acute renal failure. When the pH of his urine was measured, it was found to be pretty low, in spite of administration of large amounts of sodium bicarbonate. The patient's family stated that KR, in an effort to stay hydrated, had recently started drinking a lot of caffeine-free cola beverages. How might cola consumption have affected MTX CL_r and caused renal failure?

6. The renal clearance of MTX often decreases at high doses. Explain why this might occur.

7. Concurrent use of other weak organic acid drugs (such as nonsteroidal anti-inflammatory drugs) with MTX can result in the persistence of MTX in the body. Explain.

8. MTX is excreted to some extent in bile. What properties of MTX favor biliary excretion? Where will the drug excreted in bile end up?

Additional Readings

Dipiro JT, Spruill WJ, Wade WE, Blouin RA, Pruemer JM. Concepts in Clinical Pharmacokinetics, 5th ed. American Society of Health Systems Pharmacists, 2010.

Ritschel WA, Kearns GL. Handbook of Basic Pharmacokinetics, 7th ed. American Pharmaceutical Association, 2009.

Rowland M, Tozer TN. Clinical Pharmacokinetics and Pharmacodynamics: Concepts and Applications, 4th ed. Lippincott Williams & Wilkins, 2010.

Shargel L, Yu A. Applied Biopharmaceutics and Pharmacokinetics, 5th ed. McGraw-Hill/Appleton & Lange, 2004.

CHAPTER 10

Drug Metabolism

In Chapter 9, we learned that the body eliminates a drug from plasma by either putting it in a waste fluid such as urine or bile (excretion), or by chemically changing the drug into one or more different compounds called metabolites. In general, metabolism (also termed *biotransformation*) describes enzyme-catalyzed biochemical reactions, in which molecules are either broken down, or used to synthesize new molecules. Many metabolic reactions are in constant progress for normal body functioning and to maintain homeostasis. Drugs can be metabolized by these same types of reactions. In this chapter, we will focus on the common organs, reactions, and enzyme systems that are involved in drug metabolism.

Excretion or Metabolism?

The physicochemical properties of a drug (lipophilicity, ionization, protein binding, and molecular weight) determine the extent to which a drug is excreted or metabolized. Many drugs are eliminated by both these pathways.

The body is very efficient at excreting some types of compounds in the urine.

Factors that favor urinary excretion of a compound are as follows:

- Low plasma protein binding
- Ionization in the plasma
- Ionization in the tubular filtrate

Drugs and other molecules that are polar, and significantly ionized in the pH range 5 to 7, can be readily eliminated in the urine unchanged (i.e., without being metabolized). On the other hand, if a compound is lipophilic, extensively bound to plasma proteins, and reabsorbed from the tubular filtrate, it is excreted very slowly in the urine, if at all. These types of compounds must usually be converted to polar metabolites that are suitable for excretion in urine. The importance of metabolism in eliminating a lipophilic drug is shown in Figure 10.1.

For extensive biliary excretion, a compound needs to have a molecular weight greater than 500. Drugs with molecular weights between 300 and 500 can be excreted to some extent in bile. Many drugs have molecular weights less than 500, and only their higher molecular weight metabolites undergo significant biliary excretion.

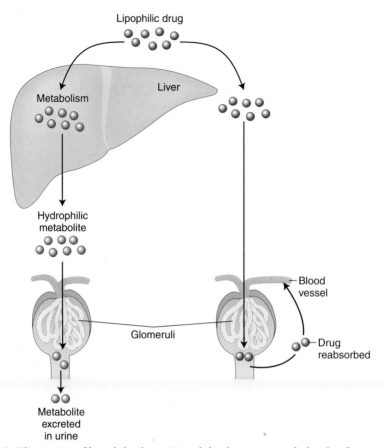

Figure 10.1. Elimination of lipophilic drugs. Lipophilic drugs are metabolized to form polar metabolites that are more easily excreted in urine.

Drugs, Metabolites, and Enzymes

The three major components of a drug metabolism reaction are the reactant (drug or *xenobiotic*), the reaction catalyst (enzyme), and the product (metabolite).

Xenobiotics

One function of a metabolic reaction is to chemically eliminate toxins, foreign molecules (collectively called xenobiotics), and other unwanted molecules from the body. When a foreign organism or macromolecule invades, our immune system interacts with and destroys the invader. However, small molecule xenobiotics do not trigger an immune response. Instead, the body's enzymes metabolize these compounds into less harmful metabolites, which are then excreted in urine or other body fluids. Metabolism becomes a particularly important elimination pathway for molecules that are difficult to excrete unchanged in urine or other waste fluids.

Xenobiotic detoxification is very important for handling the large variety of foreign materials that we are constantly exposed to, such as pesticides, environmental pollutants, and food additives. Drugs are also treated as xenobiotics, and can be metabolized by the same reactions and enzymes.

Enzymes

Enzymes are biomolecules (usually proteins) that have a variety of catalytic functions in reactions for digesting food, transmitting nerve impulses, regulating cell growth, etc. Almost all metabolic processes need to be catalyzed by enzymes to occur at significant rates; without enzymes, these reactions may be extremely slow or may not occur at all. Enzymes change the rate of a reaction without being consumed during the reaction, and can speed up reactions by a factor greater than 1,000. Enzymes are commonly classified based on the type of reaction catalyzed, as shown in Table 10.1.

Many enzymes require an additional, non-protein, molecule (called a *coenzyme*) or ion (called a *cofactor*) to catalyze reactions. Coenzymes may be covalently bound to the protein or may bind only transiently to the enzyme as it performs its catalytic function.

In Chapter 2, we saw that many cellular enzymes serve as targets for ligands and drugs to exert their action. Other enzymes catalyze xenobiotic metabolic reactions; these enzymes are found mainly in the liver and to a lesser degree in the intestinal wall, lungs, kidneys, plasma, and skin. The liver is the most important site of drug metabolism.

Enzyme Specificity

An important characteristic of enzymes is their degree of *substrate specificity*. Enzymes and their substrates must have complementary shape, charge, hydrophilic/hydrophobic characteristics, and/or stereochemistry for the reaction to occur. Our body makes thousands of different enzymes to bind to many different substrates and catalyze the numerous metabolic reactions necessary for life. Because many endogenous substrates are chiral, it follows that stereochemical factors play an important role in the action of enzymes. Some metabolizing enzymes may demonstrate stereospecificity in which one stereoisomer of the drug is metabolized more rapidly than, or to the exclusion of, others.

It would be impractical for the body to have dedicated enzymes and degradation pathways for xenobiotics that it may encounter only infrequently, or

TABLE 10.1. Classification of Important Enzymes		
Class	Reaction Catalyzed	Names
Hydrolases	Hydrolysis of substrate	Esterase
		Peptidase
		Glycosidase
Ligases	Bond formation	Carboxylase
		Synthetase
Transferases	Transfer of group between molecules	Aminotransferase
		Phosphorylase
Lyases	Elimination and addition reactions	Decarboxylase
		Aldolase
Isomerases	Rearrangement reactions	Racemase
		cis-trans isomerase
Oxidoreductases	Oxidation or reduction	Oxidase
		Reductase
		Dehydrogenase

never. A more efficient approach is to have general mechanisms that can rid the body of many different types of xenobiotics. Therefore, most xenobiotic metabolizing enzymes exhibit broad substrate specificity in that a given enzyme can metabolize a variety of chemically different compounds. Other enzymes show group specificity; that is, a large group of similar compounds (e.g., primary amines) may serve as substrates for the enzyme. The metabolism of a drug (or xenobiotic) may proceed via several reactions, each catalyzed by different enzymes, resulting in several metabolites.

Metabolites

Drug metabolites, the products of drug metabolism reactions, are usually more polar, and more likely to be ionized, than the parent drug. Consequently, they are distributed less effectively into intracellular fluid (ICF), are less plasma protein-bound, and are less likely to be reabsorbed and more likely to be secreted in the kidney. These differences enable metabolites to be excreted in the urine much more readily than the parent drug. Many metabolites also have a higher molecular weight than the parent drug, facilitating their secretion into bile.

Most metabolites are also less biologically active than the parent drug, because the altered chemical structure cannot bind to the target effectively. Therefore, metabolism usually terminates a drug's biological activity. Although most metabolites are less pharmacologically active than the parent drug, there are several exceptions. Some drug metabolites may have pharmacological activity (and toxicity) that is quite different compared to the parent drug.

Prodrugs

In some cases, the compound administered to the patient (a prodrug) is inactive,

and becomes pharmacologically active only after metabolism; i.e., the metabolite is the actual "drug" that binds to the receptor. The prodrug is usually a structural derivative of the active drug, synthesized by modifying a functional group or groups (the *promoiety*) on the drug molecule. In the body, the prodrug is cleaved to release the drug.

A popular approach involves synthesizing a prodrug that will undergo a hydrolysis reaction to release the active drug. In particular, the ester is a common prodrug form of drugs with hydroxyl or carboxylic groups. Esterases found in almost all tissues make conversion of prodrug to drug very easy. Esters can be synthesized readily with desired degrees of lipophilicity or hydrophilicity, and with controlled rates of the activating hydrolytic reaction. We will learn about hydrolysis reactions a little later in this chapter.

There are many reasons to administer a prodrug instead of active drug. The drug itself may be too polar for effective oral absorption, or for penetration into the site of action such as the brain. In such cases, a functional group that enhances membrane transport is attached to the drug. After absorption or distribution to the site of action, the group is metabolically cleaved, releasing active drug.

For example, L-DOPA is an amino acid prodrug actively transported across the blood–brain barrier and metabolized to dopamine in the brain (Fig. 10.2). Another example is *enalaprilat*, the active drug

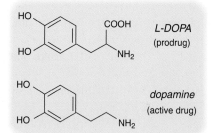

Figure 10.2. Structures of L-DOPA (prodrug) and dopamine (active drug).

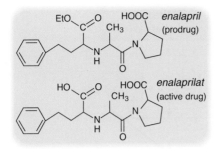

Figure 10.3. Structures of enalapril (prodrug) and enalaprilat (active drug).

that is highly ionized in the GI tract and poorly absorbed after oral administration (Fig. 10.3). Converting one of the carboxylic groups to an ester (*enalapril*) reduces ionization and improves oral absorption. An active transport system in the small intestines may also be partially responsible for the absorption of the ester prodrug (Fig. 10.3).

Other reasons for synthesizing prodrugs are poor stability or poor patient acceptability (taste, odor, gastric irritation, pain on injection, and so forth) of the active drug, or a desire to extend the half-life of the drug in the body.

Kinetics of Drug Metabolism

Enzyme-catalyzed reactions are governed by Michaelis–Menten kinetics, in which the rate of metabolism of a substrate by an enzyme is given by the equation

$$V = \frac{V_{max}[S]}{[S]+K_m} \qquad \text{(Eq. 10.1)}$$

where $[S]$ is the concentration of the substrate (drug), V_{max} is the maximum rate of metabolism, and K_m is the Michaelis constant. V_{max} depends on the concentration of enzyme available and $1/K_m$ is a measure of the *affinity* between drug (substrate) and enzyme.

The exact concentration of drug at the site of metabolism is usually not known.

However, because blood circulation carries drug to this site, it is reasonable to assume that $[S]$ is equal to drug plasma concentration $[C_p]$, which is readily measured by taking blood samples. In this situation, the Michaelis–Menten equation can be written as follows:

$$V = \frac{V_{max}[C_p]}{[C_p]+K_m} \qquad \text{(Eq. 10.2)}$$

When plasma drug concentration is low, $[C_p]<<K_m$ and Eqn. 10.2 simplifies to

$$V = \frac{V_{max}}{K_m}[C_p] = k_m[C_p] \qquad \text{(Eq. 10.3)}$$

where k_m is called the *apparent metabolic rate constant* given by V_{max}/K_m. Thus, at low plasma concentrations of drug, the rate of metabolism is directly proportional to plasma drug concentration and can be described as a first-order process.

If plasma drug concentration is high such that $[C_p]>>K_m$, the rate of metabolism becomes

$$V = \frac{V_{max}[C_p]}{[C_p]} = V_{max} \qquad \text{(Eq. 10.4)}$$

In other words, the rate has reached the maximum that the available enzyme can handle; the enzyme is *saturated*. The rate of metabolism is now independent of drug concentration, a characteristic of a zero-order process. This means any additional drug in plasma (e.g., as a result of a higher dose) will not be metabolized until more enzyme molecules become available. Such situations could result in accumulation of drug and higher plasma concentrations than expected.

The therapeutic doses of most drugs are such that plasma concentrations remain below saturation levels of the metabolizing enzyme systems. However, saturation of enzymes can occur under certain circumstances, and for certain drugs.

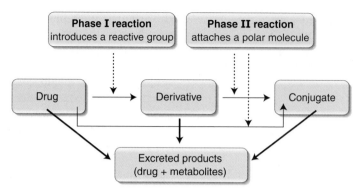

Figure 10.4. Scheme showing the phases of drug metabolism reactions.

Types of Drug Metabolism Reactions

Drug metabolism reactions are commonly divided into two groups based on the type of reaction (Fig. 10.4):

Phase I reactions: A *reactive functional group* is introduced or exposed in the drug molecule, usually in preparation for a subsequent phase II reaction.

Phase II (conjugation) reactions: A molecule provided by the body is added to the drug, or to a phase I reaction product.

The main types of phase I reactions are oxidation, reduction, and hydrolysis, which generally introduce or expose one of the following reactive groups onto the drug molecule:

- hydroxyl (–OH)
- amino (–NH$_2$)
- carboxyl (–COOH)
- sulfhydryl (–SH)

The reaction products of phase I reactions are known as *derivatives*.

Phase II reactions are called conjugation reactions because a highly polar molecule provided by the body (the *conjugating agent*) is attached or *conjugated* to the reactive group on the derivative to form a metabolite (*conjugate*). An illustration of an enzyme catalyzing the reaction between two substrates (one of which could be the drug and other the conjugating agent) is shown in Figure 10.5.

Conjugation usually results in a polar, negatively charged metabolite that can be readily excreted in urine. The conjugate also has a higher molecular weight than the parent drug or the derivative, so biliary excretion is favored as well.

Drugs that already possess one or more reactive groups can directly undergo

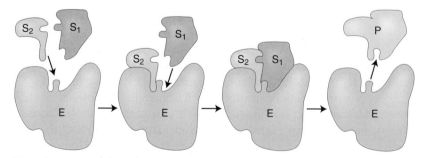

Figure 10.5. An enzyme (E) catalyzing a reaction between two substrates (S$_1$ and S$_2$) to form the product (P).

phase II conjugation without requiring a phase I reaction. Drugs that do not have a reactive group must first undergo a phase I reaction; the derivative then undergoes a phase II conjugation to make it suitable for excretion. The derivative from a phase I reaction may be sufficiently polar to be excreted without subsequent phase II conjugation. In many cases, a drug experiences all the above reactions, in which case urine will contain some unchanged drug as well as products from phase I and phase II reactions. The reaction products that appear in waste fluids are broadly called metabolites, regardless of the type of reaction that produced them.

Phase I Reactions

The major types of phase I reactions are as follows:

- Oxidation
- Reduction
- Hydrolysis

A drug may undergo more than one phase I reaction, leading to several phase I derivatives. In most cases, the reaction causes only a small structural change. Although this modest structural change usually causes drugs to lose their intended biological activity, phase I reaction may activate certain drugs or modify their activity. In particular, prodrugs are commonly activated by phase I hydrolysis reactions.

Phase I derivatives are usually of the same polarity, or only slightly more polar than the parent drug; so, many phase I derivatives need further conjugation.

Phase I Oxidation

Oxidation is the most common type of metabolic reaction because there are many different ways in which drug molecules can be oxidized, and abundant enzymes to catalyze oxidations. Most oxidations take place in the smooth endoplasmic reticulum (SER) of cells in metabolizing organs such as the liver and intestines.

Microsomal Oxidation. When metabolizing cells are isolated and homogenized during laboratory experiments, the SER becomes fragmented and forms structures called *microsomes*. Although microsomes do not exist in intact cells, enzymes contained in SER are often called **microsomal enzymes.** These enzymes are involved in many metabolic reactions, including the metabolism of a wide variety of (primarily lipophilic) xenobiotics.

The Cytochrome P450 System. Most oxidation reactions in our body are catalyzed by a group of microsomal enzymes called *the mixed-function oxidases* (MFOs); Figure 10.6 shows the wide variety of oxidation reactions catalyzed by MFOs. Many of these reactions introduce a reactive group; those that do not require a second Phase I reaction. The most important MFO system is the cytochrome P450 (abbreviated as CYP, CYP450, or P450) superfamily of enzymes. They are heme-containing mono-oxygenases that catalyze the oxidative metabolism of many structurally diverse drugs and chemicals. CYPs are located in the lipophilic membranes of the SER of cells in the liver and in other tissues.

CYP Nomenclature. CYP enzymes are subdivided into families and subfamilies based on amino acid sequence rather than on their function. *Families* include CYP enzymes with at least 40% homology in their amino acid sequences, and are indicated by Arabic numerals after the CYP root, as in CYP1, CYP2, CYP3, and so forth. Within a family, *subfamilies* have greater than 60% homology in their amino acid sequences, and are indicated by a letter after the family designation, e.g., CYP1A, CYP2B, CYP3A, and so on. For example, CYP3A is a cytochrome P450 enzyme in family 3, subfamily A.

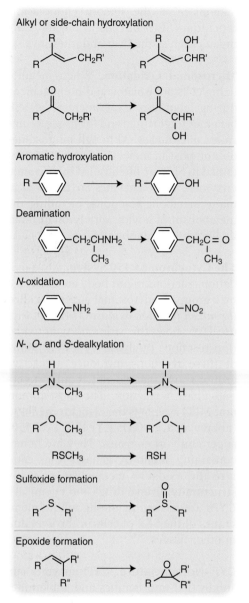

Figure 10.6. Examples of phase I oxidative metabolism reactions catalyzed by microsomal enzyme systems, particularly CYP450.

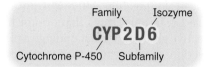

Figure 10.7. Nomenclature of cytochrome P450 (CYP) enzymes.

somewhat in amino acid sequence. They may also differ in their K_m values, substrate specificity, and exact location in the cell.

A breakdown of CYP nomenclature is shown in Figure 10.7. Genes that code for CYP enzymes are named similarly but are designated in italics as in *CYP1A2*, *CYP3A4*, and so forth.

Importance of CYP Enzymes. The CYP families 1 to 4 (particularly CYP1, CYP2, and CYP3) are very important for xenobiotic metabolism, while other CYP families are primarily involved in the metabolism of endogenous substrates such as steroidal hormones and lipids. At least 50 different isozymes in CYP families 1 to 3 have been identified, with different specificities for different types of drugs. Five of the human CYPs (1A2, 2C9, 2C19, 2D6, and 3A4) are involved in about 95% of the CYP-mediated drug oxidation reactions, representing about 75% of all drug metabolism. Table 10.2 shows examples of drugs metabolized by these CYPs.

Isozymes of CYP3A are the most abundant CYP enzymes in humans. This subfamily comprises two genes expressed in adults, *CYP3A4* and *CYP3A5*, and a third, *CYP3A7*, expressed only during fetal life. CYP3A5 plays only a minor role in drug metabolism, while CYP3A4 is arguably the single most important drug-metabolizing enzyme, involved in the metabolism of around 60% of current drugs. CYP3A4 is also the predominant P450 in human liver, where it comprises up to 60% of total P450, and is also the major P450 isozyme expressed in the human intestine.

CYP3A4 activity varies considerably between individuals, causing some individuals to be poor metabolizers of these

Arabic numerals are added sequentially when several enzymes (isoforms) within a subfamily are identified; these are referred to as *isoenzymes* or *isozymes*. For example, CYP3A has several isozymes: CYP3A1, CYP3A2, CYP3A4, and so on. Isozymes are variants of the same enzyme; they catalyze the same chemical reaction, but differ

TABLE 10.2. **Examples of Drug Substrates for the Most Important CYP Enzymes**	
Enzyme	*Substrates*
CYP1A2	Amitriptyline (Elavil®)
	Chlorpromazine
	Clozapine (Clozaril®)
	Propafenone (Rythmol®)
	Theophylline
CYP2C9	Carvedilol (Coreg®)
	Celecoxib (Celebrex®)
	Glipizide (Glucotrol®)
	Ibuprofen (Motrin®)
	Irbesartan (Avapro®)
	Losartan (Cozaar®)
CYP2C19	Clopidogrel (Plavix®)
	Diazepam (Valium®)
	Imipramine (Tofranil®)
	Omeprazole (Prilosec®)
	Phenytoin (Dilantin®)
	Sertraline (Zoloft®)
CYP2D6	Amitriptyline
	Carvedilol (Coreg®)
	Codeine
	Donepezil (Aricept®)
	Haloperidol (Haldol®)
	Metoprolol (Lopressor®)
	Paroxetine (Paxil®)
	Risperidone (Risperdal®)
	Tramadol (Ultram®)
CYP3A4	Alprazolam (Xanax®)
	Amlodipine (Norvasc®)
	Atorvastatin (Lipitor®)
	Cyclosporine (Sandimmune®)
	Diazepam (Valium®)
	Estradiol (Estrace®)
	Indinavir (Crixivan®)
	Ritonavir (Norvir®)
	Simvastatin (Zocor®)
	Sildenafil (Viagra®)
	Verapamil (Calan®, Isoptin®)
	Zolpidem (Ambien®)

Brand names, if any, are in parenthesis.

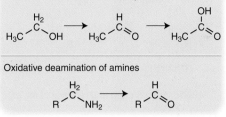

Figure 10.8. Examples of phase I oxidative metabolism reactions catalyzed by non-microsomal enzyme systems.

Non-CYP Oxidation. Although the majority of phase I oxidative reactions are mediated by the CYP superfamily, there are other, non-CYP (and non-microsomal), enzymes capable of directly oxidizing xenobiotics, or further oxidizing products formed by CYP-meditated reactions. These oxidative enzymes are present in mitochondria or cytosol of cells rather than in the SER. Many of these nonmicrosomal enzymes catalyze oxidations of endogenous substrates, but some are involved in phase I oxidation of drugs, primarily converting amines and alcohols to aldehydes and ketones (see Fig. 10.8).

Reduction

Reduction is a relatively uncommon pathway of drug metabolism, although it may be important for a few drugs. Some reductions yield active or toxic metabolites, which become important even when the metabolite concentrations are low. In general, reduction involves either adding hydrogen, e.g., across a –CO double bond, or removing oxygen and adding hydrogen, e.g., converting $-NO_2$ to $-NH_2$ (see Fig. 10.9). These reactions introduce hydroxyl and amino groups that are readily susceptible to phase II conjugations.

Reductions may be catalyzed by microsomal or non-microsomal enzymes. Many of the enzymes involved in reductive reactions are the same as those involved in oxidative reactions, but in the presence of reductive cofactors (e.g., NADPH):

drugs, while others are fast metabolizers. The extensive involvement of CYP3A4 can also result in drug interactions as a result of competition among drug substrates for the enzyme. CYP3A4 activity is increased by several drugs, such as rifampicin, phenobarbital, macrolide antibiotics, and steroids, leading to faster metabolism than expected.

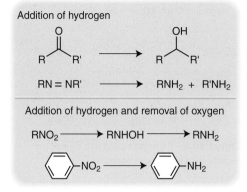

Figure 10.9. Examples of phase I reduction reactions.

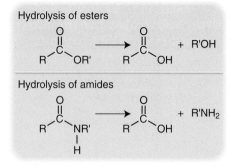

Figure 10.10. Examples of phase I hydrolysis reactions.

e.g. CYP450, CYP450 reductase, alcohol dehydrogenases, and aldehyde dehydrogenases. In fact, some products of oxidative metabolism are substrates for reductive reactions. This can result in redox cycling; the ultimate products will depend on the balance of cofactors and oxygen available.

Reductions occur in the liver and in the lumen of the lower intestines. Anaerobic intestinal bacteria carry out many reduction reactions in the large intestines, so some drugs may be metabolized even before they can be absorbed.

Hydrolysis

Hydrolysis is a common pathway of metabolism for a wide variety of drugs, particularly esters, peptides, lactones, and some amides. Examples of phase I hydrolysis reactions are shown in Figure 10.10. Hydrolysis of xenobiotic esters and amides generates carboxylic acids, alcohols, and amines, each with a reactive group that can undergo phase II conjugation. Hydrolytic enzymes are generally termed hydrolases, but have special names depending on the substrate (*esterase, lactonase, peptidase, amidase*). Hydrolases are primarily non-microsomal and are found in many tissues all over the body, such as the GI tract, plasma, liver. They are particularly important in converting ester prodrugs to their pharmacologically active metabolites.

Phase II Reactions

Phase II or conjugation reactions involve combination of the drug (or phase I derivative) with a conjugating agent provided by the body. They also require energy to be supplied by the body. The *conjugating agent* is often (but not always) a carbohydrate, an amino acid, or a molecule derived from them. The conjugating agent can combine directly with the drug if it has a suitable reactive group, or with a phase I derivative of the drug after a reactive group has been introduced.

Just as a drug may undergo several phase I reactions, it may undergo more than one phase II reaction. All these reactions proceed in parallel, at different rates depending on the K_m and V_{max} of each. The outcome is an array of drug metabolites excreted in urine, other body fluids, and/or feces.

Phase II reactions are generally significantly faster than most phase I oxidations, so that the initial (phase I) oxidation reaction is often the rate limiting step in drug metabolism.

There are six types of conjugation reactions involved in the metabolism of xenobiotics:

- Glucuronidation
- Sulfation
- Glutathione conjugation
- Amino acid conjugation
- Acetylation
- Methylation

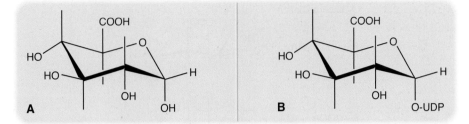

Figure 10.11. A. Structure of glucuronic acid (GA). B. Structure of uridine diphosphate glucuronic acid (UDPGA).

Glucuronidation, sulfation, and glutathione conjugation are the most prevalent types of phase II reactions for drugs. Phase II reactions are generally cytosolic, with the exception of glucuronidation, which is microsomal.

The conjugates are biologically inactive and usually less lipid soluble than the parent compound, although exceptions exist. Many conjugates are polar weak acids that are predominantly ionized at physiological pH. Therefore, transcellular passive diffusion of many phase II conjugates across membranes is poor, and carrier-mediated mechanisms are required for transport out of metabolizing cells.

Conjugation makes a drug suitable for excretion in urine, because it favors tubular secretion and reduces tubular reabsorption. Many conjugates are also high enough in molecular weight so they can be secreted in bile for biliary excretion.

Glucuronidation

Glucuronidation, also called glucuronide conjugation, is the most common phase II reaction and accounts for most conjugated metabolites seen in urine. The conjugating agent is *glucuronic acid* (GA) in its activated form of *uridine diphosphate glucuronic acid* (UDPGA), shown in Figure 10.11. Most glucuronidation reactions are catalyzed by a class of microsomal enzymes called *UDP-glucuronosyltransferases* (*UGTs*).

GA is derived from glucose and is therefore available in ample supply in the body. This is one reason for the predomi-

nance of glucuronidation over other conjugation reactions. The drug or phase I derivative reacts with UDPGA by displacing and taking the place of UDP.

UDPGA is not selective and can combine with molecules containing several reactive groups, such as alcoholic and phenolic hydroxyl groups, amines, carboxyl, sulfhydryl, and carbonyl. This also explains why glucuronidation is so common. Figure 10.12 shows examples of common glucuronidation reactions.

The metabolites (called *glucuronides*) are large molecular weight, polar weak acids (as a result of GA), and are extensively ionized (anionic) at physiological pH. In general, glucuronides of MW <500 are excreted primarily in urine, while those with MW >500 are mostly excreted in bile. Glucuronides secreted in bile will not be absorbed from the GI tract because of their ionization and polarity. However, some glucuronides may be cleaved in the GI tract and undergo enterohepatic recirculation.

Sulfation

Conjugation with a sulfate group is a common phase II pathway for aromatic hydroxyl compounds (such as phenols and catechols), and some amines; it occurs to a lesser extent with aliphatic alcohols. A sulfate group (from sulfur-containing amino acids such as cysteine) combines enzymatically with ATP to form an activated sulfate compound, 3'-phosphoadenosine-5'-phosphosulfate (PAPS). PAPS then transfers the sulfate group to a drug or a

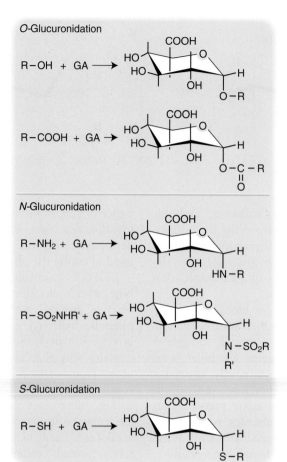

Figure 10.12. Examples of phase II glucuronidation reactions.

phase I derivative to form the sulfate conjugate (see Fig. 10.13).

The reaction is catalyzed by *sulfotransferases* (*SULTs*), cytosolic enzymes catalyzing sulfation of numerous xenobiotics, drugs, and endogenous compounds. SULTs are found in the liver, small intestine, brain, and kidney. The highly ionizable sulfate group makes sulfate conjugates water soluble and readily cleared in urine, and sometimes in bile. In general, sulfate conjugation occurs less frequently than glucuronidation presumably because of the limited supply of inorganic sulfate and fewer reactive functional groups that can undergo this reaction. The limited supply of sulfate in the body can be exhausted during metabolism. When sulfate becomes depleted, other conjugation reactions such as glucuronidation usually take over.

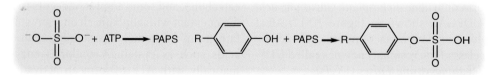

Figure 10.13. The process of sulfate conjugation. 3-phosphoadenosine-5-phosphosulfate (PAPS), generated from a sulfur-containing amino acid and ATP, reacts with the drug or a phase I derivative to form the sulfate conjugate.

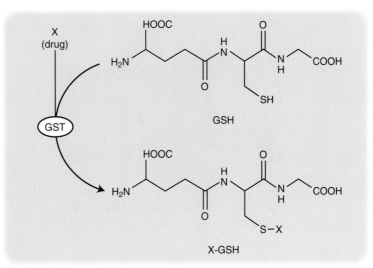

Figure 10.14. Conjugation of a drug (X) with glutathione (GSH) to give the glutathione conjugate.

Glutathione Conjugation

Glutathione conjugation is a nonspecific reaction involving the reaction of an electrophilic compound with the conjugating agent glutathione (GSH), a tripeptide of glutamic acid, cysteine, and glycine. The sulfhydryl (–SH) group of GSH combines with reactive electrophiles to give a thioether conjugate (see Fig. 10.14). The reaction is catalyzed by a class of enzymes called *glutathione S-transferases* (GSTs) found in most cells, but especially in the cells of liver and kidney where GSH concentrations are highest. GSH is present in both microsomal and non-microsomal regions of cells; cytosolic GSTs are believed to be more important in drug and xenobiotic metabolism, whereas microsomal GSTs are important in metabolism of endogenous substrates.

Conjugation with GSH protects the cell from damage by reactive electrophiles. A wide range of electrophilic heteroatoms (–O, –N, and –S) form thioether conjugates with GSH. Drugs and phase I derivatives with these heteroatoms can be conjugated by GSH.

Once formed, GSH conjugates are rarely excreted directly in urine; they usually undergo a few more metabolic reactions and are excreted as *N*-acetylcysteine conjugates. Some GSH conjugates may appear in bile because of their high molecular weight. GSH stores in cells can become quickly exhausted, leading to accumulation of the drug, or its phase I derivative, in the body.

Amino Acid Conjugation

Many endogenous amino acids (typically glycine and glutamine) can act as conjugating agents, in which their amino groups react with compounds containing a carboxylic acid group (see Fig. 10.15) to form an amide bond.

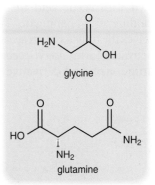

Figure 10.15. Most common amino acids (glycine and glutamine) involved in amino acid conjugation.

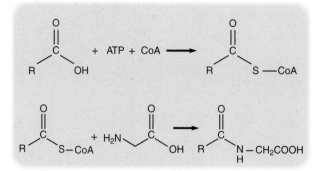

Figure 10.16. The process of amino acid conjugation. A carboxylic acid group on the drug or phase I derivative is first activated to form a CoA thioester, which then conjugates with glycine or glutamine to give the amino acid conjugate.

The carboxylic acid drugs or phase I derivatives have to be first activated by combining with ATP, and then converted to form coenzyme A (CoA) thioesters; the catalytic enzymes are *acyl CoA synthetases*. The CoA thioesters are then conjugated with glycine or glutamine, forming a peptide or amide bond between the amino acid and drug (or phase I derivative); this reaction is catalyzed by *N-acetyltransferases* (see Fig. 10.16). Amino acid conjugates are more water soluble than the original carboxylic acids and are readily excreted in urine; they may be secreted in bile, if molecular weight is high enough.

Acetylation

Primary alkyl and aromatic amines can be conjugated with acetic acid to form the corresponding acetyl conjugate. The reaction involves the transfer of an acetyl group (in its activated form, *acetyl coenzyme A*) to the drug (or phase I derivative), and is catalyzed by enzymes called *N-acetyltransferases (NATs)* (see Fig. 10.17). Acetylation occurs primarily in the liver.

Although most conjugation reactions yield more water-soluble metabolites, acetylation often gives conjugates that are less water soluble than the parent because it converts an ionizable amine into a non-ionizable amide. Nevertheless, acetylation does serve to deactivate the drug by converting it to a non-ionizable compound. Many amine drugs have to be in their cationic conjugate acid form to bind to their receptors; losing the ability to take on a proton at physiological pH results in a loss of affinity for targets, leading to a loss of biological activity.

Methylation

O- and *N*-methylation (addition of a $-CH_3$ group) is an important biochemical pathway for synthesis and metabolism of endogenous compounds but is of only

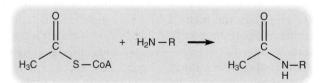

Figure 10.17. The process of acetylation. Acetyl CoA reacts with an amine drug or phase I derivative to give the acetyl conjugate of the drug.

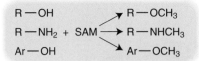

Figure 10.18. The process of methylation. The methyl group comes from activated methionine (SAM), which reacts with the drug or phase I derivative (an alcohol, phenol, or amine) to give the corresponding methyl conjugate.

minor importance in drug metabolism. Nevertheless, some drugs such as epinephrine and isoproterenol are readily methylated, accounting for their short duration of action (see Fig. 10.18). The methyl group comes from the amino acid methionine, which is first activated to *S-adenosylmethionine* (SAM). The compound to be metabolized (such as an alcohol, phenol, or amine) combines with SAM to give the corresponding methyl conjugate; the reaction is catalyzed by *methyltransferases*. Methylation, like acetylation, results in conjugates less polar than the original compound.

Sites of Metabolism

Enzymes capable of metabolizing drugs are present in cells of most tissues and organs. Some enzymes, such as digestive enzymes, are extracellular and carry out reactions outside cells. Significant drug metabolism occurs only in organs that contain high concentrations of enzymes, and receive a large fraction of administered drug. Metabolizing organs are structurally designed to maximize these reactions.

The liver, because of its structure and location, is the most important organ for drug metabolism. It has an abundance of microsomal enzymes, particularly the CYP superfamily, as well as nonmicrosomal enzymes. We will discuss the liver in detail, and then follow with a brief discussion of other metabolizing organs and tissues.

Metabolism in the Liver

The liver is the largest gland in the body and performs a wide variety of tasks that impact all body systems. Three fundamental roles of the liver can be classified as follows:

- Vascular: such as formation of lymph and the hepatic phagocytic system
- Metabolic: control of carbohydrate, lipid, and protein metabolism
- Secretory and excretory: synthesis and secretion of bile

The metabolic and secretory/excretory functions also make the liver a critical organ for drug elimination. One consequence is that hepatic disease has a huge impact on drug therapy, as well as on virtually all other body functions.

Liver Structure and Function

The liver receives approximately 30% of resting cardiac output and is therefore a very vascular organ. Blood enters the liver through two major vessels—the *hepatic artery* carrying arterial blood and the *portal vein* bringing blood from the GI tract. The hepatic artery carries oxygen to the liver and is responsible for about 25% of liver blood supply. The portal vein carries nutrients to the liver and accounts for 75% of liver blood flow. All of the venous blood returning from the small intestine, stomach, pancreas, and spleen converges into the portal vein. This means that drugs and nutrients absorbed from the GI tract into the bloodstream have to first pass through the liver before entering the general circulation. Circulation of blood among these organs is illustrated in Figure 10.19.

The functional hepatic unit is the *liver lobule* illustrated in Figure 10.20; a human liver contains about a million such lobules. Each lobule consists of liver cells (hepatocytes) arranged in plates that radiate out from the central vein, which carries blood out of the liver. Liver capillaries called

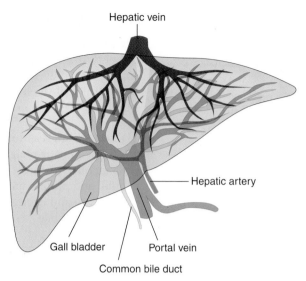

Figure 10.19. Diagram showing blood circulation in the liver. Blood enters the liver via the hepatic artery and the portal vein and leaves via the hepatic vein. The liver also makes bile that is stored in the gall bladder and emptied into the duodenum as needed.

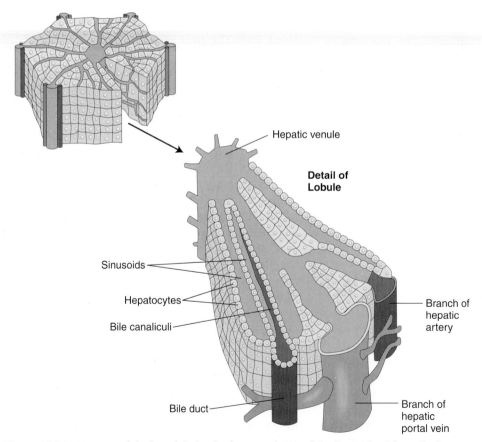

Figure 10.20. Diagram of the liver lobule, the functional unit of the liver. Blood from the hepatic artery and portal vein enters sinusoids and "bathes" hepatocytes.

sinusoids, containing blood from both the portal vein and hepatic artery, separate the plates from one another. The region between the sinusoids and hepatocytes is known as the *space of Disse*. Hepatocytes have *microvilli* that enter the space of Disse, maximizing the surface area of contact between blood and hepatocytes.

The discontinuous sinusoidal endothelium in the liver permits free transport of solutes, including proteins and protein-bound substrates, from blood in sinusoids into the space of Disse.

In this way, drugs and other molecules in the portal and systemic circulations come into close contact with hepatocytes. Lipophilic drugs are readily transported into hepatocytes by transcellular diffusion. Polar or ionized drugs have a more difficult time entering hepatocytes, and may require carrier-mediated processes and specific transporters. Several transporters are present in hepatocytes to transport substrates in and allow transport of other substances, including metabolites, out. Hepatic enzymes can metabolize free drug (not bound to plasma proteins), and even some plasma protein-bound drugs.

A secretory function of hepatocytes is to produce bile, as we saw in the Chapter 9. Bile is important for the digestion of dietary fats, and also serves an excretory role for polar, large molecular weight compounds.

Thus, drugs entering the liver from the general circulation or the portal circulation are exposed to the action of the many metabolic enzymes in hepatocytes. Depending on the K_m and V_{max} of the reactions, a portion of the drug is metabolized into one or more metabolites as blood flows through the liver. The liver may remove larger molecular weight metabolites from the circulation and secrete these into bile for eventual excretion in feces. The remaining unmetabolized drug, and metabolites, leave the liver via the hepatic vein. The blood empties into the vena cava, carrying drug and its metabolites to the general circulation.

Hepatic Clearance

The concept of clearance can be applied to elimination of a drug by the liver. Hepatic clearance, CL_h, is defined as the volume of plasma flowing through the liver that is completely cleared of drug per unit time. Factors affecting hepatic clearance of a drug are as follows:

- Hepatic extraction ratio of the drug
- Blood flow to the liver
- Plasma protein binding of drug

Hepatic Extraction Ratio. Consider a drug administered by intravenous injection. The drug distributes into the systemic circulation and into tissues, according to its volume of distribution. It enters the liver via the hepatic artery, and a portion of the drug is removed from plasma by either biliary secretion or metabolism. As a result, the drug concentration in plasma leaving the liver via the hepatic vein is less than the arterial concentration that entered the liver. The hepatic extraction ratio (ER_h) of the drug is defined as the fraction of drug removed from plasma in one pass through the liver:

$$ER_h = \frac{C_a - C_v}{C_a} \quad \text{(Eq. 10.5)}$$

where C_a and C_v are drug plasma concentrations in the hepatic artery and vein, respectively. ER_h values range from 0 to 1.0; an ER_h of 0.2 means 20% of the drug in plasma was removed by the liver in one pass.

The hepatic extraction ratio depends on the efficiency of liver enzymes to metabolize the drug, and the extent to which the drug is secreted in bile.

Metabolic Efficiency. The efficiency by which a drug is metabolized in the liver depends on several factors, including the drug's physicochemical properties, and the K_m and V_{max} of the particular reactions that occur in the hepatocytes. Drugs must enter hepatocytes to be metabolized, and this could be a passive diffusion or carrier-mediated process. The number of reactions a drug can undergo, the affinity of the drug for enzymes, and the concentration of these enzymes will control the rate of metabolism.

Biliary Secretion. Only a small number of drugs are eliminated in bile in their unchanged form; most drugs are first metabolized and it is the larger molecular weight metabolites that can be excreted in bile. Therefore, we often assume that drug elimination by the liver is primarily due to metabolism rather than excretion, and hepatic extraction is mostly due to hepatic metabolism rather than biliary secretion. Of course, there are some important exceptions, such as the "statin" drugs used to lower serum cholesterol.

Liver Blood Flow. It is apparent that drug can be eliminated by the liver only as fast as drug is delivered to the liver by blood. If blood flow to the liver is expressed as Q (mL/min or L/hr), hepatic clearance is given by

$$CL_h = Q \cdot ER_h \quad \text{(Eq. 10.6)}$$

For drugs with a high ER_h (>0.7), the liver can remove drug almost as fast as the blood flows through the liver. Thus, changes in liver blood flow can change hepatic clearance of such drugs significantly. If blood flow increases, hepatic clearance increases.

On the other hand, drugs with low ER_h (<0.2) are less affected by changes in Q than are drugs with high ER_h. Hepatic clearance of low ER_h drugs is limited primarily by the efficiency of the enzyme system; bringing drug to the liver faster or slower does not change the clearance of low a ER_h drug significantly.

Plasma Protein Binding. The effect of plasma protein binding on hepatic clearance is complex. For some drugs, hepatic enzymes are able to metabolize only the free drug in plasma; these drugs are said to exhibit *restrictive metabolism*. Thus, their metabolism is affected by the extent of plasma protein binding. In general, these are drugs with low ER_h (<0.3). Other drugs (especially those with ER_h >0.7) are metabolized so rapidly by the liver that their metabolism is not significantly affected by plasma protein binding; they exhibit *unrestrictive metabolism*. Here, the enzymatic reactions are so efficient that the enzymes are able to "pull" the drug off plasma proteins. Drugs with intermediate extraction ratios show mixed behavior, with plasma protein binding having some small effect on metabolism.

Plasma protein binding affects biliary secretion in a variable manner, like metabolism. For drugs that have a high affinity for biliary transporters, plasma protein binding has only a small effect. For drugs that are moderately secreted, only the free drug is available for secretion into bile.

A detailed discussion of restrictive and nonrestrictive hepatic extraction is outside the scope of this book.

Metabolism in Other Organs

Drugs may be metabolized in organs other than the liver; collectively, this is often called *extra-hepatic metabolism*. Significant concentrations of metabolizing enzymes are found in epithelial cells lining the intestinal tract, lung, kidney, brain, skin, and nose. Metabolism in these organs becomes particularly important when drug is administered or absorbed via the particular organ, such as during oral, nasal, inhalation, or dermal delivery. A clearance and extraction ratio can be defined for each of these sites of metabolism.

Presystemic Metabolism

The entire dose of a drug administered intravenously enters the systemic circulation. On the other hand, when drugs are given by other routes, only a portion of the administered dose may reach the systemic circulation. One reason is incomplete absorption, as we already learned. Another is because of potential metabolism in epithelial cells during absorption. For orally administered drugs, the pattern of portal blood circulation creates another opportunity for drug loss before systemic distribution. In general, the metabolism of a drug before it can enter the systemic circulation is called **presystemic metabolism**.

This phenomenon is especially important for oral drug administration, so let us consider that in some detail. There are two main regions where presystemic metabolism occurs: in the small intestines, and in the liver.

Metabolism in the Intestines. The intestines, both small and large, play a role in the metabolism of some drugs. The small intestinal lumen contains many digestive enzymes that can metabolize a drug, especially if it is administered with food. Peptides and polypeptides are particularly susceptible. Bacterial flora present in the intestine and colon also secrete enzymes that can contribute to drug metabolism. In both cases, a portion of the administered dose is lost before the drug is absorbed. Intestinal glucuronidase can hydrolyze glucuronide conjugates secreted in the bile, releasing free drug which can undergo enterohepatic recirculation.

Metabolism may also occur during absorption. The intestinal epithelium (or *gut wall*) contains enzymes that catalyze phase I microsomal oxidation and phase II glucuronidation or sulfation. Hydrolases are also abundant in intestinal wall leading to the hydrolysis of many prodrugs. The highest concentration of enzymes is found in the duodenal epithelium, with a gradual decrease further down the intestinal tract. As the drug dissolves in the GI tract and begins absorption through the epithelial cells, these enzymes act on the drug during its passage from the intestinal lumen into the capillaries in the villi. Therefore, the capillaries receive some unchanged drug, but also some metabolites.

We can define a gut wall extraction ratio, ER_{gut}, just like we did for hepatic extraction; it is the fraction of drug removed due to metabolism during absorption through the intestinal epithelium. For some drugs, gut wall metabolism can be extensive, seriously limiting the amount of parent drug absorbed. For such drugs, oral administration may not be appropriate and an alternative route may be necessary.

First-Pass Metabolism. The pattern of blood flow to the liver via the portal vein is such that all orally administered drugs first pass through the liver after absorption before entering the systemic circulation, and before being distributed into vascular and extravascular fluids. If the liver extracts the drug during this first pass, then less drug reaches the general circulation.

For drugs with a high hepatic extraction ratio ($E_h > 0.7$), a large fraction of the administered dose is lost due to metabolism (or rarely to biliary secretion). Loss of drug due to metabolism during first pass through the liver is called hepatic **first-pass metabolism**. High E_h drugs, given by other routes, also pass through the liver eventually, but only after distribution to the rest of the body. Therefore, a lower concentration of drug enters the liver via the hepatic artery, and thus a smaller amount (but same ER_h) is extracted. First pass loss can sometime be compensated for by giving a larger dose of drug, if the metabolites are nontoxic. If a larger dose is not possible, the drug may have to be administered by a non-oral route.

All drugs subject to hepatic extraction will suffer some loss during first pass through the liver after oral administration. For low ER_h drugs, this loss is small and considered insignificant. Therefore, we reserve the term "first-pass metabolism" only for drugs with high extraction ratios.

Many prodrugs are activated by first-pass metabolism; the inactive prodrug is absorbed and converted to the active metabolite as it passes through the liver.

Total Body Clearance

Total body clearance, CL_{tot}, is defined as the volume of plasma that is completely cleared of drug per unit time. A drug can be cleared from plasma by excretion of unchanged drug in urine and bile, or by metabolism in the liver and in other organs. All these pathways contribute to the total clearance of drug from plasma. The total clearance is given by the sum of individual clearances:

$$CL_{tot} = CL_r + CL_m + CL_b + CL_{other}$$
$$\text{(Eq. 10.7)}$$

Here, CL_r is renal clearance, CL_m is hepatic metabolic clearance, CL_b is biliary clearance (of unchanged drug), and CL_{other} represents other clearance pathways. For most drugs with molecular weights under 500, the renal excretion and hepatic metabolism pathways are the most significant, and the equation simplifies to

$$CL_{tot} = CL_r + CL_m \qquad \text{(Eq. 10.8)}$$

Total clearance can be measured by monitoring plasma drug concentration as a function of time, and measuring the decrease in drug concentration. Renal clearance is fairly easy to measure by monitoring the concentration of drug appearing in the urine as a function of time. In general, we assume that the difference between the total clearance and the renal clearance is equal to the hepatic metabolic clearance for most drugs.

$$CL_m = CL_{tot} + CL_r \qquad \text{(Eq. 10.9)}$$

Obviously, for drugs cleared significantly in bile or metabolized in other tissues, we need to include these terms in the equation.

Rate Versus Extent of Clearance

Hepatic clearance (CL_h) of a drug is a measure of the *rate* at which the liver can remove a drug from plasma by metabolism (CL_m) or biliary secretion. The higher the CL_h, the faster the drug is removed, and the lower the CL_h, the slower the drug is removed. As drug is being cleared by the liver, it may also be simultaneously excreted by the kidneys or eliminated by other mechanisms. The relative contributions of each of these pathways depend on the physicochemical properties of the drug, liver and kidney function of the patient, and other drugs or endogenous materials competing for these elimination processes.

A drug with a low CL_m may still be 100% cleared by hepatic metabolism, especially if its properties make it unsuitable for renal excretion. It just means that the drug is metabolized slowly and will remain in the body for a long time.

Factors Altering Drug Metabolism

Metabolizing enzymes are continually produced and decomposed in the body. The rates of these processes are equal under normal conditions, keeping enzyme concentrations constant and appropriate to normal body functioning. However, changes in enzyme levels can alter the rate of metabolism and consequently result in higher or lower drug plasma concentrations than expected. If left uncorrected, this can lead to increased side effects or failure of therapy. Consider some general situations that alter the rates of drug metabolism.

Enzyme Inhibition

If a substance interferes with the ability of an enzyme to bind to its substrate, the affinity between the enzyme and substrate decreases, causing an increase in K_m and a consequent decrease in rate of metabolism. The interfering substance is called an **enzyme inhibitor**. Enzyme inhibition is also a mechanism by which some drugs produce their pharmacological effect, as we will see in the Chapter 13. An inhibitor of a metabolic enzyme can be another drug, a drug metabolite, or even a food substance. There are two types of enzyme inhibition: competitive and noncompetitive.

Competitive Inhibition

An enzyme inhibitor is said to be *competitive* if it is

- also a substrate for the enzyme
- not a substrate for the enzyme, but combines reversibly with the enzyme.

Most competitive inhibitors have structures similar to that of the drug whose metabolism they are inhibiting, and therefore bind at the same active site of the enzyme. Thus, inhibitor and substrate compete for the same binding site and the same quantity of enzyme. The result is that the affinity of enzyme available for the substrate is decreased, and so is the rate of metabolism of the substrate.

The inhibitor may be a substrate itself, in which case it is metabolized by the enzyme. If the inhibitor is not a substrate for the enzyme, it merely occupies the active site in a reversible fashion. Both processes are reversible because the inhibitor can dissociate from the enzyme.

The degree of competitive inhibition depends on relative affinities of substrate and inhibitor for the active site, and on the relative concentrations of the inhibitor and substrate. If the inhibitor concentration is very large compared with substrate concentration, the inhibitor will occupy almost all the enzyme active sites and the substrate will not be metabolized. Conversely, if substrate concentration is made large enough, it will be able to compete with and displace the inhibitor from the active site. Thus, competitive inhibition is less pronounced at high substrate concentrations. Mathematically, the Michaelis–Menten equation for the rate of reaction of a substrate in the presence of a competitive inhibitor is

$$V = \frac{V_{max}[C_p]}{[C_p] + K_m(1 + [C_i]/K_{m(i)})}$$

(Eq. 10.10)

Note that the equation now includes the plasma concentration of the inhibitor, $[C_i]$, and its Michaelis constant, $K_{m(i)}$.

Many drugs metabolized by the same metabolic enzymes behave as competitive inhibitors of one another. This is a particular problem for drugs oxidized by CYP enzymes because a few isozymes are responsible for metabolizing so many different drugs. Foods and endogenous substrates can also competitively inhibit the metabolism of drugs, because the same enzymes are often involved in their metabolic reactions.

Noncompetitive Inhibition

Compounds significantly different in structure from the substrate can also act as inhibitors. In this case, the inhibitor binds to the enzyme, not at the active site but at another *allosteric* site. This inhibitor–enzyme binding causes a change in conformation of the active site such that the substrate can no longer bind to it. This is called noncompetitive inhibition because the substrate cannot compete with and displace the inhibitor at any concentration. Noncompetitive inhibition can be reversible, in which inhibitor will dissociate from the enzyme, or irreversible, in which inhibitor will remain bound to the enzyme for the life of the enzyme molecule. Mathematically, the Michaelis–Menten equation for the rate of reaction of a substrate in the presence of a noncompetitive inhibitor is

$$V = \frac{V_{max}[C_p]}{([C_p] + K_m)(1 + [C_i]/K_{m(i)})}$$

(Eq. 10.11)

Consequences of Enzyme Inhibition.
Inhibitory effects usually occur soon after the inhibitor is administered. Inhibition of drug-metabolizing enzymes can be undesirable and even dangerous, because it will reduce drug clearance, raise plasma levels of drug, and keep the drug in the body longer than expected. Another factor that plays into the actual clinical consequence of enzyme inhibition is the contribution of that particular enzymatic reaction in the overall clearance of the drug. If the inhibited reaction is a major clearance pathway, the clinical consequence is substantial. On the other hand, if the drug is also cleared renally, and by other metabolic reactions, the clinical consequence may be small.

Inhibitors of a particular metabolic reaction may be classified as strong, moderate, or weak based on their influence on the overall elevation of plasma levels and decrease in total clearance of drug.

- *Strong inhibitor:* >5-fold increase in AUC or >80% decrease in clearance.
- *Moderate inhibitor:* >2-fold increase in AUC or 50% to 80% decrease in clearance.
- *Weak inhibitor:* >1.25-fold but <2-fold increase in AUC or 20% to 50% decrease in clearance.

AUC here refers to *area under the curve*, which is a measure of how much drug is in the systemic circulation. We will learn about AUC in the Chapter 11.

Some examples of drugs and other substances that are strong CYP inhibitors are listed in Table 10.3. Note that the extent to which an inhibitor affects the metabolism of a drug depends on the dose as well as the ability of the inhibitor to bind to the enzyme. For example, sertraline (Zoloft®) is a moderate inhibitor of CYP2D6 at a dose of 50 mg (and therefore not listed in Table 10.3), but if the dose is increased to 200 mg, it becomes a strong inhibitor.

Although inhibition of drug metabolism is generally a problem, it can sometimes be exploited to improve therapy. If a drug is prone to very rapid metabolism resulting in low plasma levels and a very short duration of action, metabolism can be intentionally slowed down by simultaneously administering an inhibitor of drug metabolism. For example, ritonavir (Norvir®), a strong CYP3A4 inhibitor, is added to lopinavir (Kaletra®) to boost plasma levels in patients with HIV.

The effect of enzyme inhibition on a prodrug (such as tramadol or losartan) will be exactly the opposite. If an enzyme inhibitor is administered with a prodrug, therapeutic failure is very likely because of little or no conversion to the active drug.

Enzyme Induction

Some enzymes have a unique characteristic; their ability to metabolize drugs can be increased or stimulated by substances called enzyme inducers. It is believed that inducers increase production rate of the enzyme, so more enzyme is available to catalyze the reaction.

One type of enzyme induction is *self-induction*, in which a drug stimulates its own metabolism. This is the body's way of adjusting to its environment. Continued dosing of a self-inducing drug results in progressively decreasing plasma levels and therapeutic activity. An example is carbamazepine (Tegretol®), a strong self-inducer; treatment must be initiated at a low dose and then increased at weekly intervals as its clearance gradually increases over time.

Since induction is related to an increase in enzyme synthesis, it may take 7–14 days to develop after giving the inducer. Additionally, the effect of enzyme induction can persist for several days after the inducer is discontinued. This is because the inducer may remain in the body for a while before it is completely eliminated, and because the excess enzyme needs

TABLE 10.3.	Examples of Strong Inhibitors and Inducers For CYP Enzymes	
Enzyme	*Inhibitors*	*Inducers*
CYP1A2	Ciprofloxacin (Cipro®) Fluvoxamine (Luvox®) Propafenone (Rythmol®)	Carbamazepine (Tegretol®) Rifampin (Rifadin®) Tobacco
CYP2C9	Amiodarone (Cordarone®) Fluoxetine (Prozac®) Metronidazole (Flagyl®)	Carbamazepine (Tegretol®) Phenytoin (Dilantin®) Rifampin (Rifadin®)
CYP2C19	Fluvoxamine (Luvox®) Omeprazole (Prilosec®) Ritonavir (Norvir®)	Carbamazepine (Tegretol®) Phenytoin (Dilantin®) Rifampin (Rifadin®)
CYP2D6	Fluoxetine (Prozac®) Paroxetine (Paxil®) Quinidine	No significant inducers
CYP3A4	Clarithromycin (Biaxin®) Itraconazole (Sporanox®) Ketoconazole (Nizoral®) Ritonavir (Norvir®) Telithromycin (Ketek®) Grapefruit juice	Carbamazepine (Tegretol®) Phenytoin (Dilantin®) Rifampin (Rifadin®) St. John's Wort

Brand names, if any, are in parenthesis.

to be decomposed through natural processes.

As with inhibition, the degree of induction also depends on the dose of the inducer.

Many drugs, pesticides, herbicides, and food components are self-inducers or induce the metabolism of other drugs; select examples are listed in Table 10.3.

Induction of enzymatic reactions that release an active metabolite from a prodrug may cause an exaggerated therapeutic effect or adverse effect.

Genetic Variability

Genetic factors contribute significantly to interindividual variability in drug metabolism. Genes and gene products reg-ulate all enzymes involved in drug metabolism. Evolutionary and environmental influences have resulted in significant variations in these genes throughout the population. Mutations in a gene can result in enzyme variants with higher, lower, or no activity compared with the norm, with higher or lower levels of enzymes, or with no enzyme at all in certain individuals. It is not unusual to find a 10-fold difference in rates of drug metabolism of the same drug among patients, solely related to genetic differences. More than 50% of patients carry genetic variations in *CYP1A2, 2C9, 2C19,* and *2D6* genes that can dramatically alter the patient's ability to metabolize the drug, and for which DNA testing can be ordered. Chapter 17 on Pharmacogenomics will examine genetic variability in all aspects of drug response.

Key Concepts

- Metabolism is a necessary first step before excretion of lipophilic drugs.
- Drug metabolism occurs primarily in the liver, but may occur in other tissues.
- Phase I reactions convert the drug into a suitable derivative for further conjugation in phase II reactions.
- Most drugs are metabolized by phase I oxidation by a select group of isozymes of the CYP450 superfamily.
- The rate of metabolism is governed by Michaelis–Menten kinetics, and metabolizing enzymes are subject to saturation, inhibition, and induction.

- Metabolites are usually more polar than the drug and suitable for excretion in the urine.
- Large molecular weight metabolites can be excreted in bile.
- Hepatic clearance is a component of total body clearance of a drug.
- Hepatic clearance depends on the extraction ratio of a drug, and liver blood flow.
- Orally administered drugs are subject to presystemic metabolism, reducing drug concentration in the systemic circulation.
- Enzyme inhibition and induction can cause significant changes in the plasma levels and clearance of a drug.

Review Questions

1. What physicochemical properties make drugs unsuitable for urinary excretion as unchanged drug? How does metabolism solve this problem?
2. Why are metabolites more likely to be excreted in bile than the parent drug?
3. Why are phase I reactions often necessary before a conjugation reaction can occur? What types of drugs do not require a phase I reaction to precede a phase II reaction?
4. Which is the most common type of phase I reaction? Why?
5. Which enzyme system is most important in drug metabolism? Why?
6. Under what conditions does Michaelis–Menten kinetics approximate a first-order process? A zero-order process? What happens to the rate of metabolism when metabolizing enzymes are saturated?
7. What is meant by hepatic extraction ratio and hepatic clearance?
8. Under what circumstances does first-pass metabolism occur? What is the consequence?
9. What are the other pathways of presystemic metabolism?
10. What is meant by inhibition of drug-metabolizing enzymes? How might this affect plasma concentrations and clearance of drugs?
11. What is meant by induction of drug-metabolizing enzymes? How might this affect plasma concentrations and clearance of drugs?
12. What are prodrugs? How is the therapeutic effect of a prodrug affected by enzyme inhibition and induction?

Practice Problems

1. A new drug was developed and found to be primarily eliminated by hepatic metabolism; i.e., the drug was not excreted in urine or secreted into bile. The K_m of the metabolic reaction is 2 mg/L and its V_{max} is 125 mg/d. Using the Michaelis–Menten equation, calculate the rate of metabolism when the plasma drug concentration [C_p] is as shown in the table below.

[C_p] mg/L	Rate of Metabolism (mg/d)
0.025	
0.050	
0.10	
0.20	
0.5	
1.0	
2.0	
4.0	
10	
20	
40	
60	

   Plot a graph with concentration on the X-axis and rate of metabolism on the Y-axis. Note how the reaction rate increases proportionately with plasma concentration at low concentrations (first-order kinetics), and then approaches saturation (V_{max}) at high concentrations.

2. A new drug (MW 215) is administered orally as a 150 mg tablet. During absorption, 75% of the dose dissolves and enters the intestinal epithelium. The drug undergoes some gut wall metabolism with a gut wall extraction ratio (ER_{gut}) = 0.22. It is also extracted in the liver with a hepatic extraction ratio (ER_h) = 0.75. The V_d of the drug = 0.6 L/kg and it is 85% plasma protein bound.

   a. Would you expect significant biliary secretion for this drug? Is the hepatic extraction ratio due to metabolism, biliary excretion or both? Would you say that the drug undergoes significant first-pass metabolism?

   b. When the 150 mg oral tablet is administered, calculate the number of milligrams that
   - enter the gut wall
   - enter the portal circulation
   - enter the systemic circulation

   c. About 25% of the oral dose is found in the feces. Explain why.

   d. If 150 mg of the drug were to be given intravenously, would you expect the number of milligrams reaching the systemic to be lower, higher, or the same as the number calculated in part b? Explain your rationale.

3. Mitoflomacin (MW = 331) is a new antibiotic given both orally and intravenously. After IV dosing, 88% of the dose is excreted in the urine (50% as

unchanged drug, and 38% as metabolites) and 12% is found in the feces (4% as unchanged drug and 8% as metabolites).

a. Explain the source of the drug found in feces.
b. Estimate the % of the IV dose eliminated by renal excretion, metabolism, and biliary excretion.
c. After oral administration, 70% of the oral dose is absorbed. How many milligrams of a 100 mg oral dose will be found in the feces and in the urine? Break this down as unchanged drug or metabolites.

CASE STUDY 10.1

Which Statin is Best For Me?

The "statins" are a family of drugs used to lower serum cholesterol as a means of reducing risk for cardiovascular disease. Their primary action is to inhibit HMG-CoA reductase, an enzyme required for cholesterol biosynthesis; statins bind to the active site of the enzyme, sterically preventing the substrate from binding. A significant percentage of the cholesterol in our body is synthesized by liver hepatocytes, and this is the site of action of statins.

We will compare two common statins (pravastatin and simvastatin) for this case; structures are shown below.

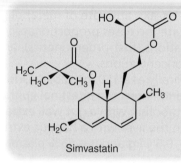

Simvastatin

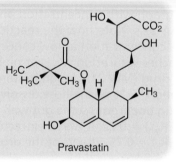

Pravastatin

The pharmacophore is the hydroxy acid group in the upper right hand of the structure. Pravastatin (Pravachol®) is administered in its active hydroxy acid form, while simvastatin (Zocor®) is a lactone prodrug that is enzymatically hydrolyzed in vivo to the active hydroxy acid form. The other properties of these statins are as shown in the following table.

	Simvastatin	Pravastatin
Molecular weight	419	447
pK_a	Nonelectrolyte	4.7
P_{app} (pH 7)	+++++ (High)	+ (Low)
% of oral dose absorbed	80%	34%
Bioavailability	4%	14%
Plasma protein binding	>95%	50%
Hepatic extraction ratio (ER_h)	0.95	0.60

Questions

1. Given the ionization behavior of the two drugs, explain why the apparent partition coefficient (P_{app}) at pH 7 is higher for pravastatin than for simvastatin.

2. Explain how the higher apparent partition coefficient of simvastatin at physiological pHs accounts for differences in its absorption, plasma protein binding, and hepatic extraction properties compared to pravastatin.

3. Based on the information in the table, suggest a reason why the bioavailability of these two drugs is significantly less than the % of drug absorbed after oral dosing. Calculate the expected bioavailability based on % absorbed and ER_h for both drugs. Are these numbers consistent with the observed bioavailability?

4. Even if the systemic bioavailability of statin drugs is low and hepatic extraction is high, they are still effective. Explain.

5. Simvastatin is a prodrug of its corresponding active hydroxy acid (simvastatin acid). Suggest a reason for developing a prodrug of simvastatin acid.

6. What type of metabolic reaction might convert the prodrug simvastatin into simvastatin acid? Indicate the site of conversion on the structure. Where in the body might the conversion from simvastatin to simvastatin acid occur? What types of enzymes are involved?

7. The elimination behavior of absorbed pravastatin and simvastatin is summarized below.

a. Hepatic extraction of drugs can be due to both hepatic metabolism and biliary secretion. Which process(es) are important for simvastatin? For pravastatin? Explain your reasoning.

b. Based on their physicochemical properties, explain why pravastatin is eliminated unchanged in the urine to some extent, but simvastatin is not.

8. Simvastatin and simvastatin acid both undergo extensive metabolism by CYP3A4, converting them to inactive metabolites. Simvastatin acid is also metabolized by CYP2C8.

a. What types of reactions are catalyzed by CYPs? Explain the difference between these reactions and the reaction that converts simvastatin to simvastatin acid.

b. Ritonavir (an HIV drug) and itraconazole (an antifungal drug) are strong CYP3A4 inhibitors. What does a "strong inhibitor" mean? How will concomitant use of these drugs affect the metabolism and elimination of pravastatin and simvastatin?

c. A major toxicity of most statins is myopathy (severe muscle weakness), seen when there is higher than expected concentration of a statin in the body. A patient with HIV has been taking ritonavir chronically. His recent blood test showed a high cholesterol level, so his physician wants to put him on a statin. Which of the two statins we have discussed would you recommend to minimize myopathy, and why?

	Simvastatin	Pravastatin
Hepatic extraction ratio (ER_h)	0.95	0.6
Elimination as unchanged drug	~0% (urine)	25% (urine)
	~0% (feces)	75% (feces)
Elimination as metabolites	16% (urine)	~0% (urine)
	84% (feces)	~0% (feces)

Additional Readings

Coleman M. Human Drug Metabolism: An Introduction. John Wiley and Sons, 2005.

Curry SH, Whelpton R. Drug Disposition and Pharmacokinetics: From Principles to Applications. Wiley Blackwell, 2011.

Gordon Gibson G, Skett P. Introduction to Drug Metabolism, 3rd ed. Stanley Thornes Pub Ltd, 2001.

Rowland M, Tozer TN. Clinical Pharmacokinetics and Pharmacodynamics: Concepts and Applications, 4th ed. Lippincott Williams & Wilkins, 2010.

CHAPTER 11

Pharmacokinetic Concepts

The aim of drug therapy is to achieve and maintain an optimal concentration of drug at the site of action. The drug concentration at the receptor depends on the dose administered, as well as its absorption, distribution, metabolism, and excretion (ADME) behavior. The drug can exert its action only when the desirable concentration is achieved. If the concentration is too low, there is no action; if it is too high, there may be other unwanted side effects. The duration of action of the drug will depend on how long the appropriate drug concentration is maintained at the receptor.

In practice, it is next to impossible to measure or know the drug concentration at the receptor in a patient. Instead, we monitor drug concentration in the plasma, which is relatively easy to measure from blood samples. The plasma concentration can then be used to inform us about the extent and duration of drug action. In this chapter, we will integrate ADME concepts from previous chapters to understand how plasma concentration of drug changes with time after dosing, and touch upon the relationship of plasma concentration to pharmacological effect.

Pharmacokinetics and Pharmacodynamics

The relationship between drug concentration at the receptor and the resulting pharmacological response is referred to as *pharmacodynamics (PD)*. We can view PD as a description what the drug does to the body, and the mechanism by which this occurs.

Pharmacokinetics (PK) describes what the body does to the drug. In other words, it is a quantitative description of the relationship of the dose, the concentration of drug in various body fluids, and time. PK helps us to understand the temporal (when) and spatial (where) distribution patterns of a drug in the body.

The PK and PD of a drug are often correlated (Fig. 11.1), helping us determine the dose and dosing frequency to get desired the therapeutic response with minimal side effects.

Drug Concentrations in Body Fluids

Drug concentrations in various tissues, including the site of action, depend on

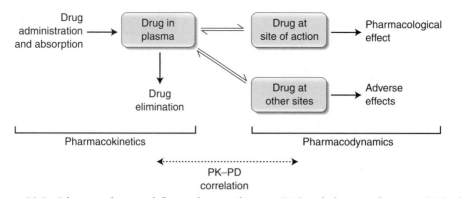

Figure 11.1. Schematic diagram defining pharmacokinetics (PK) and pharmacodynamics (PD) of a drug, and showing the concept of PK–PD correlation.

the relative *rates* of ADME processes after administration. Although we have discussed absorption, distribution, excretion, and metabolism pathways separately, it is important to remember that all these processes are proceeding simultaneously after drug administration. Absorption allows the drug to enter the bloodstream, while distribution from blood enables it to reach the receptor and other tissues. Simultaneously, metabolism and excretion processes remove the drug from the bloodstream. The net effect of these dynamic processes determines whether and for how long optimal drug concentration is achieved and maintained in the bloodstream and, therefore, at the receptor.

Drug Concentrations in Plasma

The easiest and most direct approach of obtaining PK information is by administering the drug and then measuring drug concentrations in the blood as a function of time. Drug concentration assays often use serum or plasma rather than whole blood. *Plasma* is the clear, yellowish fluid portion of blood in which blood cells are suspended. It differs from *serum* in that plasma contains fibrin and other soluble clotting substances that are absent in serum. When whole blood is allowed to clot, serum is the supernatant liquid after centrifugation; if an anticoagulant is added to the blood before centrifugation, plasma is the super-

natant. For all practical purposes, plasma concentrations and serum concentrations of a drug are identical. Blood concentrations may be higher because some drugs may enter blood cells.

Drug Concentrations in Tissues

Plasma perfuses all tissues and carries drug to various regions of the body. Drug in plasma can exist as either free drug or bound to plasma proteins. Partitioning into blood cells or binding to blood cells may also be quite significant for some drugs. Free (unbound) drug can readily leave capillaries in most tissues and equilibrate with interstitial fluid (ISF). If physicochemical properties allow, the drug can further distribute into intracellular fluid (ICF).

During early drug development, studies in animals may allow sampling of these body fluids to measure drug concentrations. Clearly, it is inconvenient and often impossible to take samples of these body fluids in humans. Therefore, we usually estimate tissue concentrations based on plasma concentration and on the drug's physicochemical properties.

The rate of drug distribution depends on tissue perfusion, as we learned in Chapter 8. Distribution of drug to well-perfused tissues (heart, liver, kidney, and brain) is rapid, and we assume that drug in plasma is in dynamic equilibrium with drug in the extracellular fluid (ECF) of these tissues at all times. This means that the concentrations of free drug in plasma and in the tissue ECF are equal. As plasma concentrations decline owing to elimination, tissue concentrations also decline.

Drug distribution to poorly perfused tissues (such as muscle and fat) is slower, and distribution equilibrium may not be reached for some time after drug administration. Tissue concentrations in poorly perfused regions will continue to increase for some time despite declining plasma concentrations. Once distribution equilibrium is reached, plasma and tissue concentrations of free drug can be considered equal, and will subsequently decline in a parallel manner.

Therefore, changes in drug plasma levels after distribution equilibrium reflect corresponding changes in drug tissue levels in the body. Plasma drug concentrations can be readily measured, giving us a convenient estimate of tissue drug levels and consequently of drug concentration at the receptor.

Pharmacokinetic Compartments

Drug disposition after absorption is the result of a complex set of dynamic processes that depend on the drug and the physiology of the patient. One objective of PK is to use plasma concentrations to develop simple mathematical models that describe drug disposition (distribution and elimination) after administration. For this purpose, the body is divided into a few (usually one to three) imaginary compartments that can be viewed as well-stirred, interconnected tanks. Drug is assumed to move between these compartments at defined rates. Tissues into which drug distributes at the same rate are grouped together in the same compartment.

A one-compartment model assumes that the body is composed of a single, homogeneous compartment (the *central compartment*) into which drug distributes rapidly and uniformly, e.g., a compartment consisting of plasma and well-perfused tissues. A two-compartment model divides the body into a central compartment as before, with a second *peripheral compartment* of poorly perfused tissues. After absorption, all drugs first distribute rapidly into the central compartment before distributing more slowly into peripheral compartments. Figure 11.2 shows a schematic diagram of one- and two-compartment models. If a drug distributes and equilibrates rapidly, primarily into well-perfused tissues, then the simple one-compartment model is usually sufficient to model its PK behavior. A more detailed discussion of compartmental PK is beyond the scope of this book.

Plasma Level Curves

The plasma level curve (also called a *plasma level vs. time curve* or a *blood level curve*)

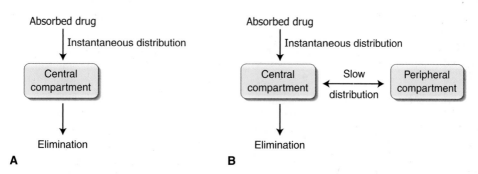

Figure 11.2. Schematic diagram of compartmental modeling. A. One-compartment model. B. Two-compartment model. Note that elimination occurs out of the central compartment.

is a graph showing drug concentration in plasma as a function of time after dosing. Data for this type of graph are obtained by administering a known dose of drug to an individual and taking blood samples at various times after administration. The concentration of drug (and sometimes metabolites) in the plasma samples is measured, and results are plotted with time of sampling on the X-axis and corresponding plasma concentration on the Y-axis. In most cases, the concentration measured is the *total* concentration of drug (free and bound) in plasma.

Pharmacokinetic Features of a Plasma Level Curve

Simply, plasma concentration is determined by two rate processes: the rate at which drug appears in plasma and the rate at which drug is eliminated from plasma. The shape of a plasma level curve depends on the route of administration and the rates of ADME processes for the drug. Figures 11.3 and 11.4 show typical plasma level curves after a single intravenous (IV) or oral dose of a drug, respectively. We will restrict our discussion to drugs that

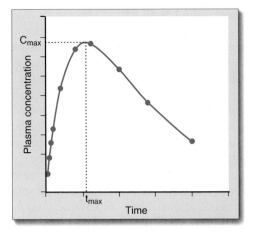

Figure 11.4. Typical plasma level curve after oral dosing of a drug product. The maximum plasma concentration (C_{max}) is reached at a time t_{max} after administration.

follow a one-compartment model, i.e., those that distribute rapidly into a single central compartment. This simple model is sufficient to describe the PK behavior of many drugs.

Rate and Extent of Absorption

The first step after systemic administration of a drug is absorption into the bloodstream. Consider a single dose of a drug given orally. After administration, the drug begins to be released from the oral dosage form, dissolving in gastrointestinal (GI) fluids. Dissolved drug can be absorbed from the small intestines, usually by passive transcellular diffusion. The absorption rate is a measure of how quickly the drug enters the bloodstream, while extent of absorption tells us about how much of the administered dose enters the bloodstream. One drug may be absorbed rapidly, but incompletely. Another drug may be absorbed slowly, but completely. Both rate and extent of absorption depend on the route, dosage form properties, and drug properties.

When a drug is administered intravenously (or rarely intra-arterially), the entire dose is placed in the bloodstream, so there is no absorption step. Thus, the

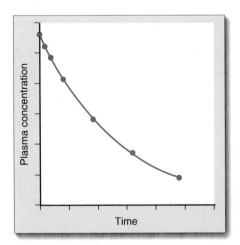

Figure 11.3. Typical plasma level curve after administration of an IV bolus dose. Note that the maximum plasma concentration occurs at time = 0, immediately after dosing.

rate of appearance of drug in plasma (input) depends on the rate of administration. When a drug is given by *IV bolus*, the entire dose is placed in the bloodstream at once, so input is instantaneous; plasma concentration reaches a maximum instantaneously. IV administration can also be an *infusion*, where the drug solution is slowly dripped into a vein; in this case, the input rate is the infusion rate. Plasma concentration rises gradually as drug is infused.

For all other systemic routes, the drug must be absorbed into the bloodstream, and this process may be slow and incomplete. The rate of appearance of drug in plasma (input) is determined by how quickly it is absorbed.

When drug products are given topically (non-systemically), absorption is not a necessary step for efficacy. However, some drug may still be absorbed into the circulation and distributed in the body. In fact, absorption often leads to unwanted side effects. The principles governing absorption from topical administration are the same as for systemic administration.

For drug products where the drug is already dissolved (e.g., drug solutions), rate and extent of absorption are controlled by the physicochemical properties of the drug (partition coefficient, pK_a, molecular size), and the permeability of the epithelial membrane. We learned these principles in Chapter 6.

For products in which the drug exists as a solid (tablets, suspensions, etc.), the drug must first dissolve at the site of absorption before it can be absorbed. Thus, rate and extend of absorption vary with dissolution rate, as we saw in Chapter 7. Dissolution rate of a drug depends on several factors such as particle size, crystallinity, and excipients. Thus, the same drug, in the same strength but in different formulations can give different rate and extent of absorption. In other words, absorption is characteristic of a particular *drug product* rather than a particular *drug*. This is a very important distinction.

Absorption Rate Constant

Absorption is generally a first-order process, a concept we learned in Chapter 6. Most drugs are absorbed by passive transcellular diffusion. The rate of absorption depends on the concentration gradient and the physicochemical properties of the drug, as well as on the permeability of the epithelial membrane at the absorption site. For a particular membrane, absorption rate is proportional to the concentration of dissolved, un-ionized drug available for absorption, and on the partition coefficient of the drug. Although the *absorption rate* varies with concentration, the absorption process can be characterized by a first-order absorption rate constant k_a, as follows:

$$\text{Absorption rate} = k_a \cdot C_a \quad \text{(Eq. 11.1)}$$

where C_a is the concentration of dissolved, un-ionized drug at the absorption site and k_a is the absorption rate constant. The value of k_a depends on many factors related to the specific epithelial membrane and the physicochemical properties of the drug.

Some drugs may be absorbed by carrier-mediated processes if appropriate transporters are present in the cell membranes of the epithelial cells at the absorption site. Absorption then is controlled by Michaelis–Menten kinetics, as we learned in Chapter 6. In such cases, the absorption rate is first order when dissolved drug concentrations are low

$$\text{Absorption rate} = \frac{V_{\max}}{K_m} C_a = k_a \times C_a$$

$$\text{(Eq. 11.2)}$$

but may approach zero order at higher doses if the transporters become saturated

$$\text{Absorption rate} = V_{\max} = \text{constant}$$

$$\text{(Eq. 11.3)}$$

Bioavailability

The extent of drug absorption from a product is characterized by a parameter called bioavailability, defined as the percentage (or fraction) of the administered dose that reaches the systemic circulation intact.

For IV administration, bioavailability is 100% because the entire dose is placed directly in the systemic circulation. For drug products administered by other routes, bioavailability may be less than 100%, implying that only a portion of the administered dose reaches the systemic circulation. This may be due to problems with the absorption process such as

- Incomplete dissolution of drug from the dosage form
- Insufficient time for absorption of all the drug
- Decomposition of the drug at site of administration or absorption
- Poor permeability of drug through epithelial tissue at the absorption site
- Efflux from epithelia cells at absorption site.

Drugs that dissolve rapidly from their dosage forms and have good permeability across absorption epithelia tend to be almost completely absorbed. Low bioavailability is most common with products of poorly water-soluble, low-permeability drugs. Poor permeability could be related to a low partition coefficient, an unsuitable pK_a, or large molecular size.

Incomplete or slow dissolution of a drug from a poorly designed dosage form will prevent a portion of the drug from being available for absorption. In such situations, the dosage form could be altered to increase dissolution rate, which could increase both absorption rate and bioavailability.

Insufficient time for absorption contributes to low bioavailability of some drugs. For example, orally administered drugs are exposed to the GI tract for about 24 to 48 hours at most, and to the small intestine for about 4 hours. If the drug dissolves slowly or has poor permeability across the intestinal epithelium, this length of time at the absorption site may be insufficient. In such cases, bioavailability tends to be low as well as highly variable.

If poor drug absorption is due to very poor permeability or efflux, alterations in the dosage form cannot improve absorption; the drug may have to be dosed by a different route, or converted into a prodrug.

A drug may be unstable and decompose at the absorption site, reducing the amount of intact drug available for absorption. For example, drugs can hydrolyze at the acidic pH of the stomach or be metabolized by digestive enzymes or intestinal bacteria. Some of the dissolved drug in the GI tract may be unavailable for absorption because of binding or complexation with food or other substances in the GI tract. In some of these cases, the dosage form can be modified to minimize this problem (e.g., enteric coating of acid-labile drugs).

Even if a drug is completely absorbed after oral administration, other factors may reduce bioavailability, such as

- Presystemic metabolism
- Physiological problems pertaining to the patient
- Interaction of the drug with food or with another drug.

Presystemic metabolism was discussed in detail in Chapter 10. Many epithelial tissues at absorption sites contain enzymes that can metabolize drugs before they enter the systemic circulation. Each route of administration has its own level of presystemic loss of drug. In particular, gut wall metabolism and hepatic first pass effect are notorious for reducing bioavailability of oral drug products. Other absorption sites where a drug may be partially metabolized are the lung and nose.

The patient's health may influence absorptive ability of many tissues. Finally, food and drug interactions may also reduce the amount of a given drug that is absorbed.

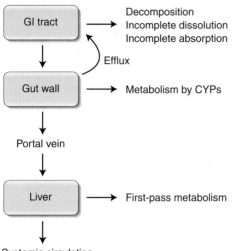

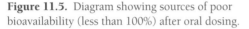

Figure 11.5. Diagram showing sources of poor bioavailability (less than 100%) after oral dosing.

Thus, the overall bioavailability of a drug from a product depends on a complex set of parameters including properties of the drug, route, dosage form, and patient.

Sources of poor bioavailability after oral administration are summarized in Figure 11.5.

C_{max} and t_{max}

When drug begins to enter the circulation during absorption, plasma concentration increases. As absorption continues, plasma concentration keeps increasing until it reaches a maximum designated as C_{max}. The length of time taken to reach C_{max} is called t_{max}. These two parameters provide a rough measure of the absorption rate of the drug from the drug product. C_{max} is high and t_{max} is short when the drug is absorbed rapidly.

As soon as drug enters the bloodstream, it is distributed quickly to the central compartment and starts being eliminated from plasma by metabolism and excretion. (If one or more peripheral compartments exist, there is further slower distribution into these tissues.) Absorption causes plasma concentration of drug to increase, whereas elimination causes it to

decrease. Elimination is also a first-order process, so elimination rate increases as plasma concentration increases.

The maximum plasma concentration C_{max} is reached when the rate of elimination becomes equal to the rate of absorption. Absorption predominates before t_{max} when there is a large concentration gradient driving absorption. As drug concentration at the absorption site declines, absorption rate decreases, and eventually becomes zero when all available drug has been absorbed. After this time, elimination processes alone control plasma concentration of drug.

If drug is administered as an IV *bolus* (the dose is given all at once), the entire dose enters plasma almost instantaneously, and there is no detectable absorption phase. The maximum plasma concentration is attained almost immediately after administration (at time zero), and plasma concentration then declines as elimination processes begin.

Rate of Distribution

Once a drug enters the bloodstream, its behavior is controlled solely by its physicochemical properties and not by the drug product formulation. Distribution equilibrium of one-compartment drugs is achieved immediately after the drug enters the bloodstream. The large cardiac output moves blood rapidly throughout the body so that distribution to well-perfused tissues is complete almost as soon as drug is absorbed. For example, the initial plasma concentration after an IV bolus dose reflects the drug concentration after distribution equilibrium has been reached. As discussed in Chapter 8, the volume of distribution, V_d, of a drug is given by

$$V_d = \frac{X}{C_{p(0)}} \qquad \text{(Eq. 11.4)}$$

where X is the IV bolus dose of drug in milligrams and $C_{p(0)}$ is the initial (and also the maximum) plasma concentration.

Equation 11.4 can be rearranged to give an expression for initial plasma concentration

$$C_{p(0)} = \frac{X}{V_d} \qquad \text{(Eq. 11.5)}$$

Equation 11.5 shows that the initial plasma concentration after IV bolus dosing of a one-compartment drug depends on the dose administered and volume of distribution of the drug; the higher the volume of distribution, the lower the initial plasma concentration. The subsequent decline in concentration is related to elimination processes only.

Distribution equilibrium is reached more slowly for drugs that distribute further to poorly perfused tissues in peripheral compartments. For such multi-compartment drugs, the decline in plasma concentration after a single IV dose reflects both distribution and elimination processes.

Rate of Elimination

How fast a drug is eliminated from the body depends on how efficiently the body can remove the drug from plasma (as measured by its clearance), and how much of the drug is in plasma and available to the clearing organ (as measured by its volume of distribution). A large V_d means a lot of the drug is in extravascular space, and less is in plasma. Drug in the tissues is "protected" from hepatic and renal elimination. It follows that the rate of drug elimination is also dependent on V_d. The elimination rate constant also depends on the efficiency of excretion and metabolism, i.e., on the total clearance (CL_{tot}) of drug by these processes.

Kinetics of Elimination

Elimination begins immediately after drug enters the blood, distributes, and rapidly reaches the highly perfused eliminating organs (liver and kidney). The drug may be excreted in its unchanged form in urine or other body fluids, and/or metabolized

by enzymatic reactions. Both processes reduce plasma concentration of the drug, and the rate of elimination is defined as the decline in plasma drug concentration over time. As drug is eliminated from plasma, drug from tissues redistributes back into plasma to maintain concentration equilibrium. These processes continue until drug is eventually completely eliminated from tissues as well as plasma.

Excretion is generally a first-order processes (with a few exceptions) in that the rate is proportional to plasma concentration for a particular drug. For example, in renal excretion, glomerular filtration and secretion increase as plasma drug concentration rises, while reabsorption decreases. Thus the overall rate of excretion increases as plasma concentration rises. Exceptions occur for drugs that are extensively secreted, and if the tubular transporters involved in secretion get saturated.

Metabolism is controlled by Michaelis–Menten kinetics, which can be approximated as a first-order process at the typical therapeutic concentrations of most drugs (generally much lower than the K_m). However, there are a few drugs where metabolic enzymes become saturated at drug high doses, and we see zero-order kinetics.

For most drugs, the overall rate of elimination is also first-order. When plasma concentrations are high, more drug is removed from plasma; when concentrations decline, the rate declines. However, for a given drug, the *fraction* (or percentage) eliminated per unit time remains a constant regardless of plasma drug concentration.

Elimination Rate Constant

Thus, as elimination (excretion and metabolism) begins, plasma concentration decreases in a first-order manner; the concentration at any time after dosing is given by

$$C_t = C_0 e^{-k_e t} \qquad \text{(Eq. 11.6)}$$

where C_t is plasma concentration at time t after dosing, and k_e is the first-order elimination rate constant for the drug, with units of *time*$^{-1}$. The elimination rate constant k_e can be viewed as the fractional decrease in plasma concentration in a given time interval. For example, $k_e = 0.05$ hr^{-1} means that plasma concentration decreases by 5% of its value every hour.

The elimination rate constant k_e is a useful mathematical parameter to describe drug elimination. Let us now examine the factors that determine the value of k_e and its relationship to the volume of distribution and clearance of a drug.

We know that CL_{tot} of a drug is given by

$$CL_{tot} = CL_r + CL_m + CL_b + CL_{other}$$

$$(Eq.\ 11.7)$$

A high total clearance means that the drug is capable of being eliminated rapidly. However, the rate of elimination is also proportional to plasma drug concentration, which in turn is related to the volume of distribution of the drug. A large volume of distribution will slow down elimination, because less of the drug is in plasma and passing through the liver and kidneys.

Thus, the elimination rate constant is related to volume of distribution and total clearance by the following expression:

$$k_e = \frac{CL_{tot}}{V_d} \qquad (Eq.\ 11.8)$$

CL and V_d of a drug do not change with dose, route of administration, or formulation characteristics. They are the two fundamental PK parameters of a drug. These parameters may change somewhat from patient to patient due to interindividual variability in physiological processes. They may change substantially in patients with liver, kidney disease, or cardiovascular disease, or with body weight and hydration.

Half-Life

Elimination of drug from the bloodstream is often characterized by a secondary parameter called half-life ($t_{1/2}$ or $t_{0.5}$), defined as the time required for plasma drug concentration to decrease by one half of its value. Half-life is given by the expression

$$t_{1/2} = \frac{0.693}{k_e} \qquad (Eq.\ 11.9)$$

Thus, k_e and $t_{1/2}$ give us the same information, and one can be readily calculated if the other is known. A drug that is rapidly eliminated will have a short $t_{1/2}$, whereas one that is slowly eliminated will have a long $t_{1/2}$. Like the elimination rate constant, plasma half-life of a drug is a fundamental property of the drug and does not usually change with dose, formulation, or route of administration.

Half-life is an easier concept to grasp and is often used instead of k_e to characterize drug elimination. Table 11.1 shows the remaining plasma concentration of a drug after one to five half-lives. Once five half-lives have elapsed after dosing, only about 3% of the absorbed dose, as intact drug, remains in the body. This means that 97% of the drug has been excreted and/or metabolized. In practice, clinicians usually assume that practically all the drug is eliminated from the body after five half-lives have elapsed. Note that this is true regardless of the drug, its elimination rate constant, or the dose. If the half-life of a drug is long (e.g., 2 days), it will take a

TABLE 11.1. Percentage of the Initial Plasma Concentration Remaining After IV Bolus Dosing of a Drug	
Number of Half-Lives Elapsed	*% Drug Remaining in Plasma*
0	100.00
1	50.00
2	25.00
3	12.50
4	6.25
5	3.13
6	1.56

The initial plasma concentration is designated as 100%.

long time (~10 days) to completely eliminate an administered dose. If the half-life of a drug is shorter (e.g., 5 hours), it will take a short time (~1 day) to completely eliminate an administered dose.

Area Under the Curve

The relative rates of ADME processes are usually in the order: distribution > absorption > elimination. Distribution is almost instantaneous for one-compartment drugs. Absorption is slower, but still usually much faster than elimination; otherwise, drug would be eliminated before it has a chance to achieve therapeutic concentrations.

The area under the curve (AUC) is a measure of the total amount of drug that enters the body after administration. It is the actual area calculated from a plasma concentration–time curve, as shown in Figure 11.6. The units of AUC are concentration × time (e.g., mg hr L^{-1}).

AUC depends on the amount of the administered dose that reaches the systemic circulation (X), and the rate of drug removal from the body (given by CL_{tot}) as shown in the following equation:

$$AUC = \frac{X}{CL_{tot}} \qquad (Eq.\ 11.10)$$

If a higher dose, X, of a drug is administered, plasma concentrations and, consequently, AUC, rise. AUC also depends on total clearance; a drug that is cleared rapidly will give low plasma concentrations and thus have a small AUC.

If the drug is administered intravenously, the entire dose enters the systemic circulation, and X in Eqn. 11.10 is equal to the administered dose. When the drug is given orally, or by some other route, the amount of drug that actually enters the systemic circulation is often less than the dose administered. Consequently, IV dosing gives the maximum AUC possible for a given dose of a particular drug. If the same dose is given orally, the AUC may be less because of incomplete dissolution, incomplete absorption, or presystemic metabolism, as discussed earlier.

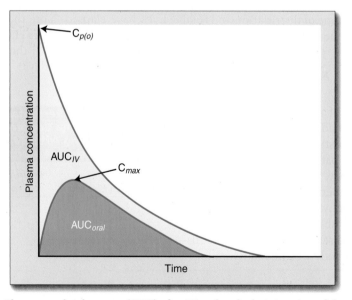

Figure 11.6. The area under the curve (AUC) after IV and oral administration of the same dose of a drug; shaded regions show the AUC for each. Note that the AUC and maximum plasma concentration are much higher with IV dosing than with oral dosing.

AUC can also be calculated as the area under the drug plasma concentration–time curve by integrating Eqn. 11.6 from $t = 0$ to $t = \infty$:

$$AUC = \int_0^\infty C_t dt \qquad \text{(Eq. 11.11)}$$

Absolute Bioavailability

The bioavailability of a drug product is generally measured by comparing the AUC after administering the product, with the AUC obtained after giving the *same dose* intravenously. Because we are comparing the drug product to IV dosing, this type of measurement is often called the absolute bioavailability of the drug product.

For example, the fractional absolute bioavailability of an oral product is given by the following equation:

$$F = \frac{AUC_{oral}}{AUC_{iv}} \qquad \text{(Eq. 11.12)}$$

where AUC_{oral} and AUC_{iv} are the areas under the curve after oral and IV administration of the same dose, respectively. Absolute bioavailability is often represented as a percentage

$$F = \frac{AUC_{oral}}{AUC_{iv}} \times 100 \qquad \text{(Eq. 11.13)}$$

Formulation or toxicity considerations often make it impractical or inappropriate to give the same dose of drug orally and IV; usually, a smaller dose is used for IV administration. In this situation, Eqn. 11.13 must be modified to account for the difference in doses to

$$F = \frac{AUC_{oral}}{AUC_{iv}} \times \frac{dose_{iv}}{dose_{oral}} \qquad \text{(Eq. 11.14)}$$

As stated before, F is equal to 1 or 100% for IV administration. For all other routes, F is less than or equal to 100% for reasons we have discussed earlier.

Effect of Route and Delivery System

The route of administration and formulation influence the shape of the plasma level curve. We have already noted the differences between plasma level curves obtained after oral and IV administration. Plasma level curves will be altered when the same dose of drug is given via different routes primarily because of differences in the absorption process.

Figure 11.7 illustrates the influence of formulation design on plasma level curves for two tablet formulations, A and B, containing the same dose of the same drug. The C_{max} and t_{max} values are different for the two formulations, presumably because the drug dissolves faster from product A than from B, resulting in a faster absorption rate for A. The AUCs of these two formulations are different as well, indicating that the bioavailability of the drug is lower from product B than product A.

Relationship Between Pharmacokinetics and Pharmacodynamics

One goal of pharmacokinetic analysis of a drug is to help understand the clinical effects of the drug in patients. An assumption made in PK analysis is that tissue drug concentrations (including concentration at the receptor) are directly related to plasma concentrations; consequently, pharmacological effect and side effects can often be correlated to plasma concentration of drug. If such a correlation between PK and PD exists, it can help to understand drug action and drug safety, and to establish an optimal dose and dosing schedule for the drug. The relationship between PK and PD is illustrated in Figure 11.8.

For drugs that are intended to work locally (nonsystemically), it is the local concentration at or near the site of administration rather than the plasma concentration

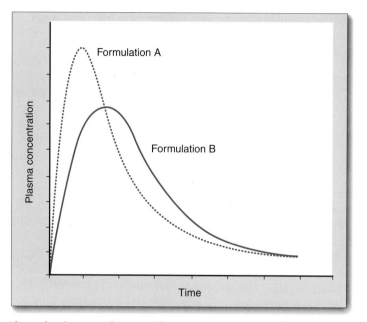

Figure 11.7. Plasma level curves of two oral formulations containing the same dose of a drug. Note that the maximal concentration (C_{max}) and time to reach maximal concentration (t_{max}) of the two curves are different. The AUC values of the two curves may also be different.

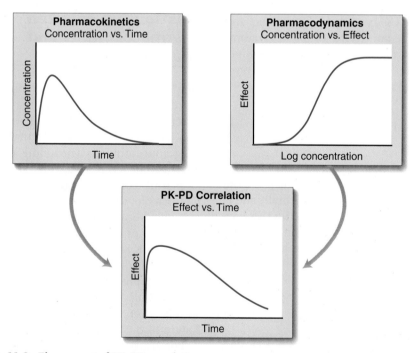

Figure 11.8. The concept of PK–PD correlation.

that controls efficacy. In such cases, plasma concentrations will not be correlated with efficacy. However, some of the drug could still be absorbed into the bloodstream, and distributed and eliminated by the same principles governing systemic drugs. Plasma concentrations of nonsystemic drugs are still important to monitor, because they are often correlated with side effects due to the drug reaching unintended tissues.

Pharmacological Features of a Plasma Level Curve

If there is a PK–PD correlation, plasma concentrations of a systemically acting drug can be related to certain pharmacodynamic parameters, and therefore to the clinical effectiveness of the drug. After administering various doses of a drug, plasma concentrations are measured, and drug action and side effects are monitored simultaneously. A graph is then constructed to show the relationship, if any, between concentration and pharmacological action. Figure 11.9 is a typical oral plasma concentration–time curve, showing how plasma concentration can be related to therapeutic response and side effects.

The minimum effective concentration (MEC) is the lowest plasma concentration at which the drug's therapeutic effect is observed. Concentrations below this are usually ineffective. The maximum safe concentration (MSC), also known as the *minimum toxic concentration (MTC)*, is the plasma concentration above which side effects and toxicity are seen.

After administration of a single dose of a drug product, therapeutic effect is first seen when plasma concentration reaches the drug's MEC; this is the time required for onset of action. Therapeutic effectiveness lasts as long as plasma concentration remains above MEC; this length of time is the duration of action of the drug product. The intensity of effect often depends on how high the plasma concentration reaches above MEC.

Plasma levels will depend on the dose of drug given. A larger dose will shift the curve higher, giving a higher C_{max} and greater intensity of effect. If the C_{max}

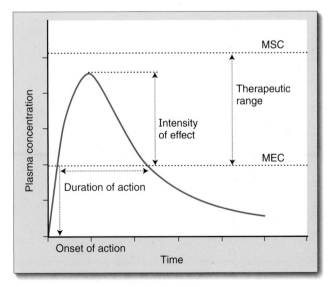

Figure 11.9. Plasma level curve after oral administration showing typical pharmacological features. Onset of action occurs when the plasma level reaches the minimum effective concentration (MEC). The duration of action is the time period for which the plasma level is at or above the MEC. The intensity of effect depends on how high the maximal concentration (C_{max}) is above the MEC. The plasma levels should remain below the maximum safe concentration (MSC) to minimize adverse reactions.

exceeds the MSC, a higher incidence of side effects will also be seen.

The aim of drug therapy is to maintain plasma concentration in the range between MEC and MSC as long as necessary; this range of concentrations is known as the therapeutic range or therapeutic window of a drug. The standard dose of the drug is designed to give concentrations in the therapeutic range. The wider the therapeutic range, the safer the drug; in other words, doses or plasma levels have to be much higher than standard values to cause side effects.

Multiple Dosing

We have examined the features of plasma level curves after a single dose. Most clinical applications require achieving and maintaining a therapeutic drug concentration over a long time, and therefore require multiple dosing. An initial effective concentration can be reached with the appropriate dose; maintaining the concentration in the therapeutic range for an extended period is a challenge. A thorough knowledge of the PK of a drug allows scientists and clinicians to design appropriate multiple-dosing regimens, where both the dose and the dosing frequency are tailored to maintain effective but nontoxic drug concentrations for an extended time. The goal is to administer drug at the same rate that it is eliminated from the body so that a fairly consistent plasma concentration in the therapeutic range is achieved.

In a multiple-dosing regimen, each successive dose is administered before the preceding dose is completely eliminated. The result is accumulation of the drug in the body, yielding a higher maximum plasma drug concentration (C_{max}) with each dose. This accumulation phenomenon, however, does not cause the plasma concentration to rise indefinitely. The C_{max} eventually reaches a consistent value, as does the minimum plasma concentration, C_{min}. In PK language, the drug has reached steady state, giving the same C_{max} and C_{min} after each dose (Fig. 11.10). A detailed discussion of multiple dosing is outside the scope of this book.

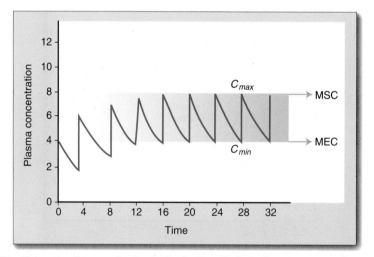

Figure 11.10. Plasma level curve after multiple dosing of a drug showing accumulation of drug and the approach to steady state. In this example, the same dose of drug is given by IV bolus at 4-hour dosing intervals. For the first five doses, there is an accumulation of drug with each dose, seen by the progressive increase in maximum concentration (C_{max}) and minimum concentration (C_{min}). After reaching steady state at the fifth dose (16 hours), C_{max} and C_{min} remain consistent with subsequent dosing, within the therapeutic range of the drug.

Key Concepts

- Compartmental PK modeling is used to quantitatively describe the disposition and time course of a drug in the body.
- The shape of a plasma level curve depends on the relative rates of absorption, distribution, and elimination of the drug.
- Absorption rate and bioavailability of a drug product depends on the route, dosage form properties, physicochemical and PK properties of the drug, permeability of the absorption membrane, and the physiology of the patient.
- The elimination rate constant and half-life of a drug can be calculated from a drug's fundamental PK parameters, V_d and CL.
- For drugs that work systemically, the efficacy and toxicity of the drug are usually related to plasma concentration. A minimum plasma concentration is necessary for efficacy, and too high a plasma concentration can cause toxicity.
- Drugs that have a wide therapeutic range are safer than those with a narrow range.
- The goal of drug therapy is to maintain plasma concentration in the therapeutic range for the desired time, usually by multiple dosing of drug.

Review Questions

1. What is a pharmacokinetic compartmental model? What are the differences between a one- and two-compartment model?
2. What do the parameters C_{max}, t_{max}, k_e, $t_{1/2}$, and AUC tell you about a drug product? Which of these are independent of the dose and the route of administration? Which depend on the dosage form and route?
3. What does the absorption rate of a drug from a product depend on?
4. What is meant by the absolute bioavailability of a drug? Why is the absolute bioavailability after IV administration equal to 100%?
5. How is the bioavailability of a drug product determined?
6. What are the reasons for less than 100% bioavailability of a drug after oral administration? How can an oral drug that is completely absorbed still have a bioavailability of less than 100%?
7. Why is it important to measure plasma concentrations of a drug? How are these concentrations related to the efficacy and toxicity of a drug?
8. What is the therapeutic range of a drug? Why is it important to maintain plasma concentrations in the therapeutic range?
9. What is PK–PD correlation? How does it help to plan the dose and dosing frequency of a drug?

Practice Problems

1. An antibiotic has a volume of distribution = 35 L and total clearance = 65 mL/min. What is its elimination rate constant? Its half-life? Calculate in units of hours and days.

2. In the average patient, Drug X has a volume of distribution = 40 L and $t_{1/2}$ = 8.7 hr.
   a. What is the total clearance of Drug X?
   b. How long will it take for all (>97%) of the drug to be eliminated from the body after administration? Does this depend on the dose administered?
   c. In a patient who has liver disease, the total clearance was reduced to 30 mL/min. Estimate the half-life of drug X in this patient. How many hours will it take for all (>97%) of the drug to be eliminated from the body after administration to this patient? Assume no change in V_d.
   d. In an obese patient with normal liver and kidney function, the volume of distribution of drug X is found to increase to 60 L, but there is no significant change in total clearance compared to the average patient. Estimate $t_{1/2}$ of drug X in this obese patient. Explain why the half-life changed in the direction it did.
   e. How long will it take for all (>97%) of the drug to be eliminated after administration of drug X to the obese patient?
   f. If plasma concentrations of drug X are related to therapeutic efficacy (PK–PD correlation exists), how might the dosing have to be adjusted in the obese individual to achieve adequate efficacy?
3. A 300 mg oral dose of a drug gave an AUC = 750 mg hr/L. A 100 mg IV dose of the same drug gave an AUC = 375 mg hr/L. What is the bioavailability of the drug from the oral product? Express as a fraction and a percentage.
4. After oral dosing, 80% of a drug from an oral tablet is absorbed. ER_{gut} = 0.2 and $ER_{hepatic}$ = 0.3. Estimate the oral bioavailability of this drug from this product as a fraction and a percentage. Assume no biliary secretion.

CASE STUDY 11.1

Heartburn no more..

Histamine is an endogenous agonist found throughout body and plays a key role in regulating many physiological processes. It binds to histamine receptors, of which there are four subtypes: H_1, H_2, H_3, and H_4. In the stomach, histamine stimulates gastric acid production by interacting with the H_2-receptors of the parietal cells. H_2-receptor antagonist drugs reduce the volume and acidity of gastric fluids by blocking the H_2-receptors. Cimetidine (Tagamet®) is a competitive histamine H_2-receptor antagonist. It is used to treat heartburn, duodenal ulcers, and gastroesophageal reflux disease (GERD).

The structure of cimetidine is

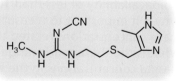

It is a weak base with a pK_a = 6.8. The typical PK parameters of cimetidine are as follows:

V_d (L/kg)	1.2
f_u	0.8
CL_{tot} (mL/min/kg)	7.1

Cimetidine is available for oral and IV administration and works effectively by both routes. A comparison of IV and oral dosing gave the following results in a group of patients:

	Cimetidine IV (300 mg)	Cimetidine Oral Tablet (400 mg)
AUC (μg hr mL^{-1})	11.3	9.1
C_{max} (μg/mL)	11.2	2.2
t_{max} (min)	60	~1

Questions

1. What are the k_e and the half-life of cimetidine?
2. How long will it take to completely eliminate an IV bolus dose after administration? What about an oral tablet dose?
3. Calculate the absolute bioavailability of the oral tablet.
4. About 20% of the oral dose was found in the feces after an oral dose of cimetidine. No degradation products or metabolites of cimetidine were found in feces. In view of this, what are the likely reasons for the <100% oral bioavailability of cimetidine?
5. Cimetidine is excreted in urine (primary pathway) and metabolized in the liver (secondary pathway). On IV dosing, 75% of the drug is excreted in urine as the parent compound and 25% is excreted in urine as metabolites. On oral dosing, 20% of the drug is found in feces, 36% is found in the urine unchanged, and 44% in urine as metabolites. Suggest why there is more metabolism after an oral dose than after an IV dose. Are the numbers consistent after you take into account the oral bioavailability?
6. Cimetidine reduces gastric acid secretion by competing with histamine in binding to H_2-receptors in the parietal cells of the stomach, which are located on the basal side of the parietal cells. The MEC of cimetidine is 0.7 μg/mL.
    a. What is meant by the MEC? Does this tell you whether the drug exerts its action systemically or locally?
    b. Look up a diagram of gastric parietal cells and note the location of the histamine receptor. Use this to explain how cimetidine works when given IV.
    c. After oral dosing, cimetidine's onset of action is 30 minutes after dosing and peak effects occur about 1 hour after administration. Explain why it takes 30 minutes before any therapeutic effect is seen, and why the peak effect occurs after 1 hour.
    d. A patient suffers from frequent heartburn right after breakfast each morning, and has been taking cimetidine during breakfast with little relief. How might you advise him to change his cimetidine dosing to get better relief? Explain your rationale.
7. Cimetidine is a very safe drug, which is one of the reasons why it is available over-the-counter without a prescription. What can you say about the MSC of cimetidine relative to the MEC?

Additional Readings

Dipiro JT, Spruill WJ, Wade WE, Blouin RA, Pruemer JM. Concepts in Clinical Pharmacokinetics, 5th ed. American Hospital Association, 2010.

Jambhekar S, Breen PJ. Basic Pharmacokinetics, 1st ed. Pharmaceutical Press, 2009.

Shargel L, Wu-Pong S, Yu ABC. Applied Biopharmaceutics and Pharmacokinetics, 5th ed. McGraw-Hill Medical, 2004.

Tozer TN, Rowland M. Introduction to Pharmacokinetics and Pharmacodynamics: The Quantitative Basis of Drug Therapy. Lippincott Williams & Wilkins, 2006.

PART IV

Drug Action

All substances are poisonous, there is none which is not a poison; the right dose differentiates a poison from a remedy
—Paracelsus

Chapter 12 Ligands and Receptors

Chapter 13 Mechanisms of Drug Action

Chapter 14 Dose–Response Relationships

Ligands and Receptors

The human body is made up of approximately 10^{13} cells. Each of these cells is capable of responding to an external signal and carrying out a specific function. Some of these functions may require a rapid response to an event or stimulus. Other functions and responses may require changes and adaptations over long periods of time. The ability of the many and diverse cells to function in a coordinated and timely fashion requires a sophisticated form of signaling or communication. The major signaling system between cells and organ systems involves ligands and receptors. Ligands, as discussed briefly in Chapter 2, are chemicals released by cells that interact with receptors. Receptors are typically large macromolecules or proteins located within or on a cell and have a specific site capable of binding the ligand in a stereocomplementarity fashion. This ligand–receptor complex, in turn, initiates a process within the cell to produce a biological response. This chapter discusses in more detail the different types of endogenous ligands and receptor systems that are present and how a biological response occurs following an interaction between a ligand and its receptor.

The Signaling Process

Cell signaling is the process by which cells release, transmit, receive, and respond to information from their environment. This information is carried by endogenous ligands (also called *cell mediators* or *signaling molecules*) made and released by cells as needed. Human cells can also detect and respond to external signals such as drugs, bacteria, viruses, and toxins.

There are three main players involved in the signaling process: the signaling cell, the ligand, and the recipient of the signal, the receptor. The term *signaling cell* refers to the cell that synthesizes and releases the ligand. The synthesis and release of a ligand is often itself the result of a ligand–receptor interaction. The binding of the released ligand to a complementary receptor initiates a cascade of biochemical reactions within the cell that ultimately results in a biological response.

The overall behavior or response of a cell depends on the signals it receives and the genetic programming of that cell. A cell may respond to one set of signals by multiplying, to another set of signals by carrying out a biochemical reaction, and to yet another set by differentiating. In addition, different types of cells require different sets of signals to carry out a process, and the same ligand often has different effects on different cell types. For example, the neurotransmitter norepinephrine can act on both blood vessels found in skeletal muscles and on cholinergic neurons, a specific type of nerve cell found in the brain. When acting on the cholinergic neuron, norepinephrine prevents the neuron from releasing its own neurotransmitter and, when acting on a blood vessel, norepinephrine will cause the blood vessel to constrict. The same ligand, in this case norepinephrine, can produce very different responses in cells based on the genetic programming of the cell. In contrast, similar functions in different cell types may require different ligands. Brain-derived neurotrophic factor (BDNF) is the ligand that promotes growth and survival of cholinergic neurons while certain blood vessels require a different ligand called vascular endothelial growth factor (VEGF) for growth and survival.

Many drugs act by competing with or taking the place of endogenous ligands or by modifying the signaling pathway in some manner. In this way, a drug can make a quantitative change in an existing physiological or biochemical process; however, most drugs do not qualitatively alter the nature of the process. That is, drugs may increase or decrease a process that is already occurring but cannot direct the cell to create a new or different process. Understanding cell signaling is important in understanding drug effects and enables scientists to design more effective drugs and identify new targets for drug action.

The major steps in the signaling process can be described as follows:

1. Signaling cells synthesize the appropriate ligand, usually based on a signal they themselves receive.
2. The signaling cells release ligand molecules, usually into the extracellular fluid.

3. Ligand molecules are transported to target cells in a variety of ways, as we will see shortly. Depending on its physicochemical properties, the ligand may remain in the extracellular fluid or enter the target cell.
4. Appropriate receptors at the target cells recognize and bind to the ligands with specificity, forming a complex. Receptors may be located either inside the target cells (intracellular receptors) or on the cell membrane (cell-surface receptors).
5. The ligand–receptor complex transforms the signal into an intracellular message and triggers a biological response in target cells.
6. The ligand is removed, terminating the response.

Endogenous Ligands

A simple or commonly accepted classification system for ligands does not exist. The number of ligands and their diversity in structure and action are so great that a single classification would be either quite complicated or incomplete. Presented below are three different classification systems based on chemical, biochemical, and anatomical perspectives.

Classification of Ligands

First, it is possible to classify endogenous ligands based on the chemistry and structure of the ligand; some ligands are small molecules whereas others are peptides and proteins; some are charged in the physiological pH range whereas others are uncharged; some are hydrophobic whereas others are polar. This classification is helpful when focusing on the physicochemical features of a molecule necessary for ligand–receptor interactions.

A second classification or perspective can be based on the site of the receptor upon which the ligand interacts. The receptor may be either an extracellular, membrane bound receptor, or an intracellular

TABLE 12.1. Examples of Various Types of Ligands Grouped by Their Hydrophilicity and Hydrophobicity[a]		
Hydrophilic Ligands (Cell-Surface Receptors)	**Hydrophobic Ligands (Intracellular Receptors)**	**Hydrophobic Ligands (Cell-Surface Receptors)**
Small molecule hormones	Steroid hormones	Arachidonic acid derivatives
Peptide hormones	Retinoids	Prostaglandins
Neurotransmitters	Thyroxins	Leukotrienes
Growth factors	Vitamin D	Platelet activating factor
Trophic factors	Cortisol	
Cytokines	Nitric oxide	
Chemokines		
Neuromodulatory peptides		

[a]Hydrophilic ligands cannot cross the cell membrane and can act only on cell-surface receptors. Hydrophobic ligands may have intracellular or cell-surface receptors.

receptor. The vast majority of ligands are polar or charged and thus unable to cross the lipid bilayer of the cell membrane. Their receptor must therefore reside in the cell membrane and be able to transmit its signal into the interior of the cell. Hydrophobic ligands such as steroids and some vitamins can cross the cell membrane by passive diffusion and enter cells. Their target receptors may be on the cell surface but often are located in the cytoplasm or the nucleus. Table 12.1 lists examples of common ligands classified by their hydrophilicity, hydrophobicity, and site of receptor. Figure 12.1 illustrates the location of receptors that interact with hydrophilic and hydrophobic ligands. As we will see later, the location of the receptor and the biochemical mechanisms associated with signaling will influence how fast the endogenous ligand or drug can produce a biological response. Therefore, a classification system focusing on the site of the receptor is useful when considering the intracellular effects resulting from ligand–receptor interactions.

A third method of classifying ligands is based on anatomy and physiology, that is, the type of cell that produces the ligand and where in the body the action takes place. For example, neurotransmitters are released from nerve cells and produce their effects on nearby cells. Hormones are released from endocrine glands and produce their effects on cells located at sites distant from the cells that release it. This systems-based classification is useful when focusing on the anatomical sources and physiological consequences associated with ligand–receptor interactions. Table 12.2 lists examples of ligands classified by cell type and locus of action.

Modes of Intercellular Signaling

Ligands are synthesized and secreted by many different types of cells and can move from the releasing cells to the target cells in a variety of ways. The major modes of

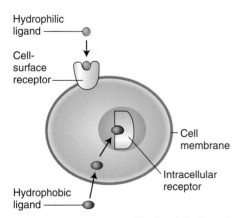

Figure 12.1. Interaction of hydrophilic ligands with cell-surface receptors and hydrophobic ligands with intracellular receptors.

TABLE 12.2. Characteristics of Modes for Intercellular Communication

	Juxtacrine: Gap Junctions	Neuronal synapse	Paracrine	Endocrine
Mode of signaling	Direct cell to cell contact	Diffusion across synaptic cleft	Diffusion through interstitial fluid	Circulating in blood stream
Local or diffuse	Local	Local	Locally diffuse	Diffuse
Signal controlled by	Anatomic localization	Anatomic localization	Anatomic localization and receptor selectivity	Receptor selectivity

signaling between cells are endocrine signaling by hormones and local signaling by a diverse group of ligands.

Endocrine Signaling

The term **gland** refers to an organ or a group of specialized cells that produces secretions. The secretions typically are transported to other sites in the body to produce an effect or aid in some process. Glands that maintain contact with the epithelial surface by a system of ducts are called *exocrine* or ducted glands. Examples include sweat and salivary glands. These glands release their secretions (sweat, tears, mucus, bile) into tubes or ducts that lead to internal or external body surfaces. Exocrine glands are typically not an important source of signaling molecules.

Endocrine or ductless glands secrete hormones, a very important class of signaling molecules involved in growth, development and homeostasis. Hormones are released directly into the blood and produce their effects at sites distant from their site of release (Fig. 12.2). Because most hormones circulate in the blood, they have a diffuse distribution and come into contact with essentially all cells. Yet,

some hormones, such as thyroid stimulating hormone (TSH), act on only one tissue (e.g., thyroid gland) whereas other hormones, such as estrogen and growth hormone, act on many tissues and cell types. The specificity of hormone action, just as we will see with drugs, is determined by the presence of specific receptors in or on those target cells.

The timing of hormone release and subsequent action are quite variable, depending on the function of the hormone. A few hormones, such as the thyroid hormones, are secreted in a relatively steady amount so that their concentration in the blood remains essentially constant under normal conditions. Other hormones are secreted on a specific cycle. For example, glucocorticoids are secreted on a 24-hour or diurnal rhythm, whereas female sex hormones are secreted on a 4-week cycle. Testosterone levels are consistent from week to week but, over a lifespan, blood levels of testosterone fluctuate from very small amounts in preadolescence, peaking in young adults followed by a gradual decline beginning at middle age. Still other hormones, such as insulin, antidiuretic hormone (ADH), and epinephrine are secreted on demand in response to internal or external stimuli and produce a response within seconds to minutes. These differences in the timing of release become important considerations when designing or using drugs to either mimic or replace the actions of endogenous ligands.

Types of Hormones. Hormones may be categorized into three structural groups, with members of each group having many properties in common.

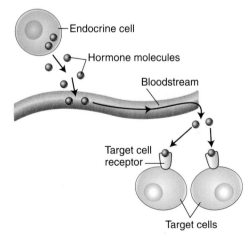

Figure 12.2. The process of endocrine signaling by hormones. Hormones released by the signaling cells enter the bloodstream and travel to the distant target cells. Here they exit the bloodstream and bind to receptors to elicit a response.

- Steroids: Steroids are lipids derived from cholesterol. Examples include the sex hormones, such as testosterone, and adrenal hormones, such as cortisol (Fig. 12.3).
- Modified amino acid derivatives: These comprise catecholamines, thyroid hormones, and melatonin. Catecholamines

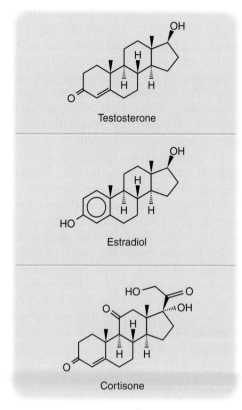

Figure 12.3. Structures of some common steroid hormones.

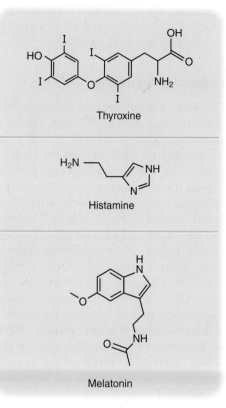

Figure 12.4. Structures of some hormones derived from amino acids.

(dopamine, norepinephrine, and epinephrine) and thyroid hormones (thyroxine and triiodothyronine) are derived from tyrosine; melatonin is synthesized from tryptophan (Fig. 12.4).

- Peptides and proteins: Peptide and protein hormones are products of translation and vary considerably in size and posttranslational modifications, ranging from peptides as short as three amino acids to large, multisubunit glycoproteins. Examples are the neuropeptides (vasopressin, oxytocin), pituitary hormones (corticotropin, gonadotropins), and gastrointestinal hormones (insulin) (Fig. 12.5).

Despite their molecular diversity, hormones can be categorized into one of two types based on the location of their receptors as either hormones with intracellular receptors or hormones with cell-surface receptors.

Hydrophobic hormones (e.g., the steroids) can cross cell membranes by passive diffusion and carry their signal into the cell. Examples are the sex hormones (androgens, estrogens, and gestagens) and the adrenal hormones (mineralocorticoids and glucocorticoids). Thus, their receptors are usually located within the cell, either in the cytoplasm or the nucleus. Thyroid hormones (e.g., thyroxin, triiodothyronine) enter the cell by facilitated diffusion and also bind to intracellular receptors. The primary mechanism of action of hormones with intracellular receptors is to modulate gene expression in target cells.

Most polar or charged hormones, such as catecholamines and the protein and peptide hormones, cannot cross the cell membrane and must rely on cell-surface receptors to

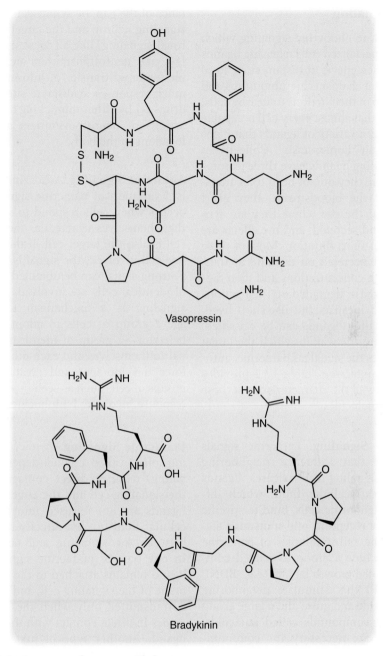

Vasopressin

Bradykinin

Figure 12.5. Structures of some peptide hormones.

convey a signal. Binding of hormone to an extracellular receptor initiates a series of events that leads to generation of so-called *second messengers* within the cell (the hormone is the first messenger) that transmit the signal inside the cell. We will examine second messengers later in the chapter.

Signaling by hormones decreases and stops as hormones are eliminated from the bloodstream. Elimination takes place by biotransformation in the liver, bloodstream, and other sites. Hormones can also be eliminated by excretion in the urine or bile.

Local Signaling

In contrast to endocrine signaling which involves specialized cells releasing ligands that produce effects at distant sites, local signaling mechanisms are ubiquitous and are limited in their actions to nearby cells. It appears that almost every cell is capable of secreting a variety of ligands that helps to maintain homeostasis. Collectively, local signaling ligands have three features in common: they do not need to be transported by the bloodstream, they exert effects near the site where they are synthesized and secreted, and the effects are typically of short duration. Most of these ligands are secreted on demand at transiently high concentrations and then rapidly removed or degraded, so their actions are not only localized but also short-lived. Local signaling ligands can be classified, according to the way in which the target cell receives the signal, as paracrine, autocrine, or juxtacrine. Table 12.2 provides an overview of the characteristics of these signaling molecules.

Paracrine Signaling. Paracrine signals are those that influence neighboring cells. A signaling cell releases ligands into the extracellular fluid, which diffuse to neighboring cells, bind to specific cell-surface receptors, and transmit a signal into the cell. Examples of paracrine ligands include a group of related compounds called growth factors (e.g., BDNF and VEGF) that stimulate neighboring cells to divide and grow, and a large group of diverse compounds called autacoids. Autacoids are necessary for communication between cells during defense and repair processes and are involved in helping the body respond to injury. Examples of autacoids are shown in Figure 12.6.

A special type of paracrine signaling is synaptic transmission associated with neurons; the ligands are called neurotransmitters. An electrical impulse triggers the release of the neurotransmitter from the neuron which then travels the short distance of the gap, or synapse, between the signaling neuron and the target cell. Neuronal signaling, like all local signaling, is fast, and neurotransmitters are responsible for rapid transfer of information and quick responses at discrete sites. Several drugs act by either mimicking or blocking actions of neurotransmitters at specific locations in the body.

Autocrine Signaling. Autocrine signaling is a variation of paracrine signaling and occurs when cells respond to substances they themselves secrete, i.e., the signaling cell is also the target cell. If there is only one cell involved, the signal is weak, but a strong signal can be obtained if a group of identical cells are involved. Autocrine signaling is a mechanism to encourage a group of cells to adopt a similar behavior—a group of identical cells signal to themselves and each other to reinforce development and create identical groups of cells such as seen in an immune response involving lymphocytes.

Juxtacrine Signaling. Juxtacrine signaling, often called contact-dependent signaling, requires direct contact between the signaling cell and the target cell. The ligands are not released into the extracellular fluid but are directly transferred between the signaling and target cells. In one type of juxtacrine signaling, the ligand remains attached to the cell membrane of the signaling cell, and the signal is transmitted only when the target cell comes in direct contact with the attached ligand. Another type of juxtacrine signaling involves direct transfer of signaling molecules from one cell to another through gap junctions between adjacent cells. Recall that gap junctions are communicating junctions that allow small molecules and ions to pass directly from the cytoplasm of one cell to another. An example of juxtacrine signaling is electrical transduction from cardiac cell to cardiac cell via the gap junction.

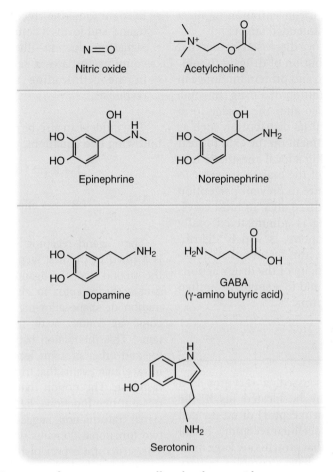

Figure 12.6. Structures of some common small-molecule autacoids.

Specificity of Actions

The ability of the body to control signaling is critical to achieving the correct response at the correct time. We have noted how some ligands (TSH, for example) are distributed throughout the body but yet seem to produce very specific actions in a very limited number of tissues or sites. In other cases, we noted how other ligands (e.g., norepinephrine) are capable of binding to several different targets (α and β receptors) located in several areas of the body but yet avoid causing widespread effects when released from a particular cell. Two different but related concepts can explain this apparent paradox. (1) The actions of the hormone TSH are limited by the hor-mone's ability to bind to only one receptor and that one receptor is found in a limited number of tissues. The complementarity between the hormone and its intended receptor is so specific, that the hormone, even though it encounters several other types of receptors, binds only to one particular type and will therefore cause a biological response in only those cells expressing that protein/receptor. (2) Other ligands' actions, however, are limited by their distribution to a very localized area. In the case of norepinephrine released from a neuron, even though norepineph-rine can bind to several receptors located in several other tissues, its release from a neuron is so close in proximity to its tar-get cell, it has little opportunity to diffuse in a high enough concentration to affect other cells or unintended targets.

In Chapter 8, we discussed factors that affect the distribution of drugs. Lipophilicity, ionization, and protein binding can affect the distribution of a drug. In some cases, we can also alter the dosage form of a drug to limit its distribution such as applying an ointment on the skin to treat a rash or injecting a local anesthetic into the epithelium of the oral cavity prior to a dental procedure to prevent perception of pain in a localized area. In most cases, however, a drug is administered orally and, like a hormone, is widely distributed. Therefore, the feature that determines the specificity of the drug's actions is its ability to bind to a single or limited number of receptors.

Receptors

As we have discussed, a receptor is a protein that may be located inside the cell (intracellular receptor) or on the cell membrane (extracellular receptor). Recall from Chapter 2 that proteins are large macromolecules that have a complex tertiary structure. The binding site for the ligand is a very discreet and specific area on the protein and is highly *stereoselective*. The ligand has to exhibit *stereocomplementarity* with the binding site of the receptor in order for an interaction to occur. A cell has numerous different receptors that can respond to various combinations of ligands. Some receptors are linked to other receptors and act in concert to strengthen or amplify the signal. Other receptors are completely independent of one another and have no biochemical or anatomical interactions with other receptors.

Ligand–Receptor Interactions

The interaction between a receptor (R) and a ligand (L) to produce a biological response can be expressed as a two-step process.

- Recognition—the receptor detects a ligand and forms a complex with it.
- Signal transduction—the ligand–receptor complex initiates a series of changes in the cell leading to a biological response.

The model can also be expressed in the following two equations:

$$L + R \rightleftarrows LR \qquad \text{(Eq. 12.1)}$$

$$LR \rightarrow \rightarrow \text{effect} \qquad \text{(Eq. 12.2)}$$

The ligand–receptor complex (LR) is formed in the first step (Eqn. 12.1). In the second step, the ligand, upon binding, causes the receptor to change its conformation or shape allowing it to physically come in contact with intracellular proteins. This interaction between the receptor and other proteins leads to a series of intracellular events that triggers a biological response. The notion that a receptor carries out two functions, ligand binding and signal transduction, suggests that there are two functional domains within a receptor. The structural aspect of having two functional domains explains two important but sometimes confusing observations about the control of cell signaling. (1) Some endogenous ligands can activate multiple receptors and yet produce very different cellular responses. In these instances, the binding domains of the receptors are similar but the signal transduction domains are different. (2) A number of different ligands can produce similar cellular responses. In these instances, the binding domains of the receptors are different but they share similar signal transduction domains.

Noncatalytic and Catalytic Receptors

Receptors that are linked to cell signaling are considered *noncatalytic*, meaning that ligand–receptor binding is reversible (as shown in Eqn. 12.1) and the ligand dissociates intact from the receptor after the effect is produced (Eqn. 12.2). This noncatalytic interaction is the basis of drug action. A ligand that interacts with a noncatalytic receptor to produce intracellular changes and causes a biological response is an *agonist*. A ligand that forms a complex with the receptor but does not produce subsequent intracellular changes or a biological response is an *antagonist*. These terms will be discussed more fully in Chapter 13.

Ligands can also bind to catalytic *enzymes* either in the cell or on the cell membrane; the ligand, in this context, is now referred to as a *substrate*. Enzymes interact with their substrates to form complexes, but unlike receptors, the enzyme catalytically transforms the substrate into chemically different products that are then released. The process can be viewed as follows:

$$S + E \rightleftarrows ES \rightarrow Product + E \quad (Eq.\ 12.3)$$

where S is the substrate and E is the enzyme. Therefore, the two major characteristics of enzymes are their ability to recognize a substrate (just like noncatalytic receptors) and their ability to catalyze a reaction or change in the structure of the substrate. By convention, when discussing a drug's pharmacological action (its ability to produce a biological response), we refer to it in the context of a drug–receptor interaction. When discussing the metabolism of the same drug, we refer to the drug as a substrate for an enzyme. The factors governing how a drug binds to a receptor and how a substrate binds to an enzyme are very similar. Both the receptor and the enzyme are proteins and the binding of the drug and the substrate require stereocomplementarity and attractive forces. And, as we will see in Chapter 13, the mathematical expressions of these binding interactions are similar. The subsequent effects of drug–receptor and substrate–enzyme interactions, however, are different and independent of each other. The drug–receptor interaction results in a biological response and the drug is released from the receptor unchanged. The substrate–enzyme interaction produces no change in cell function and the substrate is released from the enzyme in a changed form (product or metabolite).

Interestingly, some noncatalytic receptors have the potential to be active even in the absence of an agonist ligand. Such receptors are referred to as constitutively active receptors. That is, the receptor, like most organic molecules, can change shape or adopt different conformations. In some cases the conformational change is identical to that which occurs when an agonist ligand binds to the receptor. This agonist-independent activity emphasizes the concept that the receptor is responsible for conducting the signal into the cell to modulate cell function. The role of the ligand is to activate the receptor; the ligand does not determine what biological changes will occur. In some cases, a ligand can inhibit this constitutive activity *after* binding to the receptor. These ligands act as inverse agonists. Rather that activating the receptor to cause a biological response, inverse agonists do the opposite and not allow the receptor to alter cell function. The discovery of inverse agonists provides scientists another tool helpful in understanding receptor function. The concepts of agonism, inverse agonism, and constitutively active receptors will be discussed again later in Chapter 13.

Receptor Subtypes

The manner in which a cell responds is dictated by what types of receptors the cell expresses and by the kind of signal transduction machinery available for responding to the signal. As we have discovered in the last several years using cloning and molecular biology techniques, there are a multitude of receptors and receptor subtypes. Receptor subtypes are a group of receptors that have similar (but not identical) binding domains and different signal

transduction domains. As a result receptor subtypes are activated by a common
endogenous ligand but can produce different biological responses. From a physiological standpoint, the existence of receptor subtypes allows our bodies to use just
one ligand for a variety of actions by
releasing it in different locations. For
example, norepinephrine can interact
with α- and β-*adrenoreceptors*, which are
further subdivided into α_1 and α_2 and β_1
and β_2 receptor subtypes. These recep-
tor subtypes are found in different target
organs: e.g., the heart contains β_1 receptors whereas β_2 receptors are found in the
bronchial smooth muscle. Each receptor
subtype has a different function, and the
release of norepinephrine locally at each of
these sites produces a different physiological effect. Another example is acetylcholine
binding to *cholinergic* receptors that can be
classified as either *muscarinic* or *nicotinic*
subtypes; each of these is subdivided into
many different subtypes with distinct functions in different areas of the body including the brain and peripheral organs.

From drug discovery and drug therapy
standpoints, the existence of receptor
subtypes allows us to design drugs that
bind to only one receptor subtype of a
ligand. In this way, drugs can be made
very selective, that is, produce only one
desired effect. Conversely, a drug that can
bind to many subtypes of receptors could
have many uses but at the same time can
cause unwanted side effects.

Signal Transduction

We have noted that in order for a ligand
or a drug to produce a biological response,
it follows a two-step process: recognition
(ligands binds to binding domain of the
receptor) and signal transduction. When
a ligand binds to a receptor, it causes a
change in the conformation of the receptor which elicits a series of changes inside
the cell to produce a biological response.
Signal transduction refers to the processes by which an extracellular ligand–

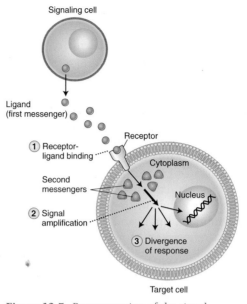

Figure 12.7. Representation of the signal-
transduction process. The signaling cell releases
a ligand that binds to a surface receptor on the
target cell. This binding initiates signal transduction, which may involve second (intracellular) messengers. The outcome is some sort of
cellular response in the target cell.

receptor interaction causes an intracellular change without the ligand entering the
cell. In other words, it is the translation
of an extracellular signal into changes
in intracellular activity. Additional cellular molecules often become involved in
transmitting the message to its ultimate
destination in the cell. Figure 12.7 illustrates this concept in general terms.

The ligand is considered the *first messenger*, carrying a signal from the signaling cell to the target cell-surface receptor.
Once the initial ligand–receptor binding
has occurred, other compounds called
second messengers play an important role
in transmitting the signal to specific intracellular sites in the cytoplasm or nucleus.
Second messengers are short-lived molecules that mediate the transduction of the
extracellular signals, and are usually generated strictly in response to a specific ligand–
receptor interaction. Particularly important
second messengers in a variety of signaling

pathways include cyclic AMP (cAMP), calcium ions, inositol 1,4,5-trisphosphate (IP_3), and diacylglycerol (DAG).

Signal transduction has several important features:

- The signal can undergo amplification, a process by which a small amount of ligand can create a large cellular response. As an illustration, consider one molecule of ligand activating one receptor. This activates 10 molecules of the enzyme adenylate cyclase, generating 100 molecules of cAMP, which activate 1,000 protein kinases, which phosphorylate 10,000 calcium channels, which allow 100,000 units of calcium to enter the cell.
- The signaling pathway may be influenced by opposing actions from different receptors. For example, β_1 receptors can activate a specific protein in the cell to activate the enzyme adenylate cyclase. However, α_2 receptors can activate a different protein that inhibits adenylate cyclase. These opposing actions are important for balance and control of cell function (Fig. 12.8A).
- Signaling pathways may converge from different receptors. Different receptors may be linked to common second messenger systems in order to enhance, reinforce, or provide redundancy to the signal (Fig. 12.8B).
- The signaling pathway can diverge such that several processes in the cell can be influenced at the same time. Some receptors are linked to a protein that can generate two different second messengers that influence different or diverging signaling systems. These pathways, while different, may serve a specific but complex cell function such as to promote growth and differentiation or they may diverge in order to coordinate multiple pathways of cell metabolism (Fig. 12.8C).
- The time course of the response of signaling pathways can vary from very fast and transient (milliseconds) to very slow and sustained (hours to days).

- Control of the signaling pathways is dynamic. Transmission of the signal can be altered according to the needs of the cell, by variation in the nature (synthetic vs. catabolic, excitatory vs. inhibitory) and amounts of the second messengers.

Protein phosphorylation is a common means of signal transduction and information transfer. Approximately one-third of the proteins present in a typical human cell may be phosphorylated (covalently bound to phosphate) at one time or another. Protein phosphorylation and dephosphorylation are controlled by two enzymes: *protein kinases* that put phosphate on a protein and *phosphatases* that remove phosphate attached to a protein. Phosphorylation can increase or decrease the biological activity of an enzyme, help move proteins between subcellular compartments, and allow interactions between proteins to occur, as well as label proteins for degradation.

The use of common second messengers in multiple signaling pathways creates both opportunities and potential problems. Input from several signaling pathways, often called *crosstalk*, may affect the concentrations of common second messengers. Crosstalk permits more finely tuned regulation of cell activity than would the action of individual independent pathways. However, inappropriate crosstalk can cause the signal carried by second messengers to be misinterpreted.

After a signaling process has been initiated and the information has been transduced to affect other cellular processes, these processes must be terminated. Without such termination, cells lose their responsiveness to new signals. Protein phosphatases are one mechanism for the termination of a signaling process; the role of protein phosphorylation and dephosphorylation is shown in Figure 12.9.

Signal transduction pathways control most cellular functions. From a drug discovery point of view, the signaling pathways provide a rich source of drug targets.

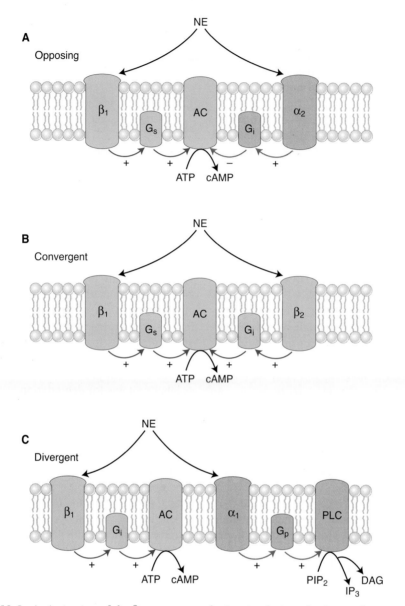

Figure 12.8. **A.** Activation of the β_1 receptor results in stimulation of a G stimulatory protein that activates the enzyme adenylate cyclase to produce the second messenger cAMP. Activation of α_2 receptor results in stimulation of a G inhibitory protein that inhibits adenylate cyclase thereby decreasing synthesis of cAMP. **B.** Activation of either β_1 receptor or β_2 receptor stimulates G stimulatory proteins, both of which can activate adenylate cyclase. **C.** The same ligand can activate two different receptors that are coupled to two different second messenger pathways leading to divergent effects. These effects of these two signaling pathways may be complementary or completely independent.

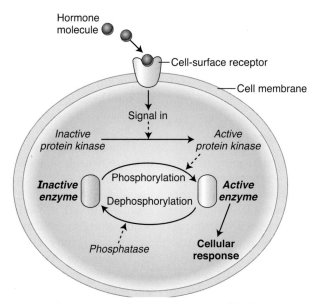

Figure 12.9. Activation and deactivation of an enzyme mediated by hormones. The binding of a hormone to its cell-surface receptor sends a signal that is transmitted into the cell interior. The signal activates a protein kinase that results in phosphorylation of another enzyme, eventually resulting in a cellular response. The active enzyme is deactivated by a phosphatase and awaits another signal.

Each step in the pathway represents a potential site of drug action.

Receptor Structure and Classification

Now that we have covered the general concepts behind the two major steps associated with receptor-mediated cell signaling (recognition and transduction), this next section will discuss and illustrate specific examples of how receptors and signal transduction pathways interact and how that plays a role in classifying receptors. A common way of classifying receptors is by the ligand that binds to them; e.g., estrogen, insulin, or acetylcholine (ACh) receptors. While this classification is useful from the perspective of identifying the ligand involved, it does not tell us much about the signal transduction mechanisms that are involved or what the effect on the cell will be. Another approach to receptor classification is based on structure, function, and

signal transduction pathway. On this basis, we can construct five broad categories of receptors:

Cell-surface receptors:

- Ion-channel receptors
- G protein-coupled receptors
- Enzymatic receptors

Intracellular receptors:
- Transcriptional regulation receptors
- Intracellular enzymes

A brief description of each of these structural classes and how they work is given below.

Cell-Surface Receptors

The primary mechanism through which a cell senses extracellular stimuli is through cell-surface receptors. Cell-surface receptors are imbedded within the membrane of the cell with the ligand binding domain oriented to the extracellular side and the signal transduction domain oriented to the intracellular side of the membrane. Because these receptors are within the membrane and are exposed to both the intracellular and extracellular sides of the cell, they are referred to as transmembrane receptors.

Ion-Channel Receptors

Many cellular functions require ions to pass through the cell membrane either into or out of the cell. Because the membrane is lipid and does not allow ionized molecules to pass through, specialized transmembrane channels are necessary for the passage of small ions (e.g., Na^+, K^+, Ca^{2+}, and Cl^-). The conformation, structure, and ionization of functional groups on the amino acids making up the channel protein allow the channel to be selective for transport of a particular ion. For example, some channels permit only Na^+ to pass through and other channels are selective for Cl^-. Conformational changes in these channel proteins can open or close the channels, regulating ion movement into and out of a cell.

Ligand-gated ion-channels are opened and closed by the binding of certain neurotransmitters with receptors. The ion channel–receptor complex is a large protein complex that includes several subunits making up the channel that traverses through the cell membrane and a discreet ligand-binding site (receptor) (Figure 12.10). Upon binding of the ligand, the channel rapidly changes conformation from a closed to an open state. Dissociation of the ligand from its receptor closes the ion channel. However, after prolonged exposure to the ligand, the receptors can become desensitized.

The signal ligands for these ion channels are neurotransmitters. Examples are the nicotinic ACh receptors (where the ligand is ACh and it regulates Na^+/K^+ channels found in skeletal muscle) and γ-aminobutyric acid (GABA) receptors (where the ligand is GABA and it regulates Cl^- channels in the brain). Neuromuscular blocking agents such as tubocurarine can block the ACh receptor on skeletal muscle preventing Na^+ from depolarizing the muscle cell and not allowing it to contract. Tubocurarine and similar neuromuscular blocking agents are used to paralyze patients prior to major surgery. Diazepam (Valium®) acts on the GABA receptor complex to prolong the opening of the Cl^- channel thereby promoting the effects of the endogenous ligand GABA. Diazepam is used to treat anxiety and acts to promote the inhibitory effect of GABA in areas of the brain that generate anxious behavior. A schematic representation of a ligand-gated ion-channel receptor is shown in Figure 12.10. Signaling by

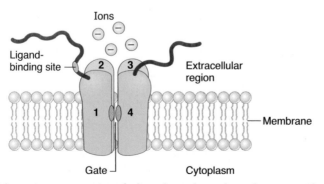

Figure 12.10. Schematic representation of a ligand-gated ion-channel receptor. The receptor is a transmembrane protein (shown here with four transmembrane segments labeled 1 to 4). The extracellular part of the protein contains the ligand-binding site. Ligand–receptor binding causes a change in the conformation of the receptor. This opens the gate, creating a pore through which ions can diffuse into the cell.

ligand-gated ion channels is very fast—on the order of milliseconds—which is very important for the rapid transfer of information across synapses.

Another type of ion channel is called a voltage-dependent ion channel. These channels are not linked to a ligand-binding site. They can be opened or closed only by generating a voltage difference across the membrane. In this case, a voltage change, rather than a ligand, causes a conformational change of the channel protein and an opening and closing of the channel. There is no ligand directly involved in the transport of ions by voltage-dependent receptors.

G Protein-Coupled Receptors

The G protein-coupled receptors (GPCRs) are a superfamily of related cell-surface receptors vital for normal cellular communication and function. GPCRs are important targets for drug design and therapy; it is estimated that more than half of all the drugs on the market today target GPCRs.

The GPCR system has three parts: the cell-surface receptor, the G protein, and the second messenger system. The receptor itself is a single polypeptide chain that has seven *transmembrane domains*, i.e., it is imbedded in the membrane and traverses the lipid bilayer seven times (Fig. 12.11A).

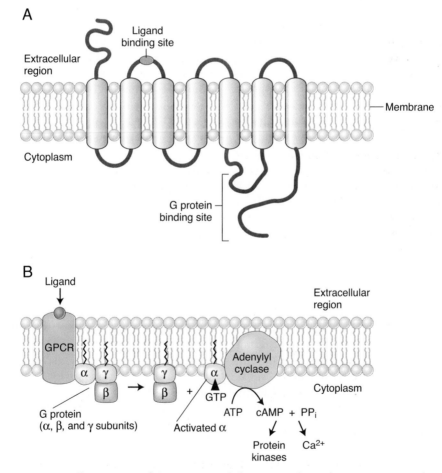

Figure 12.11. **A**. The structure of G protein-coupled receptors shows the seven-transmembrane (7TM) protein receptor with its seven transmembrane domains, and the binding sites for ligand and G protein. **B**. The signal transduction pathway after activation of a G protein-coupled receptor (GPCR) by a ligand.

The G protein is located near the intracellular surface of the cell membrane and serves as a link or coupling mechanism between the receptor and the second messenger. The second messenger eventually produces the biological response.

The term *G protein* refers to *guanine nucleotide-binding protein*. G proteins are heterotrimeric, made up of three distinct subunits termed α, β, and γ. The G proteins may link to a variety of second messenger systems such as enzymes or ion channels. Consequently, there are several isoforms of G proteins including G_s and G_i which are linked to adenylate cyclase and G_q which is linked to phospholipase C.

GPCRs bind to a wide spectrum of extracellular ligands, including hormones, neurotransmitters, and autacoids. As you would expect, the extracellular binding domain varies considerably among this family of receptors in order to recognize the different endogenous ligands. The signal transduction domain (also known as the effector domain) of this family of receptors is highly homologus (has similar amino acid sequence). The function of this domain is to physically interact with the G proteins located on the intracellular side of the cell.

The sequence of events leading to formation of the second messenger cAMP through a GPCR is depicted in Figure 12.11 and described in the following text.

1. Prior to binding of the ligand to the receptor, the α subunit is bound to both GDP and the β–γ subunit complex. The function of the β–γ subunit complex is to inhibit α subunit activity. The α and γ subunits are covalently attached to the intracellular surface of the cell membrane.
2. When the ligand binds to the extracellular domain of the receptor, the receptor undergoes a conformational change that allows the intracellular portion of the receptor to physically interact with the α subunit of the G protein in the cell. The

interaction allows for the exchange of GDP for GTP on the α subunit.
3. The binding of GTP to the α subunit allows the α subunit to dissociate from the inhibitory β–γ complex. The activated α subunit is now able to interact with and activate a second messenger system. The second messenger system depicted in Figure 12.11 is adenylate cyclase, a transmembrane protein with catalytic sites in the intracellular side of the cell. In this case, adenylate cyclase catalyzes the conversion of ATP into cAMP which ultimately produces a biological response. In other cell types, the α subunit acts through a similar mechanism to activate or perhaps inhibit other second messenger systems.
4. The α subunit contains GTPase activity which allows it to hydrolyze GTP to GDP. The presence of GDP on the α subunit causes it to reassociate with the β–γ subunit complex thereby stopping its interaction with adenylate cyclase. This "on–off" mechanism is a crucial component of controlling signaling pathways.

Keep in mind the concept of amplification. That is, one ligand will activate one receptor and one receptor is capable of activating several G proteins and each G protein is capable of activating several second messenger systems.

Enzymatic Receptors

This simple class of receptors has an extracellular portion that binds to the ligand, a single linear hydrophobic region that traverses the membrane lipid bilayer, and an intracellular portion that is located in the cytoplasm. This intracellular region may have intrinsic enzyme activity that is triggered on binding to a ligand, i.e., the receptor is itself an enzyme. Note that ligand–receptor binding in this case is reversible because the signaling ligand is not the substrate. The substrate is located inside the cell and is transformed to a product on receptor activation by the ligand.

The best understood family of enzymatic receptors is the **protein kinase receptor** family, in which the enzyme activated is a protein kinase. For example, *tyrosine kinases* selectively attach a phosphate group to the amino acid tyrosine in a protein, and *serine/threonine* kinases to serine and threonine residues. Enzymatic receptors with intrinsic protein kinase activity bind to and mediate actions of most growth factors (epidermal growth factor, nerve growth factor, platelet-derived growth factor) and are of great interest for their role in cancer.

Alternatively, the receptor may be an **enzyme-linked receptor**; when activated by a ligand these receptors bind to and activate enzymes nearby. Here, too, the signaling ligand is not the substrate. Ligand–receptor binding initiates a cascade of protein phosphorylations that result in the ultimate effect inside the cell. This class of single transmembrane (1TM) receptors is further classified according to the intracellular enzyme system that is activated after ligand binding.

Figure 12.12 illustrates an enzyme-linked receptor showing the single transmembrane

protein, the extracellular ligand-binding site, and the intracellular site associated with enzyme activity. For example, the cytokine receptor is a tyrosine kinase-linked receptor. Cytokine receptors must first be activated by their signaling ligands (cytokines, interferons, and human growth factor [HGF]), and then bind to cytoplasmic tyrosine kinases before they are able to phosphorylate their target proteins. Therefore, protein kinases are involved in the process of signal transduction in these pathways as well, as they were with GPCRs.

Intracellular Receptors

Many intracellular proteins act as receptors for signaling ligands and other compounds. Because the receptor is inside the cell, the signaling ligand has to cross the cell membrane, reach the receptor, and bind to it. Thus, the ligands must be lipophilic (like the steroid hormones) so that they can cross the cell membrane.

Transcriptional Regulation Receptors

The transcriptional regulation receptors, also known as *nuclear receptors*, constitute most of the intracellular receptor class. Transcriptional regulation receptors usually trigger an effect when the ligand–receptor complex travels from the cytoplasm into the nucleus, initiating transcription of RNA. They are further subdivided as

- Steroid receptors (e.g., receptors for corticosteroids, sex steroids, and mineralocorticoids)
- Nonsteroid receptors (e.g., receptors for thyroid hormones, retinoic acid, and vitamin D).

The process by which a hormone binds to its intracellular receptor and triggers a response is illustrated in Figure 12.13.

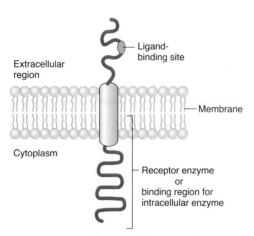

Figure 12.12. Schematic depiction of an enzymatic receptor showing the single transmembrane protein, the extracellular ligand-binding site, and the intracellular site associated with enzyme activity.

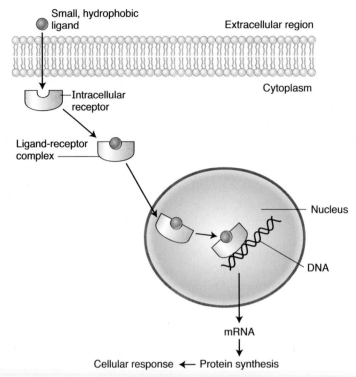

Figure 12.13. Mechanism of action of a typical intracellular hormone receptor. The receptor is located in the cytoplasm of the cell. The hormone (ligand) has to cross the lipid bilayer and enter the cell to bind to the receptor.

The hormone crosses the cell membrane by passive diffusion and binds to its receptor in the cytoplasm, thus activating the receptor. The receptor has three functional domains: a ligand-binding domain that selectively binds a given hormone or ligand; a DNA-binding domain that allows the ligand-receptor complex to bind to a specific site on the genome; activation function domain needed for regulation of transcription. The hormone–receptor complex then travels to the nucleus, where it binds to DNA and initiates transcription of mRNA. The mRNA leaves the nucleus and serves as a template for synthesis of specific proteins within the cytoplasm. This process takes time, and there is generally a lag time—up to several hours—between initial ligand–receptor binding and production of proteins. For this reason, the effect produced by hormones that act at nuclear receptors can persist long after the initial signaling event.

Figure 12.14 depicts an overview of the signaling resulting from an agonist binding to various types of receptors.

Intracellular Enzymes

Enzymes catalyze most cellular processes and reactions. Each cell requires more than 500 different enzymes to carry out all its functions, and the types and concentrations of these enzymes vary according to the needs of the cell. Given the role of enzymes in maintaining cell function, they represent an important group of drug targets. In our discussions up to this point, we focused on receptors as proteins involved in cell signaling–translating an extracellular signal to an intracellular

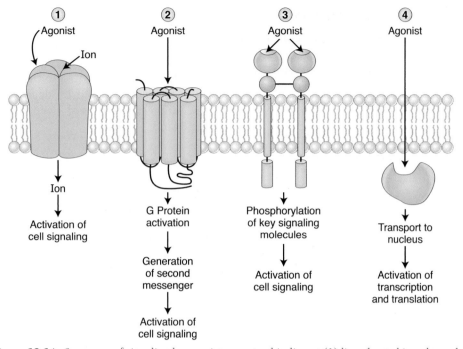

Figure 12.14. Summary of signaling by agonist–receptor binding at (1) ligand-gated ion channels, (2) G protein-coupled receptors, (3) enzyme-linked receptors, and (4) intracellular receptors.

response. Enzymes, technically, do not fit this definition because they catalyze a reaction that converts a substrate into a product; they are not directly involved in producing a biological response. They, however, play an important role in controlling cell signaling because one of the functions of enzymes is to catalyze the synthesis or break down of signaling molecules.

Enzymes may be located in the extracellular and intracellular spaces. Intracellular enzymes may be membrane-bound as we have seen already, or may be contained in the cytosol or in various intracellular structures. Many intracellular enzymes are involved in signal transduction cascades as discussed earlier with the protein kinases, and serve as intracellular drug targets. Extracellular enzymes are also important drug target. In Chapter 13, we will further discuss the similarities and differences between receptors and enzymes in relation to drug action.

Modulation of Ligand–Receptor Interactions

Ligand–receptor interactions are the body's way of maintaining homeostasis, responding to a need or a demand and defending or repairing itself. As we have seen, there is a variety of ligands, receptors, and signaling processes that allows the body to respond, in some cases, very rapidly and, in other cases, in a slow and sustained manner depending on the need. In order to work optimally in response to short- and long-term changes in our environment (diet, exercise, environmental conditions), the body must also be able to adapt. The body achieves this modulation by controlling or altering several parameters including how much ligand is present and how well the receptor and its signal transduction mechanism work. When one of these modulation mechanisms does not work optimally, the result could be a disorder or disease.

Concentration of Ligand

The concentration of ligand will in part determine how much of the ligand–receptor complex is formed and therefore the strength of the signal. Ligand concentration is controlled by

- Increasing or decreasing ligand synthesis
- Increasing or decreasing ligand release
- Altering the destruction or removal of ligand from the receptor site.

Receptor Density

Receptors also have the capacity to adapt to the changing environment to maintain homeostasis; this ability is known as receptor dynamism. The primary manifestation of this response is a constant fluctuation in receptor density or the number of receptors at a particular site. Receptor density is not fixed but is dynamic, controlled by opposing rates of receptor synthesis and receptor degeneration. The body can modify these rates by

- Increasing the number of receptors when there is a shortage of ligand, known as receptor upregulation. An example of this phenomenon is seen in Parkinson's disease in which there is progressive loss of the neurons that synthesize and release the neurotransmitter dopamine. As the disease progresses and there is less and less dopamine, the neurons respond by increasing the synthesis and density of receptors for dopamine to compensate for the deficiency of the dopamine.
- Decreasing the number of receptors when there is an abundance of ligand, known as receptor downregulation. An example of this phenomenon is seen with the over use of β agonists in the treatment of asthma. Overstimulation of the β receptors can lead to phosphorylation of the β receptor via the enzyme β-adrenergic receptor kinase (βARK). The phosphorylation causes

recruitment of β-arrestin, a protein that uncouples the receptor from the G protein and recruits enzymes that destroy second messengers. In this case, the body is adapting to the presences of excess ligand by decreasing the number or density of receptors for the ligand.

Allosteric Modulation

Allosteric effects occur when the binding properties of a protein for a ligand change as a consequence of a second molecule binding to the protein. The modulating molecule and ligand bind to different sites on the protein or even to different subunits; the modulator binding location is called the *allosteric* site. The structures of the ligand and modulating molecule can be very different because they bind to different sites. Binding of the modulator to the receptor alters the conformation of the receptor active site and either increases or decreases its affinity for the primary ligand. Thus, the presence and concentration of the modulating molecule can control ligand–receptor interactions, and the presence of an allosteric modulator provides one more means of controlling cell signaling.

Allosteric effects are important in the regulation of enzymatic reactions. Cells use allosteric activators (which enhance activity) and allosteric inhibitors (which reduce activity) to control enzyme reactions. Noncatalytic receptors can also be allosterically modulated. For example, drugs such as anesthetics, neurosteroids, neurotoxins, and alcohol can modulate the activation of ligand-gated ion channels. Similarly endogenous compounds such as the family of proteins referred to as GPCR-interacting proteins (GIPs) modulate receptor function by altering ligand affinity, promoting close association with other signaling proteins, and controlling receptor density by transferring to or removing them from the cell membrane.

Key Concepts

- Cellular communication is carried out by the appropriate release and binding of ligands to their receptors.
- Hydrophilic ligands bind to cell-surface receptors, whereas hydrophobic ligands can bind to intracellular receptors after crossing the cell membrane.
- Hormones are ligands made in endocrine glands and carried by the bloodstream to their target receptors; they act by activating enzymes or modulating gene expression.
- Ductless glands and other cells secrete autacoids for local signaling; many ligands can function as both hormones and local signals.
- Paracrine signals influence neighboring cells; autocrine signaling occurs when cells respond to substances they themselves secrete; and juxtacrine signals are those passed between two cells in contact.

- Signal transduction is the translation of an extracellular signal into changes in cell behavior by a cascade of several second messenger systems.
- Receptors may be noncatalytic (act by binding reversibly to agonists), catalytic (act by catalyzing a reaction), or constitutively active (act in the absence of an agonist).
- Cell-surface receptors (e.g., ion-channel receptors, G protein-coupled receptors, and enzyme-associated receptors) bind to ligands on the cell membrane, whereas intracellular receptors (e.g., transcriptional regulator receptors and enzymes) require the ligand to enter the cell.
- Receptors of the G protein-coupled cell-surface receptor superfamily are targets for almost half of marketed drugs.
- Ligand–receptor interactions are modulated by changes in ligand or receptor concentration or by allosteric effects.

Review Questions

1. What are the steps involved in cellular communication?
2. Describe the types of hormones secreted by endocrine glands and tissues.
3. Explain the process of endocrine signaling by hormones. What are the key features of endocrine signaling?
4. What are the similarities and differences between endocrine and local signaling by ligands?
5. List the features and differences between paracrine, autocrine, and juxtacrine signaling.
6. Explain the process of signal transduction. Why is transduction essential for polar signaling ligands?
7. What is the role of second messengers in the transduction process? How is a signal altered according to the needs of the cell?
8. Explain how one type of signaling ligand can cause different effects in different locations in the body.

9. What are receptors? Distinguish between catalytic, noncatalytic, and constitutive receptors.
10. List and briefly describe the types of cell-surface and intracellular receptors.
11. Elaborate on the mechanisms by which the body modulates and controls ligand–receptor interactions.

CASE STUDY 12.1

Steroids: How can we limit their effects?

FY is a 64-year-old male experiencing painful swelling in his knees. He has been taking Naproxen (Naprosyn®) on a daily basis for several years. Recently the swelling and pain have worsened and higher doses of Naproxen have not provided adequate relief. FY is a candidate for knee replacement surgery. Until that time, his physician has decided to administer an intra-articular injection of hydrocortisone into both knees.

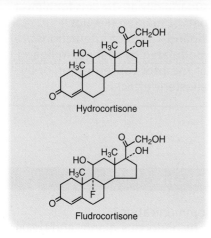

1. Hydrocortisone has a steroid structure. Explain how the chemical features of the drug plays a role in determining the class of receptors (e.g., cell surface, intracellular) the drug is most likely to act upon?
2. Hydrocortisone is an agonist. Describe, in general terms, its mechanism of action, that is, what cellular changes occur when it interacts with its receptor.

3. Describe, in general terms, the mechanism of action of an antagonist at this receptor.
4. Describe, in general terms, the mechanism of action of an inverse agonist at this receptor.
5. The drug was administered to this patient as an injection into the knee. The patient was told that relief would not be experienced until much later that day. Based on the actions of the drug, explain why there is a delay in action.
6. Hydrocortisone is also used to treat adrenal insufficiency, asthma, shock, and skin rashes and causes immunosuppression. How can hydrocortisone produce so many seemingly disparate effects?
7. Hydrocortisone can be used as a replacement for the endogenous ligand cortisol. Long-term use of hydrocortisone can lead to osteoporosis. Cite at least two reasons why, in normal people, endogenous cortisol does not cause osteoporosis.
8. Hydrocortisone also comes in several topical preparations such as creams, ointments, and lotions to treat skin rashes. But these products are not useful in treating adrenal insufficiency, asthma, or shock. How does the product change the pharmacology of the drug?
9. Fludrocortisone, when given systemically, has no anti-inflammatory actions. Its only effect is to promote sodium retention by an action at

the kidney. How can you explain why the effects of fludrocortisone are limited to the kidney? Does it involve binding domains or signal transduction domains?

Additional Readings

Foreman JC, Johansen T, Gibb A (eds). Textbook of Receptor Pharmacology, 3rd ed. CRC Press, 2010.

Gomperts BD, Kramer IM, Tatham PER. Signal Transduction. Academic Press, 2009.

Hancock JT. Cell Signaling. Oxford University Press, 2010.

Vauquelin G, von Mentzer B. G Protein-coupled Receptors: Molecular Pharmacology. John Wiley & Sons, 2007.

CHAPTER 13

Mechanisms of Drug Action

In Chapter 2, we introduced the concept that the cellular targets of most drugs used for medical treatment are proteins and associated macromolecules, and that most drugs produce their effect by binding to specific sites on the protein called receptors. Drugs usually work by competing with or taking the place of an endogenous ligand or by altering the ligand–receptor interaction in some way. Therefore, a drug generally makes a *quantitative* change in an existing physiological or biochemical process but does not *qualitatively* alter the nature of the process or create a new process.

Theory of Drug Action

Chapter 2 examined how stereocomplementarity and attractive forces between the structures of the drug and the receptor play a role in the binding of these two molecules. Chapter 12, discussed how receptors play a role in generating changes in cell activity (or producing a biological response). We now combine and expand on these concepts to account for the different effects that can be seen when a drug binds to a receptor.

One theoretical model of drug action is the two-state receptor model, illustrated in Figure 13.1. This model was originally developed to explain constitutive activity of G protein-coupled receptors (GPCRs), and is now used as a general approach to understand drug action at any receptor. The model assumes that the receptor exists in two conformations that are in equilibrium—an inactive form (the R state) and an active form (the R* state). Receptors in the R* conformation can produce changes in cell activity (or a biological response). Most receptors, when not bound to a drug or an endogenous ligand, exist in the inactive R conformation with only a small fraction in the active R* conformation. Exceptions are the constitutive receptors (discussed in the previous chapter), which have a significant fraction of receptors in the R* state even in the absence of ligand.

For a drug to influence the function of a receptor it first must have an affinity or an attraction to the receptor. (The concept of affinity will be discussed in more detail in this chapter and in Chapter 14.) The same drug, depending on its physicochemical properties, may have different affinities or equal affinity for R and R*. Drug–receptor binding can therefore influence receptor function in different ways. In general, a drug can enhance, diminish, or block the transmission of a signal when it binds to a receptor.

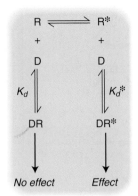

Figure 13.1. A schematic representation of the two-state receptor model. R is the receptor in the inactive state, R* is the receptor in the active state, D is the drug, and DR and DR* are the respective drug–receptor complexes. R, R*, DR, and DR* are in constant equilibrium. K_d and K_d^* are equilibrium constants defined for the dissociation of the drug–receptor complex, and are inversely related to affinities of the drug for the receptor in its inactive and active states, respectively.

Agonists and Antagonists

An agonist is a compound that binds to the active receptor state (R*) and stimulates a response characteristic of that receptor. Agonist drugs preferentially bind to R* to form the active DR* complex as follows:

$$D + R^* \rightleftarrows DR^* \rightarrow Effect \quad (Eq.\ 13.1)$$

The ability of agonists to preferentially bind to R* may vary. A drug with great selectivity for R* over R is referred to as a full agonist and is capable of producing a maximal response. A drug with only a small selectivity for R* over R is referred to as a partial agonist and will stimulate the receptor to produce a response but not to the same extent as a full agonist. Consider Eqn. 13.1 and the two-state receptor model depicted in Figure 13.1. A full agonist binds preferentially to R* to form DR* complex which leads to an effect or biological response. When DR* is formed, the equilibrium between R and R* (shown

in Fig. 13.1) will shift to favor formation of more R* and allow additional molecules of the drug to bind to R* and produce a biological response. If the drug's attraction to R* is highly preferential over its attraction to R, theoretically all receptors will shift to the activated state and elicit a full and complete response. This describes the actions of a full agonist. A partial agonist, however, has some but not total preference for binding to R*. As a result, the equilibrium will shift toward the formation of more R* and cause a biological response but the response will not be as great as that seen with a full agonist. The partial agonist's ability to shift the equilibrium to form R* will not be as great because some of the partial agonist is also bound to R.

Using this same model, we can explain the actions of an inverse agonist. As the name implies, an inverse agonist produces an action that is the opposite of an agonist. From a binding perspective, inverse agonists preferentially bind to R over R* to form the inactive DR complex. This binding drives the equilibrium between R and R* toward R, decreasing the proportion of receptors in the R* state.

$$D + R \rightleftarrows DR \rightarrow No\ effect \quad (Eq.\ 13.2)$$

The biological effects of an inverse agonist are most readily seen and understood when considering a receptor with a significant level of constitutive receptor activity. That is, if a significant number of receptors exist naturally in the R* state, an inverse agonist will shift the equilibrium from R* to R and decrease receptor signaling and thereby decrease the biological activity of the cell. If there is no significant constitutive receptor activity, inverse agonists will have no discernable action (unless it is competing with another agonist or an endogenous ligand, a concept that will be covered in Chapter 14).

The last class of drugs, in a sense, falls between agonists and inverse agonists. Antagonists do not differentiate between R and R*; they bind with equal affinity

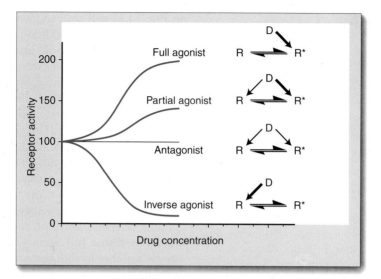

Figure 13.2. The two-state receptor model and its relationship to the mechanism of action of drugs. The heavy arrows indicate a strong affinity between drug and receptor (either in its active or inactive conformation), whereas the light arrows indicate a weak affinity. The **Y-axis** plots the activity of the receptor at 100 arbitrary units when no drug is present. The activity of the receptor (the amount in the R* state) changes based on the affinity of the drug for either R or R*. (*Source*: Brunton LL, Lazo JS, Parker KL: Goodman and Gilman's The Pharmacological Basis of Therapeutics, 11th edition. http://www.accessmedicine.com).

to both conformations and therefore do not change the equilibrium between R and R*. They do not alter receptor activity on their own, but can compete with agonists and inverse agonists for receptor binding, thereby competitively blocking the responses elicited by these drugs. The clinical utility of antagonists is to decrease the ability of endogenous ligands to produce a biological response. Figure 13.2 shows a schematic representation of how the two-state receptor model relates to the action of drugs.

An agonist and competitive antagonist for the same receptor will bind to the same site on that receptor. Therefore, it seems logical that an agonist and an antagonist for the same receptor would share some structural similarities. As discussed in Chapter 2, the pharmacophore is often times modeled after the endogenous ligand of a drug target. Many times, the endogenous ligand is a small hydrophilic molecule and the design of an agonist follows suit because both the endogenous ligand

and the agonist must fit the receptor in a nearly identical fashion in order to activate the receptor. Competitive antagonists, however, tend to be bulky and lipophilic compared to the agonist and do not always share structural similarities. In order to explain this exception to the concept of stereocomplementarity requirement for competitive antagonists, it has been suggested that antagonists bind to *hydrophobic accessory binding sites* that are located near the binding sites for agonists. In this way, the competitive antagonist is able to block access to the active site of the receptor but does not physically interact with the signal transduction domain, the receptor component that causes conformational changes and elicits a biological response. Figures 13.3 and 13.4 illustrate the hydrophilicity of and structural similarities between the endogenous ligands and agonists and the contrasting lipophilicity and structural dissimilarities of the antagonists. Examples of agonist and antagonist drugs are given in Tables 13.1 and 13.2, respectively.

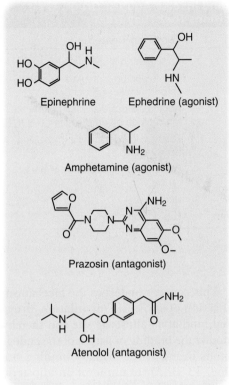

Figure 13.3. Examples of agonists and antagonists of epinephrine. Note structural similarities between epinephrine and its agonists, and the dissimilarities between epinephrine and its antagonists. Ephedrine and amphetamine are stimulants, whereas prazosin and atenolol are antihypertensives and are used to treat high blood pressure.

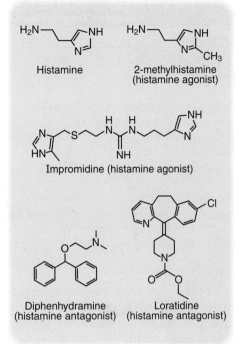

Figure 13.4. Examples of agonists and antagonists of histamine. Note the structural similarities between histamine and its agonists, and the dissimilarities between histamine and its antagonists. Histamine agonists do not have a clinical role, but are used in research. Diphenhydramine and loratadine are antihistamines and are used clinically to treat allergies.

Allosteric Drugs

The receptor model we have discussed to this point involves a direct link between the drug–receptor interaction and the biological response. A significant number of drugs currently used today work in this manner and are effective. However, our ability to control the effect or intensity of the signal is dependent on our ability to control the concentration of the drug at

Receptor	Drug	Condition Treated
α adrenoceptor	Oxymetazoline[a]	Nasal congestion
Opioid receptor	Meperidine, morphine	Pain
Glucocorticoid nuclear receptor	Dexamethasone	Inflammation
GABA$_A$ receptor	Alprazolam	Anxiety
Potassium ion channel	Minoxidil	Hair regrowth

TABLE 13.1. Examples of Agonist Drugs, Their Receptor Targets, and Conditions That They Treat

[a]Partial agonist.
GABA, γ-aminobutyric acid.

TABLE 13.2. Examples of Antagonist and Inverse Agonist Drugs, Their Receptor Targets, and Conditions That They Treat

Receptor	Antagonist Drug	Condition Treated
Calcium ion channel	Diltiazem	Angina, high blood pressure
Angiotensin receptor	Losartan	High blood pressure, heart failure, chronic renal insufficiency
β-adrenoceptor receptor	Propranolol	Angina, myocardial infarction, heart failure, high blood pressure
Mineralocorticoid nuclear receptor	Spironolactone	Edema caused by liver cirrhosis and heart failure
Estrogen nuclear receptor	Tamoxifen	Prevention and treatment of breast cancer
Serotonin transporter	Fluoxetine	Depression
Histamine H_2 receptor	Cimetidine,[a] ranitidine[a]	Gastric acidity

[a]Inverse agonist.

the site of action. Over stimulation or prolonged blockade of receptors may be problematic. There are ways, however, to intercede in receptor function that allow for a more controlled and selective "tuning" of the action of a drug on a receptor. Allosteric modulation has long been recognized as a general and widespread mechanism for control of protein function. Allosteric modulators bind to regulatory sites distinct from the receptor's active site, resulting in conformational changes (such as R to R* or vice versa) that profoundly influence ligand binding and protein function. This concept has been studied intensively and is now considered an important mechanism to control protein behavior. For example, many enzymes contain allosteric regions separate from the substrate-binding site to which small, regulatory molecules (*effectors*) may bind and thereby affect the catalytic activity.

Allosteric agonists (or activators or enhancers) are drugs that enhance agonist affinity or action of the ligand while having no effect on their own. *Allosteric inverse agonists* reduce agonist affinity or action. *Allosteric antagonists* or *inhibitors* bind to an allosteric site without affecting the binding or function of the endogenous ligand but can still block the action of other allosteric modulators that act via the same allosteric site.

This concept underlies the mechanism of action of **allosteric modulators**, drugs that bind at an allosteric site and thereby modify the binding or action of the endogenous ligand at the primary binding site (Fig. 13.5). An example of an allosteric protein that is an important drug target is the GABA receptor–chloride ion channel complex. GABA is a neurotransmitter that, upon binding to the $GABA_A$ receptor, causes the chloride ion channels to open. Also present on this receptor–ion channel complex is a separate and distinct receptor called the benzodiazepine receptor. When a benzodiazepine such as diazepam (Valium®) binds to this site, it enhances the actions of GABA by modulating the ion channel to stay open longer. In the absence of GABA, diazepam has no effect on chloride ion channels. In this way, the allosteric effect of diazepam is to fine tune or adjust GABA-mediated effects but diazepam's actions are limited based on the availability and release of GABA.

Quantitation of Drug–Receptor Interactions

One of the major difficulties in measuring drug–receptor interactions is that the structure, characteristics, and concentrations of many receptors are still unknown or not

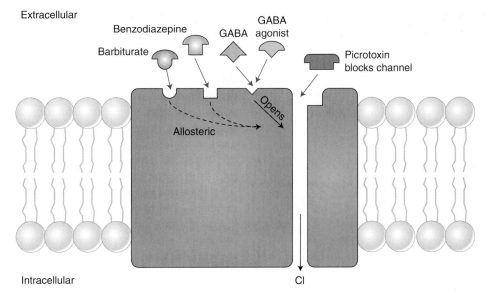

Figure 13.5. Mechanisms of allosteric and noncompetitive antagonism on the GABA receptor/chloride ion channel complex. The endogenous ligand GABA or a GABA agonist activates the receptor to open the Cl ion channel. Benzodiazepine agonists can produce a positive allosteric effect to enhance the ability of GABA to open the ion channel. Benzodiazapine inverse agonists can produce a negative allosteric effect to reduce the ability of GABA to open the ion channel. Picrotoxin is a noncompetitive antagonist. It blocks the Cl ion channel and prevents Cl ion entry even if GABA is present to open the ion channel. The benzodiazepine receptor, the picrotoxin binding site, and the GABA receptor are separate and distinct receptors located on this receptor–ion channel complex.

fully understood. Various empirical parameters and approaches are used to describe the interaction between drugs and receptors. These parameters have evolved over several decades, and each gives us different pieces of information. Modeling the actions of drugs and receptors in the ways outlined below is a powerful tool that allows us to better understand, analyze, and describe the actions of drugs. The concepts of affinity, intrinsic activity, and efficacy will help you to get a better picture of how drugs can act at receptors.

Affinity

The first step that a drug must complete in order to produce a pharmacological effect is to bind to its receptor. Affinity is a measure of a drug's ability to bind to a receptor. Affinity does not tell us about the action of the drug at the receptor, only whether or how well the drug can bind. Agonists, partial agonists, and antagonists all must have affinity for a receptor in order to produce its effects.

The affinity of a drug can be expressed in mathematical terms. Recall Eqn. 13.1 which describes the response of a drug as a function of it interacting with a receptor.

This concept of drug–receptor interaction is based on the Law of Mass Action which states that the rate of a chemical reaction is proportional to the concentrations of each reacting substance. This equation can be expressed as

$$[\text{Enzyme}] + [\text{Substrate}] \rightleftharpoons [\text{E} - \text{S}] \rightarrow \text{Product}$$

(Eq. 13.3)

Applying the Law of Mass Action to the drug–receptor interaction, we can slightly revise Eqn. 13.1 and then mathematically define the equilibrium constant for the "reaction" between a drug and its receptor where K_A is the association constant and K_D is the dissociation constant. [D] refers to the concentration of the free or unbound drug; [R] refers to the concentration of unbound receptors; [DR] refers to the concentration of drug–bound receptors.

$$[D] + [R] \underset{K_2}{\overset{K_1}{\rightleftharpoons}} [DR] \quad (Eq. 13.4)$$

$$K_A = \frac{k_1}{k_2} = \frac{[DR]}{[D][R]} \quad (Eq. 13.5)$$

$$K_D = \frac{1}{K_A} = \frac{[D][R]}{[DR]} \quad (Eq. 13.6)$$

Affinity, the ability of a drug to bind to its receptor, is more influenced by the "off rate" (k_2) than by the "on rate" (k_1). Therefore, K_D is the customary measure of affinity. The unit of measure for affinity is concentration such as μM. Based on these equations, we see that a drug with a strong affinity has a low K_D value. That is, a low concentration of the drug (or a small amount) is needed to bind to the receptor because its attraction to the receptor is great. If the drug has weak attraction for the receptor, then higher concentrations of the drug are needed and the drug, therefore, has a high K_D value.

When describing this relationship, the following assumptions are applied:

- All receptors are identical and equally accessible to the drug.
- One molecule occupies one receptor.
- The formation of the drug–receptor complex is reversible.
- The total amount of drug bound to receptor is negligible relative to the total amount of drug present. That is, [D] does not significantly decrease as [DR] is formed.

Occupation Theory

The occupation theory is based on the notion that a drug must bind to or occupy a receptor in order to produce its pharmacological or biological effect. Taking this reasoning further, the occupation theory also states that the magnitude of the pharmacological effect is directly proportional to the fraction of *occupied receptors*. The implications are that maximum drug effect occurs from the occupation of all possible receptors, 50% maximal effect results from occupation of 50% of the receptors, and so on. This theory is based on the following series of equations.

Assumption: The concentration of free or unbound receptors is equal to the concentration of total receptors minus the concentration of receptors bound to drug. $[R] = [R_T] - [DR]$

Substitute $[R_T] - [DR]$ for [R] in Eqn. 13.6

$$K_D = \frac{[D]([R_T] - [DR])}{[DR]} \quad (Eq. 13.7)$$

Multiply both sides by [DR]

$$K_D[DR] = [D][R_T] - [D][DR] \quad (Eq. 13.8)$$

Add [D][DR] to both sides and simplify

$$[DR](K_D + [D]) = [D][R_T] \quad (Eq. 13.9)$$

Rearrange the equation

$$\frac{[DR]}{[R_T]} = \frac{[D]}{K_D + [D]} \quad (Eq. 13.10)$$

In this equation $[DR]/[R_T]$ defines the fraction of receptors occupied by the drug. If the concentration of the drug at the receptors is equal to the K_D value for that drug, then, according to the equation, half of the receptors are occupied. Therefore, K_D is not only a measure of affinity but also defines the concentration of the drug needed to occupy half of the receptors. Note that Eqn. 13.10 is very similar to the Michaelis–Menten equation (Eqn. 13.11). Just as $K_M = \frac{1}{2}\ V_{max}$, $K_D = $ half the occupancy.

$$\frac{[V]}{[V_{max}]} = \frac{[S]}{K_M + [S]} \qquad \text{(Eq. 13.11)}$$

According to the occupation theory, the response is directly proportional to the fraction of receptors occupied. Using this reasoning, we substitute $[DR]/[R_T]$ with E/E_{max} in Eqn. 13.9 where E refers to the given effect and E_{max} is the maximal effect that can be attained when all receptors are occupied. From this, we can derive Eqn. 13.12.

$$E = E_{max}\frac{[D]}{K_D + [D]} \qquad \text{(Eq. 13.12)}$$

Eqn. 13.12 implies that at high drug concentrations, where [D] is much greater than K_D, and therefore, $K_D + [D]$ $\sim [D]$, E is essentially equal to E_{max}, suggesting that drugs produce maximum effect when all available receptors are fully occupied. However, this is not always the case. We have already seen in the previous chapter that the relationship between receptor binding and response can lead to a complex set of biochemical events involving G proteins, enzymes, and second messengers. Agonist–receptor binding is only the first step in a series of biochemical events that ultimately produce a pharmacological effect. A deficiency of the occupation theory is that it does not provide any information about the ability of the drug to produce a response after binding to the receptor. In particular, it cannot distinguish between full agonists, partial agonists, and antagonists, all of which can occupy receptors fully.

Two concepts—intrinsic activity and efficacy—were introduced to address shortcomings of the occupation theory.

Intrinsic Activity

It was postulated that two factors govern the effect of a drug: affinity and intrinsic activity. Affinity is a measure of drug–receptor binding as discussed above. Intrinsic activity (denoted by α) describes the ability of the drug to evoke a maximal effect upon binding to the receptor. Therefore, both agonists and antagonists have affinity for their receptors, but only agonists have intrinsic activity.

A full agonist, which by definition gives a maximum response when all receptors are occupied (because it binds preferentially to the R* form), is assigned an α value of 1. Partial agonists elicit less than maximal response even when all receptors are occupied (because they bind to both R and R* receptor forms), and have α values less than 1. Antagonists, which have no intrinsic activity (because they do not alter the equilibrium between R and R*), have an α value of 0.

It is proposed that drug effect (E) is related to intrinsic activity and the concentration of the drug–receptor complex is as follows:

$$E = \alpha[DR] \qquad \text{(Eq. 13.13)}$$

We can also say that

$$E = \alpha \cdot E_{max}\frac{[DR]}{R_T} \qquad \text{(Eq. 13.14)}$$

These equations indicate a linear relationship between drug effect E and *fractional receptor occupancy* $[DR]/[R_T]$, until $[DR]/[R_T] = 1$. This suggests that a full agonist ($\alpha = 1$) will exhibit maximal effect when all the receptors are occupied ($[DR] = [R_T]$). A partial agonist ($0 < \alpha < 1$) will not show maximum effect even when all receptors are occupied.

The assumption so far has been that the maximum effect requires the complete occupation of receptors. This, however, is not always the case. There are situations when two full agonists ($\alpha = 1$)

can elicit a maximum response ($E = E_{max}$) while occupying different fractions of the available receptors. That is, agonist A may be able to produce a maximal effect by occupying 40% of the receptors and agonist B requires 80% occupancy to achieve a maximal effect. This is thought to occur because the two agonists activate the receptors to different extents. Such a nonlinear relationship between drug effect and receptor occupancy cannot be explained by this approach.

Efficacy

It was postulated that occupancy of receptors by an agonist first produces a stimulus, S, in the receptor, and this stimulus eventually produces the effect E. The efficacy e of an agonist is a measure of how efficiently it stimulates the receptor; an agonist with a higher efficacy has the ability to produce a stronger stimulus. In molecular terms, the stimulus is a measure of the degree to which the agonist–receptor complex can assume its active conformation (DR*). Note that in this context, the term *efficacy* has a different meaning than in a clinical context, in which efficacy refers to how effectively the drug treats the disease or symptoms.

The concept of efficacy explains the apparent ability of agonists to give maximum effect while occupying different fractions of receptors. Different agonists may produce stimuli of different strengths even when they occupy the same fraction of receptors, resulting in different degrees of effect E. Conversely, two drugs can produce the same effect while occupying different fractions of receptors.

Expressing the concept of efficacy mathematically, we can write that the effect of an agonist is a function of the stimulus produced after drug–receptor binding

$$E = f(S) \qquad \text{(Eq. 13.15)}$$

where f is the function that converts receptor stimulus into response, E is the effect as before, and S is the stimulus. The strength of the stimulus depends on the efficacy e of the drug and on the receptor occupancy, as follows:

$$S = e \frac{[DR]}{[R_T]} \qquad \text{(Eq. 13.16)}$$

The definition of efficacy says that maximum effect can be observed when only a fraction of the receptors are occupied, provided the drug–receptor complex produces a strong enough stimulus. Thus, a highly efficacious drug can stimulate a maximum response while occupying only a small fraction of the receptors. Conversely, a drug with low efficacy may show a submaximal response even at 100% receptor occupancy because of a small stimulus.

Efficacy (e) and intrinsic activity (α) describe two approaches of explaining how a drug modulates pharmacological effect. Although these are two different concepts, they are often used interchangeably in the literature.

Spare Receptors

The above approaches show that the drug effect depends on the total number of occupied receptors. However, maximum effect is frequently seen before the drug occupies all available receptors. The excess receptor sites beyond that required for a maximum response are called spare receptors, or the *receptor reserve*, i.e., it is the fraction of receptors that are unoccupied by an agonist when the maximal agonist response is obtained.

We can better understand the concept of spare receptors using GPCRs as an example. One agonist-occupied GPCR can activate many G proteins. At a certain degree of receptor occupation all available G proteins in the cell are activated, and a further increase in the occupancy of GPCRs will not lead to a subsequent increase in G protein activation and pharmacological effect.

Thus, the spare receptor theory is a hypothesis to explain the particularly high efficiency of some receptor-modulated signaling pathways. The assumption is that spare receptors increase *sensitivity* to a drug, i.e., if a response is produced by occupancy of a certain number of receptors, increasing the number of available receptors allows the same response with a lower concentration of drug. This can be understood by referring to Eqn. 13.1; a higher concentration of receptors (and, therefore, R*) means that a lower concentration of D can give the same concentration of complex DR*.

Mechanisms of Antagonism

So far, we have mainly dealt with agonist drugs. However, receptor antagonists are very important in drug therapy. Antagonists are compounds that reduce or prevent the effect of agonists. They can be classified as

- Competitive antagonists
- Noncompetitive antagonists
- Functional antagonists
- Chemical antagonists

Competitive Antagonists

Competitive antagonists are compounds that have an affinity for and bind to the same receptor as the agonist. However, the antagonist does not have intrinsic activity and cannot generate a stimulus that leads to a biological response. One way to think of competitive antagonists is that they are "silent" ligands, i.e., agonists and antagonists bind to similar sites on the receptor, but whereas agonists stimulate a response, antagonists do not. According to the two-state receptor model, the lack of intrinsic activity of antagonists is a result of the antagonist having similar affinities for both the inactive (R) and active (R*) forms of the receptor. Thus the equilibrium between R and R* is not changed, and there is no "perceived" effect of the antagonist. Refer back to the models and equations that include intrinsic activity and efficacy and recall from Chapter 12 that a receptor consists of a binding domain and a signal transduction domain. Competitive antagonists have affinity; they bind to the same binding domain as the agonist. The competitive antagonist, because it does not bind to or interact with the signal transduction domain, lacks intrinsic activity or efficacy and is, therefore, unable to produce a stimulus or biological response. Figure 13.6 provides a simplified depiction of agonist and competitive antagonist binding.

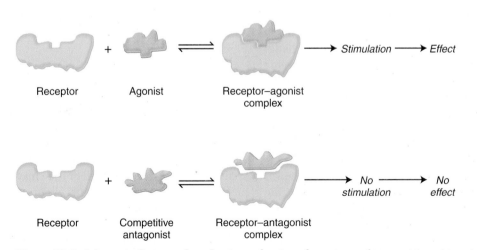

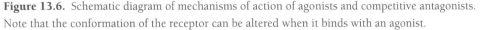

Figure 13.6. Schematic diagram of mechanisms of action of agonists and competitive antagonists. Note that the conformation of the receptor can be altered when it binds with an agonist.

Two important characteristics of competitive antagonism is that (1) the antagonist and the agonist compete with each other for the same receptor and (2) an antagonist does indirectly produce a biological response when it prevents the actions of an agonist such as an endogenous ligand or a drug. Because the competitive antagonist and the agonist are competing for the same site, the concentration of each drug and their relative affinities for the receptor are important considerations. In Chapter 14, we will provide a mathematical model describing the interactions between competitive agonists and antagonists. It is important to keep in mind that competitive antagonism can always be reversed by increased concentrations of the agonist; conversely, increasing the concentration of the antagonist drug relative to ligand will favor the antagonist binding with the receptor.

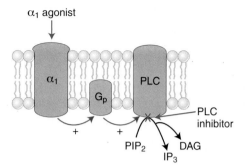

Figure 13.7. Mechanism for noncompetitive antagonism in drug–receptor interactions. The α agonist activates the α_1 receptor to activate a G protein leading to activation of phospholipase C (PLC). PLC catalyzes the conversion of phophatidyl inositol 4,5 bisphosphate (PIP_2) to the second messengers inositol triphosphate (IP_3) and diacyl glycerol (DAG). A drug that inhibits PLC will act as a noncompetitive antagonist to α_1 receptors. See Figure 13.5 for another mechanism for noncompetitive antagonist.

Noncompetitive Antagonists

A noncompetitive antagonist can reduce or prevent the activity of an agonist in one of several ways. As the name implies, noncompetitive antagonists do not compete with the agonist for the same binding site. They may act at other sites to impede the process somewhere in the chain of events that begins with activation of a receptor and ends with a biological response. For example, the antagonist may bind to an allosteric site on the same receptor, changing the conformation of the receptor site in a way that interferes with the binding of the agonist. This type of noncompetitive antagonism is called allosteric antagonism, discussed earlier in this chapter. Another way that a noncompetitive antagonist may exert its effect is by interfering with events after the agonist–receptor complex is formed, thereby interrupting the series of changes necessary to generate the biological response. For example, consider an endogenous ligand that interacts with a GPCR to increase synthesis of the second messenger diacyl glycerol

(DAG). A drug that blocks synthesis of the DAG would prevent the actions of the endogenous ligand in a noncompetitive manner. For noncompetitive antagonism, increasing the agonist concentration does not result in a reversal of the effects of the antagonist. The two agents are not competing for the same site and adding more agonist cannot change or alter how the noncompetitive antagonist binds or produces its effects. The mechanisms of noncompetitive antagonism are illustrated in Figure 13.7.

Functional Antagonists

Functional antagonists are actually agonists that produce effects that oppose one another. Usually, functional antagonists interact with different and independent receptor systems found on the same cell or they may produce opposing effects at the organ or systems level. For example, at the receptor/cellular level, isoproterenol, a β_1 receptor agonist, and methacholine, a muscarinic agonist, produce an increase and a decrease in heart rate, respectively. Stimulation of a β_1 receptor allows the receptor to interact with a G stimulatory protein which in turn activates the enzyme adenylate cyclase causing an increase in the second messenger cAMP. Stimulation of the M_2 muscarinic receptor allows the receptor to interact with a G inhibitory protein which in turn inhibits the enzyme adenylate cyclase causing a decrease in the second messenger cAMP in the same cardiac cell. Although working at different receptors, the two drugs' pathways converge within the cell to oppose one another. Other functional antagonists may work at separate organ systems (e.g., heart and blood vessels to control blood pressure) or at the same organ but at receptors that do not share a common signaling pathway (e.g., amphetamine as a stimulant and diazepam as a depressant of the central nervous system).

Chemical Antagonists

A chemical antagonist reacts with the agonist chemically to change its structure so that it cannot complex with the receptor, making the drug inactive. These types of antagonists actually decrease the concentration of the agonist at the receptor site, and are useful in treating overdoses and poisonings. An example is protamine sulfate, a chemical antagonist of the anticoagulant drug warfarin. Too much warfarin can cause excessive bleeding and hemorrhage. Protamine sulfate (a weak base) can bind to warfarin (a weak acid) in such a manner that does not allow heparin to bind to its receptor. The concept is not dissimilar to that of a competitive antagonist except that the target for the chemical antagonist is the drug and not the receptor. The end result is the reversal of warfarin's action.

Stereoselectivity in Drug Action

We have seen in Chapter 2 that the stereochemistry of a molecule has profound consequences on its ability to bind to the active site of proteins. This is particularly true in drug–receptor interactions, where several scenarios are possible with a chiral drug:

- *Enantiomer 1 is active; enantiomer 2 has the same activity:* There is little difference in anticonvulsant activity of the enantiomers of various barbiturates, or anticoagulant activity of the enantiomers of warfarin.
- *Enantiomer 1 is active; enantiomer 2 is inactive:* The profen class of nonsteroidal anti-inflammatory drugs (NSAIDs; e.g., ibuprofen, ketoprofen, and flurbiprofen), only the (S)-enantiomer has the desired activity.
- *Enantiomer 1 is an agonist; enantiomer 2 is an antagonist of the same receptor:* In dihydropyridines and dihydropyrimidones, the (R) enantiomers have the desired calcium channel antagonism, whereas the (S) enantiomers are calcium channel agonists.
- *Enantiomer 1 is active; enantiomer 2 has a separate, desirable activity:* In β-blockers, the (l) enantiomers block β-adrenergic receptors whereas the (−) enantiomers have beneficial effects on blood lipids.
- *Enantiomer 1 is active; enantiomer 2 is toxic:* Both enantiomers of bupivacaine have the same local anesthetic activity, but the (R) enantiomer is cardiotoxic.

The examples and observations given above are important on a number of levels. The activity, inactivity, or change in activity associated with different enantiomers can tell us a great deal about the function of these receptors in both normal conditions and in disease states. Very small changes in the receptor or ligand structure can result in significant changes in function. In addition, these observations demonstrate the difficulty and complexity associated with drug development. In order to enhance the efficacy and safety of many racemic drugs, the development of a single enantiomer rather than a racemate is the goal of drug research. Technology is now available to synthesize single enantiomers in a pure form on a large scale, and most new chiral drugs in development are being designed as single isomers. However, it is sometimes difficult to design a synthetic pathway to produce a single enantiomer; in such cases, the drug is first made as a racemate and then separated into enantiomers. One approach to avoiding the complication introduced by chiral drugs is to specifically design *achiral* drugs, compounds that do not have asymmetric centers. However, this approach may limit drug design and increase unwanted effects or toxicities.

Interaction of Drugs with Enzymes

Enzymes are proteins that catalytically change a substrate into a product by enhancing a chemical reaction. Cells in our bodies require hundreds of enzymes to carry out their normal functions, such as cell signaling (synthesis of neurotransmitters, hormones, and autacoids), metabolism (breakdown of fats, carbohydrates, and proteins for energy), and replication (transcription and translation). Malfunctions in these processes can lead to illness. Similarly, infectious bacteria require enzymes to survive and multiply. Many diseases and illnesses are treated by specifically interfering with the action of certain human or bacterial enzymes. Although enzyme activation could be exploited therapeutically, most effects are produced by enzyme inhibition.

Enzyme Inhibitors

An enzyme inhibitor is a compound that can bind to the enzyme and decrease or abolish its catalytic activity. Most inhibitors work either by decreasing the affinity of the enzyme for its natural substrate, by decreasing the amount of enzyme available for catalysis, or by a combination of both of these effects.

The first enzyme inhibitor drugs developed were antibacterial agents and antitumor agents whose goal was to inhibit cellular replication by blocking enzymes in pathways essential for cell growth. Drugs such as 5-fluorouracil (5FU) and 6-mercaptopurine (6MP) block enzymes involved in synthesis of pyrimidine and purine nucleotides, respectively, which are essential for DNA and RNA synthesis. Cephalosporins are effective antibiotics because they inhibit the enzyme associated with bacterial cell wall synthesis at a concentration that does not significantly affect human enzymes.

A large number of current drugs exert their action by inhibiting a target human enzyme. This becomes a useful approach for new drug design when the natural substrate of the enzyme is a beneficial substance that is depleted in a certain disease, or when the products of an enzymatic reaction are harmful.

Consider a disease that results from a deficiency of a certain compound, and that this compound is a substrate for the target enzyme. Using a drug that inhibits the target enzyme will slow or prevent the degradation of the substrate, thereby increasing its concentration and treating the disease. An example is Parkinson's disease, a condition that arises from low levels of dopamine in the brain. Inhibition of catechol-O-methyltransferase (COMT), an enzyme that degrades dopamine, is the mechanism of action of the anti-Parkinson drug tolcapone (Tasmar®).

Conversely, if an excess of a certain compound leads to disease, then inhibiting an enzyme that catalyzes its synthesis will be a useful approach. For example, angiotensin-converting enzyme (ACE) is an important target for antihypertensive drugs. Angiotensin I is converted by ACE to angiotensin II, which is responsible for increases in blood pressure. Inhibiting

ACE and thus lowering the concentration of angiotensin II reduces blood pressure. ACE inhibitors such as captopril, enalapril, and lisinopril are very effective antihypertensive drugs.

Enzyme inhibitors can be classified as reversible or irreversible.

Reversible Enzyme Inhibitors

Most inhibitors are reversible enzyme inhibitors, meaning that noncovalent interactions are involved in inhibitor–enzyme complex formation, and that the complex can subsequently dissociate. Reversible enzyme inhibitors can be further classified as *competitive* or *noncompetitive* depending on their mechanism of binding to the enzyme.

Competitive Enzyme Inhibitors

Competitive inhibitors bind at the same enzyme active site as the natural substrate. The inhibitor and substrate can therefore displace each other from the binding site depending on their relative affinities and concentrations. Such inhibitors are highly specific for a particular enzyme and have a structure similar to either the substrate or product of the target enzyme. Most enzyme inhibitor drugs are *competitive and reversible.*

Binding of an enzyme E to its substrate S and reversible competitive inhibitor I can be represented by the following set of equations:

$$E + S \rightleftarrows ES \rightarrow \text{Product}$$
$$E + I \rightleftarrows EI \rightarrow \text{No product}$$

(Eq. 13.17)

The free enzyme is capable of reacting with the substrate to give an ES complex, or with the inhibitor to give an EI complex. The ES complex can continue on to form the desired product whereas the EI complex cannot.

Recall that the rate of an enzymatic reaction for converting a substrate to product is mathematically described by the Michaelis–Menten equation:

$$V = \frac{V_{max}[S]}{K_m + [S]} \quad \text{(Eq. 13.18)}$$

and that the affinity, K, of the enzyme for the substrate is given by

$$K = \frac{1}{K_m} = \frac{[ES]}{[E][S]} \quad \text{(Eq. 13.19)}$$

The presence of a competitive inhibitor blocks the active site on some enzyme molecules and therefore decreases the concentration of the [ES] complex. This lowers the apparent affinity of the enzyme for substrate, increasing K_m. V_{max} can still be attained, although a higher concentration of substrate will be needed to achieve this.

Generally, a competitive inhibitor merely binds at the enzyme's active site without further reaction. However, in some cases, the competitive inhibitor may be an alternative substrate for the enzyme and is converted to alternative products after binding to the enzyme.

A reversible inhibitor, whether competitive or noncompetitive, is effective only as long as its concentration at the site of action remains high enough to prevent the enzyme–substrate complex from forming. Thus, additional doses of the inhibitor are necessary to maintain the pharmacological effect.

The sulfonamides, a class of antibacterial drugs, are good examples of competitive enzyme inhibitors. Sulfonamides specifically inhibit the enzyme dihydropteroate synthetase, which is responsible for biosynthesis of tetrahydrofolate, a compound necessary for the replication of bacteria. Thus, sulfonamides are bacteriostatic and are used to treat bacterial infections.

Another example is the group of statin drugs (lovastatin, mevastatin, and simvastatin) that are competitive inhibitors of the enzyme 3-hydroxy-3-methylglutaryl coenzyme A (HMG-CoA) reductase, one of the enzymes that catalyze cholesterol biosynthesis. Inhibition of this enzyme results in a decrease in cholesterol biosynthesis in the body and lowers plasma cholesterol levels.

Noncompetitive Enzyme Inhibitors

Noncompetitive enzyme inhibitors usually bind at an allosteric site on the enzyme, different from the active site where the substrate binds. These inhibitors are generally structurally unrelated to the substrate, but their binding results in a conformational change in the active site so that it can no longer bind effectively with the substrate to convert it to the product. The substrate and inhibitor are capable of binding to the enzyme at the same time to create a ternary complex, but this complex is inactive. This is illustrated in Figure 13.8. Noncompetitive inhibition can be represented by the following set of equations:

$$E + I \rightleftarrows EI$$
$$EI + S \rightleftarrows EI \rightarrow \text{No product}$$
$$E + S \rightleftarrows ES \rightarrow \text{Product} \quad \text{(Eq. 13.20)}$$
$$ES + I \rightleftarrows EIS \rightarrow \text{No product}$$

Notice that the enzyme–inhibitor–substrate (EIS) complex can be produced by two routes, but the final result is the same—an inactive complex and no product formation.

The rate of enzyme catalysis is decreased because the catalytic site is influenced by the inhibitor. V_{max} is thus reduced, but because the binding site is not affected, K_m remains unchanged. Because binding occurs at different sites on the enzyme, an excess of substrate cannot displace noncompetitive inhibitors, and thus substrate concentration does not influence the degree of inhibition.

Irreversible Enzyme Inhibitors

Most interactions between an enzyme and substrate are reversible in that the enzyme remains unchanged after the reaction and is available to bind to more substrate molecules. If the interaction of an inhibitor with the enzyme is of a covalent nature, the compound is called an irreversible enzyme inhibitor or enzyme inactivator; an example of this is shown in Figure 13.9. Irreversible inhibitors can sustain their action for a long time because they do not dissociate from the

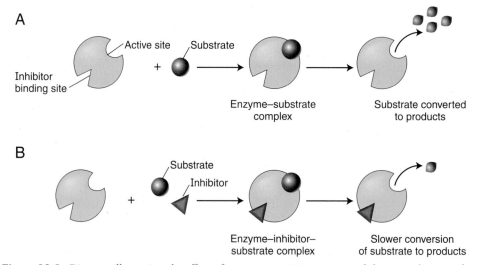

Figure 13.8. Diagram illustrating the effect of a noncompetitive enzyme inhibitor on the rate of an enzymatic reaction. A. Reaction without inhibitor. B. Reaction with inhibitor.

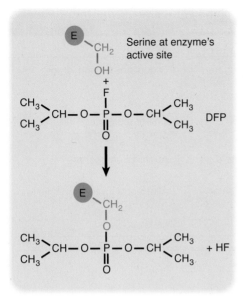

Figure 13.9. Example of covalent bond formation between an enzyme and an irreversible inhibitor. The reaction shown is of the competitive irreversible inhibitor, diisopropyl fluorophosphate (DFP), which can react with serine groups at the active site of an enzyme to form a covalent adduct.

enzyme. However, this does not mean that additional doses of inhibitor are not needed. As the enzyme loses activity, the body synthesizes more molecules of the enzyme, requiring more inhibitor to sustain the action. Synthesis of new molecules of the enzyme can take hours or days, so that the effect of such an inhibitor is of long duration.

Many poisons are harmful to cells because they are potent irreversible inhibitors and denature the enzyme. Examples are heavy metals (mercury, lead, and arsenic) and cyanide.

Many drugs also work by irreversible enzyme inhibition. A familiar example is aspirin's irreversible inhibition of the enzyme prostaglandin synthetase. Antimicrobial drugs such as antibiotics are irreversible enzyme inhibitors as well; for example, penicillins bind to and inactivate the bacterial enzyme transpeptidase, an essential enzyme for synthesis of bacterial cell walls. Other irreversible inhibitors such as the nitrogen mustards are used in anticancer therapy.

Selectivity of Enzyme Inhibition

Selectivity in enzyme inhibition is desirable so that beneficial effects are not accompanied by unwanted side effects. As scientists continue to learn more about enzyme activity and structure, the design of more specific inhibitors becomes possible. Both reversible and irreversible enzyme inhibitors can be made selective. A good example of improving selectivity is seen in the class of drugs called NSAIDs. These drugs were known to be effective analgesics before the discovery that they worked by inhibiting cyclooxygenase (COX), a component involved in the production of prostaglandins. These ligands cause the pain and swelling of arthritis.

However, all NSAIDs also caused disruption of the gastric mucosa, resulting in severe gastric side effects and bleeding. Scientists later discovered that there are two forms of COX: COX-1, which is primarily responsible for unwanted effects on the stomach, kidney function, and platelet aggregation, and COX-2, which is responsible for fever, pain, and swelling. These enzymes are about 60% homologous.

Older NSAIDs (aspirin, ibuprofen, and naproxen) inhibited both COX-1 and COX-2 and therefore had serious side effects such as gastric bleeding, and kidney and liver toxicity. Selective COX-2 inhibitors such as celecoxib (Celebrex®) and rofecoxib (Vioxx®) were then found by selective screening. These drugs are effective COX-2 inhibitors without anti-COX-1 activity. New data indicate an increased risk of major fatal and nonfatal heart attacks in

TABLE 13.3. Comparison of Terms and Events in Enzymatic and Receptor Processes

Event	Enzyme	Receptor
Compound bound at active site	Endogenous substrate, drug	Endogenous ligand, drug
Complex	ES or ED	LR or DR
Number of binding sites	One or more sites	One or more sites
Binding affinity	K_m	K_d
Molecules that also bind to protein	Activators, inhibitors	Agonists, antagonists
Regulation	Allosteric activation or inhibition	Allosteric activation or inhibition
Outcome	Product formed	Response

ED, enzyme–drug; ES, enzyme–substrate; K_m, Michaelis constant; K_d, dissociation constant; DR, drug–receptor; LR, ligand–receptor.

clinical trial participants taking COX-2 inhibitors. Rofecoxib has been withdrawn from the market, and celecoxib is to be used with utmost caution.

Similarities Between Receptors and Enzymes

Whether a drug works by binding to a cellular receptor or an enzyme, there are many similarities in the principles of binding and processes that affect the function of the protein. These similarities are summarized in Table 13.3.

Nonreceptor-Based Drug Action

Not all drugs act on discrete receptors or at active sites of specific enzymes in the body. Some drugs act extracellularly, and their actions are aimed at noncellular constituents of the body. Still other drugs may act at cellular sites or at membranes, but their actions are primarily the result of their physicochemical properties rather than a specific interaction with a receptor or enzyme. These types of drugs are said to work by *nonspecific* mechanisms of action. There are several examples that fit into this category. Gastrointestinal drugs, such as antacids, laxatives, and cathartics, have nonspecific actions in the gastrointestinal tract. Blood plasma substitutes are macromolecules used in cases of blood loss. Various agents applied to the skin such as sunscreens also fall into this group.

The activity of many nonspecific drugs is related to their physicochemical properties. For example, one theory describing how inhalation anesthetics with a variety of chemical structures (nitrous oxide and various organic volatile substances such as chloroform and ether) all produce similar actions on the brain is by dissolving in the lipid bilayer of neurons and altering ion channel function. Chemical disinfectants and germicides act by nonspecifically destroying living membranes and tissue. These actions are irreversible and the functional integrity of the cells is permanently destroyed. In all these cases, activity can be correlated with the physicochemical properties of the drug rather than through an action at the receptor.

Key Concepts

- Drugs either enhance the natural activity of a ligand (agonists) or reduce it (antagonists, inhibitors). A few drugs work by nonspecific mechanisms that do not require binding to a receptor or enzyme.
- Agonists interact with the active receptor state to stimulate an effect characteristic of that receptor. Full agonists have a greater selectivity for the active receptor form, whereas partial agonists have a smaller selectivity for the active receptor and show a lesser effect than a full agonist.
- Competitive antagonists compete with agonists for the same receptor depending on their relative concentrations and affinities; competitive antagonism can be reversed by excess agonist.
- Noncompetitive antagonists reduce the effect of an agonist by binding at an allosteric site or by interfering in signal transduction. This antagonism cannot be reversed by excess agonist.

- The intensity of a drug effect can be characterized by several factors such as affinity, intrinsic activity, and efficacy. Each measures, in different ways, how a drug modulates pharmacological effect.
- Enzyme inhibitors decrease the target enzyme's activity either by reducing the affinity of the enzyme for its natural substrate or by reducing the amount of enzyme available for catalysis, or a combination of both.
- Competitive enzyme inhibitors bind at the same enzyme active site as the natural substrate; this inhibition can be reversed by excess substrate. Noncompetitive enzyme inhibitors bind at an allosteric site on the enzyme; this inhibition cannot be reversed by excess substrate. Irreversible enzyme inhibitors generally work by binding covalently to and inactivating the enzyme.

Review Questions

1. How do agonists, antagonists, partial agonists, and inverse agonists differ in their interactions with receptors?
2. Explain the occupation theory of receptors. What are its deficiencies? How are these addressed by the concepts of intrinsic activity?
3. Describe how the concepts of stimulus and efficacy explain the ability of drugs to give maximum effect while occupying different fractions of receptors.
4. How do competitive and noncompetitive antagonists work? What are the differences in their mechanisms?
5. How can drug administration cause upregulation or downregulation of receptors? What are the consequences?
6. Explain how enzyme inhibitors work as drugs.
7. Distinguish between the mechanisms of binding and action of competitive, noncompetitive, and irreversible enzyme inhibitors.
8. Elaborate on nonspecific mechanisms of drug action.

CASE STUDY 13.1

Running with β-blockers

LT is a 45-year-old male. Despite being an avid runner and possessing a body mass index in the normal range, he has high blood pressure (160/110) and normal resting heart rate (70). He was prescribed the selective β_1 receptor antagonist metoprolol.

After 4 weeks on the drug, his blood pressure was in the normal range and resting heart rate was 40. LT complained that during his runs he felt very fatigued and did not seem to have the same endurance. Over the course of the next 8 weeks, the physician worked with a pharmacist to alter the dosing of metoprolol. Lowering the dose helped reduce LT's fatigue but the drug no longer provided an appropriate control of blood pressure.

The pharmacist suggested changing to labetalol (Normodyne®), a nonselective β receptor antagonist with partial agonist activity. After 4 weeks of therapy, LT's blood pressure was in the normal range and resting heart rate was 70.

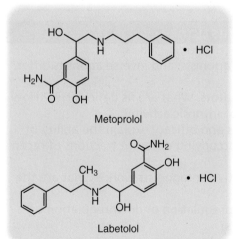

Metoprolol

Labetolol

1. Why is a selective β_1 receptor antagonist potentially a better drug than a nonselective β receptor antagonist? Do selective antagonists block the receptor better?

2. Labetalol is said to have intrinsic sympathomimetic activity (ISA). Explain how the terms ISA and partial agonist represent the same concept.

3. Explain how affinity and efficacy are similar or different when comparing metoprolol, labetalol, and the endogenous ligand norepinephrine.

4. In this case, the partial agonist labetalol lowered LT's resting heart rate. How did it do that?

5. Labetalol is classified as having low lipophilicity and metoprolol as having moderate lipophilicity. What advantages and disadvantages are associated with changes in lipophilicity?

6. LT claimed that metoprolol caused a decline in his running performance. Is this possible? Explain why or why not. Based on the principles of competitive antagonism, could he overcome this?

7. Long-term use of antagonists can alter receptor number or density. If LT were to use metoprolol for several months and then abruptly stop taking metoprolol, how would this affect his heart rate? Would this effect be similar with long term use and then abrupt withdrawal of labetalol?

Additional Readings

Brunton L, Lazo J, Parker K (eds). Goodman & Gilman's The Pharmacological Basis of Therapeutics, 11th ed. McGraw-Hill Professional, 2005.

Harvey RA, Champe PC, Finkel R, Cubeddu L. Lippincott's Illustrated Reviews: Pharmacology, 4th ed. Lippincott Williams & Wilkins, 2008.

Katzung BG (ed). Basic and Clinical Pharmacology, 11th ed. McGraw-Hill/Appleton & Lange, 2009.

Rang HP, Dale MM. Rang and Dale's Pharmacology, 5th ed. Churchill Livingstone, 2003.

CHAPTER 14

Dose–Response Relationships

We now understand the mechanisms by which drugs work at the molecular level in the body. This mechanistic knowledge must be translated into practical concepts for effective drug therapy. In particular, clinicians should be able to compare various drugs in terms of their effectiveness, selectivity, and safety, and to understand how these parameters are related to the dose of the drug. It is also important to know how to adjust the drug dose in a particular patient to achieve efficacy without toxicity. Understanding the relationship of response to dose is one of the most challenging tasks in new drug development.

In Chapter 13, we learned that most drugs work by binding to receptors or enzymes, and that the response is related to the concentration of drug available at the active site of the target protein. Let us proceed from there to understand the relationship between the dose of a drug and the response it generates.

Concentration–Response Relationships

Using the concepts discussed earlier, we can describe a concentration–effect relationship for the interaction of an agonist and antagonist (or inhibitor) with a receptor. Most of these relationships are derived from in vitro experiments on enzymes, cells, and isolated organs, in which it is possible to know the precise concentration of the drug at the active site. Later in the chapter, we will discuss dose response curves as they relate to studies in animals and humans.

Binding and Response Curves

Figure 14.1 shows a *concentration–effect* or *concentration–response* curve for a full agonist and a partial agonist acting at the same receptor. To generate such a curve, a known amount or concentration of a single drug is placed in an in vitro experimental system (such as a tissue bath, cell culture, or well plate) and a measurement is taken such as contraction of a muscle, release of a signaling molecule, or phosphorylation of a protein. The experiment is repeated several times using multiple concentrations of the drug in order to demonstrate a range of effects from very small responses to the maximal response. The dose, expressed as concentration, is the independent variable and is plotted on the horizontal or x-axis. The effect (E/E_{max}) is the dependent variable and is plotted on the vertical or y-axis. Concentration–response

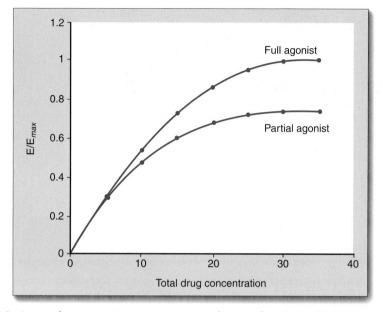

Figure 14.1. A typical concentration–response curve showing the relationship between total drug concentration and the fractional response (E/E_{max}) for a full and partial agonist at a receptor site.

curves are usually governed by the following equation, which was introduced in Chapter 13:

$$E = \alpha \cdot E_{\text{max}} \frac{[DR]}{[R_T]} \qquad \text{(Eq. 14.1)}$$

In addition to the concentration–response curve, we can also generate concentration-binding curves, which share similarities to the concentration–response curves. Recall that an agonist and a competitive antagonist for a given receptor will bind at the same site on the receptor. Both drugs have affinity for the receptor but only the agonist has efficacy, which allows it to cause a change in receptor conformation to produce a change in cell activity. The antagonist does not have efficacy and therefore cannot directly alter cell activity. Therefore, because an antagonist cannot produce a change in cell activity, we measure its "effect" based on its ability to bind to or occupy receptors at different concentrations. A concentration–response curve measures the fraction or percent of the maximal response, corresponding to

E/E_{max}. A concentration-binding curve measures the fraction or percentage of the total number of receptors bound that corresponds to $[DR]/[R_T]$. Concentration-binding curves provide important information when describing the selectivity of a drug for a particular receptor. The concept of selectivity will be discussed later in this chapter.

Notice a few important and interesting details of the concentration–response curves shown in Figure 14.1.

• At low doses the curve is very steep. Small changes in the concentration produce large changes in the response making it almost impossible to use the graph to accurately match the concentration with the effect.

• At high doses, when the effect is approaching maximal, the problem is the opposite. Large changes in the concentration produce very small changes in the response, making it difficult to evaluate.

• The relationship between the concentration and the response is not proportional, i.e., the concentration needed for 100%

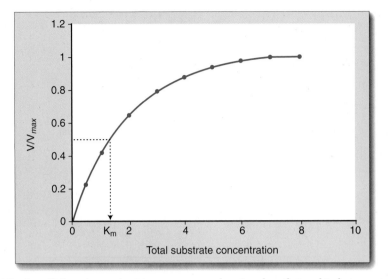

Figure 14.2. A typical concentration–response curve showing the relationship between total substrate concentration and the fractional response (V/V_{max}). The Michaelis constant (K_m) is the substrate concentration at which the rate of the reaction is 50%.

response is not double the concentration for 50% response, it is much larger. As noted earlier, the initially steep concentration–response curve accounts for a significant portion of the effect.

- The catalytic response of an enzyme–substrate interaction shown in Figure 14.2 is very similar to the graphs depicting concentration–response and concentration-binding curves. Thus, our discussion earlier about agonists applies to substrates of enzymes as well.

Logarithm Scales

Concentration–response curves are better and more commonly represented with the *logarithm* of the drug concentration on the x-axis, because this allows a broader range of agonist concentrations to be shown. When plotted in this manner, as in Figure 14.3 for an agonist, a sigmoid or S-shaped log concentration–response curve with a center of symmetry at 50% response is obtained. This midpoint represents the concentration that gives 50% of the maximum response and is called the median effective concentration (EC_{50}). Another advantage of using

a logarithmic concentration scale is that the curve is essentially linear around the EC_{50} (between about 20% and 80% maximal response), making mathematical analysis easier. Therefore, at intermediate agonist concentrations there is a linear relationship between relative response and log concentration. The slope is the highest in this region of the curve, and small changes in agonist concentration can produce large changes in response.

The same type of sigmoid curve is obtained for enzyme–substrate systems; here, V/V_{max} is plotted against the logarithm of the substrate concentration. The midpoint concentration of this curve, representing 50% maximum response, is K_m.

The concentrations of endogenous ligands in the body usually lie near the EC_{50} or K_m of the drug–protein interaction, i.e., in the linear portion of the concentration–response curve. By making small changes in ligand concentration, the body can precisely control cellular behavior.

Antagonists and Inhibitors

In Chapter 13, we discussed the mechanism of action of antagonists and inhibitors.

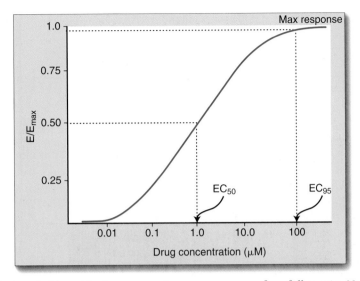

Figure 14.3. A typical logarithmic concentration–response curve for a full agonist. Note the logarithmic x-axis and the characteristic sigmoid shape of the curve. The EC_{50} is the drug concentration that gives 50% maximal response ($E/E_{max} = 0.50$). Also note the linearity of the curve between approximately 20% and 80% maximal response.

Antagonists are drugs that reduce or prevent the effect of agonists at a receptor. Enzyme inhibitors are drugs that prevent or decrease the rate of the reaction converting substrates to products. In general, antagonists and inhibitors can be classified into two categories: competitive and noncompetitive. *Competitive* antagonists or competitive inhibitors have affinity for and bind to the same site on the target protein as the agonist (substrate). The agonist and competitive antagonist compete for the same active site, and can displace each other from the site depending on their relative concentrations and affinities. On the other hand, *noncompetitive* antagonists or inhibitors usually bind to an allosteric site on the target protein; a site different and distinct from the site the agonist binds.

Competitive Binding

Figure 14.4 shows the concentration-effect curve for an agonist (or substrate) in the absence and presence of two different concentrations of a competitive antagonist (or inhibitor). In the absence of the antagonist (curve 0), the agonist produces a maximal effect of 1.0 and has an EC_{50} value of 1.0 μM. That is, it produces a half maximal effect at a concentration of 1 μM. In the presence of a low concentration of the competitive antagonist (curve 1), the concentration of the agonist needed to produce a response is greater, although, if enough agonist is given, the same maximal effect can be produced. When an even higher concentration of the competitive antagonist is given (curve 2), the curve shifts further to the right but the same maximal response can be obtained by increasing the amount of agonist present.

Three important points can be determined from this series of concentration–effect curves:

1. Competitive antagonists produce a change in the apparent K_d (or the EC_{50}). Just as in enzyme kinetics when a competitive inhibitor changes the apparent K_m, a competitive antagonist changes the apparent K_d, the concentration at which half of the receptors are occupied, which correlates to the EC_{50}.

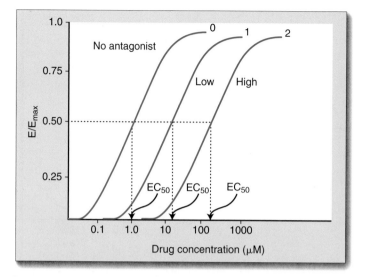

Figure 14.4. Concentration–response curve for a full agonist in the absence and presence of a competitive antagonist. Curve 0 shows the relationship when no antagonist is present. Curves 1 and 2 show the shift in the relationship in the presence of low and high concentrations of the competitive antagonist respectively. Note there are changes in the EC_{50} values but no changes in the E/E_{max} values.

2. Competitive antagonists do not produce a change in the maximal effect. The same E_{max} can be obtained with a competitive antagonist. If enough agonist is given, it can eventually out compete the antagonist for binding at the active site and produce the full effect.

3. Competitive antagonists produce a parallel shift to the right in the concentration–effect curves. The slope of the curves remains the same as the mechanism of the drug–receptor interaction is not altered by the competitive antagonist.

Because competition between agonist and antagonist depends on their relative concentrations and affinities for the receptor, the shift to the right is greater for an antagonist present at a higher concentration, or with a greater affinity. The extent of this shift is a useful way of comparing antagonists and is best expressed as a *concentration ratio.* This is the factor by which the agonist concentration must be increased to restore the original response in the presence of an antagonist. This also

illustrates the concept that the effect of a competitive antagonist can be reversed by high agonist concentrations.

The same discussion holds true for enzyme substrates and their competitive inhibitors.

Noncompetitive Binding

Figure 14.5 shows concentration–response curves for an agonist in the absence and presence of different concentrations of a noncompetitive antagonist. In the absence of the antagonist (curve 0), the agonist produces a maximal effect of 1.0 and has an EC_{50} value of 1 μM. In the presence of a low concentration of the noncompetitive antagonist (curve 1), the curve is shifted down and to the right. The maximal effect is reduced; no matter how much more agonist is added. When a higher concentration of the noncompetitive antagonist is used (curve 2), the E_{max} is further reduced.

Three important points can be determined from this series of concentration–effect curves:

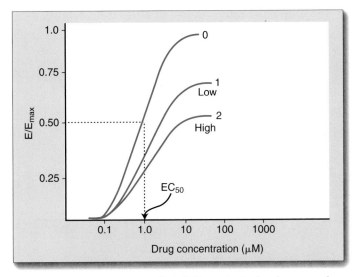

Figure 14.5. Concentration–response curve for a full agonist in the absence and presence of a noncompetitive antagonist. Curve 0 shows the profile when no antagonist is present. Curves 1 and 2 show the shift in the curve in the presence of low and high concentrations of the noncompetitive antagonist respectively. Note there are no changes in the EC_{50} values but the E/E_{max} values change.

1. Noncompetitive antagonists do not produce a change in the apparent K_d (or the EC_{50}). As shown in Figure 14.5, the EC_{50} is not changed in the presence of a noncompetitive antagonist—similar to an unchanging K_m associated with noncompetitive enzyme inhibitors. (Note: the determination of the EC_{50} is based on the E_{max} associated with the agonist + noncompetitive antagonist curve and not the original E_{max} associated with the agonist alone.)
2. Noncompetitive antagonists produce a change in the maximal effect. The agonist and the noncompetitive antagonist do not compete for the same site. As a result, not matter how much agonist is added to the system, it cannot overcome the antagonism or inhibition caused by the antagonist.
3. Noncompetitive antagonists produce a downward and rightward shift in the concentration–effect curves. The slopes of the curves change because the mechanism of the drug–receptor interaction is altered by the noncompetitive antagonist.

Irreversible Binding

In Chapter 13, we introduced the concept of spare receptors—a maximal response can occur with only a fraction of all receptors occupied. It is hypothesized to occur in certain receptor systems that have a very efficient coupling mechanism between the receptor and the intracellular signaling pathway. If we were to construct a series of concentration–effect curves in this type of system using an antagonist that binds to and forms a covalent bond (in effect, irreversible) at the active site, we would see a series of curves as shown in Figure 14.6. In the presence of a low concentration of an irreversible receptor antagonist (curve 1), the curve is shifted to the right in a parallel fashion, suggesting a competitive interaction. In a system without spare receptors, we would predict the curve to be shifted downward as well as to the right. (Even though the antagonist is binding at the same site as the agonist, the interaction is regarded as noncompetitive because the covalent bond formed between the antagonist and

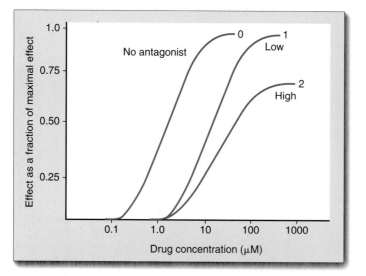

Figure 14.6. Concentration–response curve for a full agonist in the absence and presence of an irreversible noncompetitive antagonist. Curve 0 shows the profile when no antagonist is present. Curve 1 depicts the effect of an irreversible inhibitor in a system with spare receptors. Curve 2 depicts the effect of adding more irreversible inhibitor resulting in depletion of spare receptors.

the receptor does not allow the antagonist to dissociate from the receptor making it impossible for the agonist to displace it.) In a system with spare receptors, the curve is consistent with competitive inhibition because even with the reduced number of receptors, there are still an adequate number of receptors (spare receptors) available to produce the maximal effect. As the dose of the irreversible antagonist is increased (curve 2), enough receptors are now blocked to not allow a full response. The curve now reflects noncompetitive antagonism.

Dose–Response Relationships

When dealing with animals or humans, the exact concentration of drug at the receptor is not known. However, this concentration is related to the dose of drug administered; the higher the dose administered, the greater the concentration at the receptor. Therefore, if the drug dose is known and the pharmacological response can be measured, a *dose–response* or *dose–effect relationship* can be established. Dose–

response relationships are a common way to portray data in both experimental and clinical sciences.

From discussions in earlier chapters we know that drug dose is only one of the factors that determine concentration of drug at the receptor active site, and subsequent pharmacological response. The drug's absorption, distribution, metabolism, and excretion (ADME) behavior is also important; ADME determines drug plasma concentration, which in turn affects concentration at the receptor (site of action) and in other tissues. Thus, the same dose of drug administered by a different route, or by different formulations with the same route, can give varying pharmacological responses.

In Chapter 11, we examined the relationship between plasma concentration and response. In most situations, a higher dose of drug gives a proportionately higher plasma concentration (up to a limit), all other conditions being the same. It is in this context that one should understand the discussion of dose–response relationships.

A dose–response curve (DRC) is usually constructed using the *logarithm* of

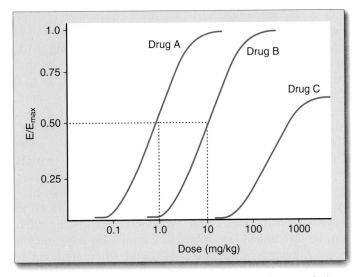

Figure 14.7. A typical graded dose–response curve for three drugs (A, B, and C) acting at the same receptor. The dose is expressed as milligram per kilogram of body weight. Note the logarithmic x-axis and the sigmoid shape of the curve. Drug A is 10 times more potent than drug B. Drug C is less potent than drug A or B. Both drug A and drug B reach the same maximal effect and have the same efficacy, whereas the efficacy of drug C is lower than that of drug A or B.

the dose on the x-axis. The y-axis shows the response, presented either as intensity of effect in a graded DRC, or as frequency of effect in a quantal DRC.

Graded Dose–Response Curves

A graded dose–response curve is useful in representing the dose–effect relationship in an individual. The assumptions are that the response varies continuously with dose and that a higher dose gives a greater response. An example is shown in Figure 14.7; note that the graded DRC is sigmoid with a center of symmetry at 50% response. The threshold dose is defined as the lowest dose that produces a measurable response. The slope of the curve near its center of symmetry also has significance; a steep slope shows that a small increase in dose produces a large increase in response.

Potency, Affinity, and Efficacy

The potency of a drug is the dose needed to produce a certain defined response. The response could be a variety of measurements ranging from the cellular level (change in membrane voltage) to the systems level (change in blood pressure). Affinity is a measure of the drug's ability to bind to a receptor. It is measured in vitro and is expressed as the K_d. Both measures are useful parameters that allow comparisons of different drugs that act at the same target site. The smaller the dose required to produce the defined effect, the more potent the drug; alternatively, the more potent the drug, the less of it is required to produce a given effect. Potency is, therefore, related to the affinity of a drug for the receptor; the greater the affinity, typically the more potent the drug.

When administering a drug to an individual, potency also depends on how much of the dose reaches the receptor after administration. The fraction of the dose that arrives at the receptor site depends on the drug's ADME behavior. Thus, a drug with the greatest affinity in vitro may not be the most potent because less of it may reach the receptor site due to ADME processes. Moreover, differences in ADME are often responsible for variability in potency of the same drug in different individuals.

Efficacy, on the other hand, is a measure of the maximum response a drug can produce regardless of the dose, and is often related to the intrinsic activity of the drug; drugs with high intrinsic activity usually give a greater maximal efficacy. This parameter is also useful in comparing two drugs with the same action.

The potency of agonists can be compared by their position on the x-axis, and their efficacy can be determined from the maximum response exhibited, by the position on the y-axis. For example, Figure 14.7 shows that

- Drug A has a higher potency than drugs B or C.
- Drug B has the same maximal effect as drug A but is less potent.
- Drug C will never achieve the efficacy of drug A, even at high doses.

Potency is useful in determining drug doses when changing from one drug to another, but does not provide any information about effectiveness or safety. Thus, the most potent drug may not necessarily be the best drug. Potency is clinically important only when drugs are very potent (difficult to administer safely because very small changes in the dose can cause very large changes in the effects) or very weak (difficult to administer conveniently because the tablet or capsule may be too large to take). Efficacy is more important than potency for therapy because it focuses on the effectiveness of a drug rather than on the size of the dose.

Quantal Dose–Response Curves

Not all patients respond to a drug in the same way or to the same extent. Very few individuals show the desired effect at low doses, whereas almost all show the

desired effect at very high doses. This illustrates the problem of *biological variability* when dealing with individuals. The variability may be the result of differences in receptors or in the amount of drug reaching the receptor site, or some other reason. We shall discuss the various factors responsible for this behavior in Chapter 15.

To measure this variability in individual dose–response, the DRC can be constructed to show the *frequency* of a certain response (e.g., the number of individuals exhibiting a defined response to a minimum dose) on the y-axis. This is useful when studying the effect of a drug on a patient population rather than in an individual patient. For such analysis, the response needs to be well defined, both qualitatively and quantitatively. This is because the measurement of response is *quantal*, not continuously variable; the patient either shows the defined response or does not, such as falling asleep or lowering blood pressure by 10 mmHg.

To obtain these data, the population is given increasing drug doses until virtually all patients respond. In essence, one is finding the threshold dose for each individual in the group. The graphs are usually bell-shaped, following a Gaussian or normal distribution as shown in Figure 14.8. This type of curve, called a quantal dose–response curve, is useful in describing the DRC in a group of subjects.

Another way of showing quantal dose–response is to plot the data as the *cumulative* frequency responding to a certain dose, illustrated in Figure 14.9. As the dose is increased more individuals exhibit the defined effect; all individuals show the response at the highest dose. Notice that we again have a sigmoid curve with a center of symmetry at 50% response. The dose at the center of symmetry of a cumulative quantal DRC is called the ED_{50} or the *median effective dose*. The ED_{50} is defined as the dose that produces the desired effect in half of the individuals studied.

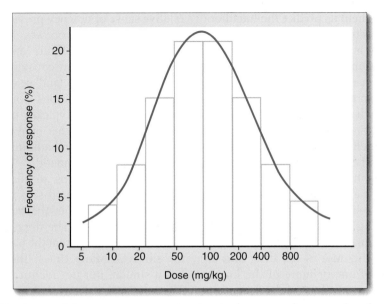

Figure 14.8. A quantal dose–response curve showing the frequency of response (number of patients responding) as a function of the minimum dose administered.

One way to compare the potency of two drugs that produce the same response is to compare their ED_{50} values; the lower the value, the more potent the drug. Similarly, we can define ED_{95} as the dose at which 95% of individuals show an effect, and so on.

Dose-Related Selectivity and Toxicity

DRCs and concentration-binding curves can be used to determine the selectivity of a drug for a receptor or an effect. These

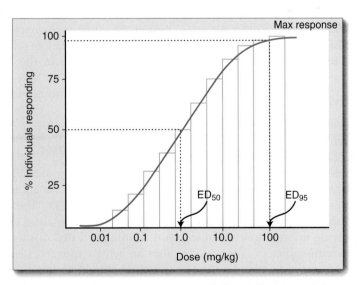

Figure 14.9. A typical quantal dose–response curve with dose milligram per kilogram of body weight on the logarithmic x-axis and the cumulative percentage of individuals responding on the y-axis. The ED_{50} and ED_{95} are the doses at which 50% and 95% of individuals, respectively, show the defined response.

curves also help us predict the likelihood for side effects and toxicity.

Most if not all drugs produce side effects or unintended effects. These side effects often result from the drug acting at more than one receptor and are related to how much of the drug is given; that is, they are dose-related side effects. Sometimes these effects cause serious problems (*toxicity*), whereas in other cases they may be relatively harmless. In a few situations, a drug's side effect may even be desirable. Undesirable side effects are also known as adverse drug reactions (ADRs).

Most common types of ADRs are related to the dose of the drug and are the result of one or more of the known pharmacological effects of the drug; these account for about 80% of ADRs seen in practice. Dose-related ADRs are frequently predictable and can be avoided. Examples are drowsiness after taking antihistamines or an elevated heart rate after using β-agonists. Other types of side effects are not related to the dose or even directly to the drug's biological action. These are generally called "*idiosyncratic reactions*" or *allergic* effects. We will discuss this type of side effect in Chapter 15.

Just as we can construct quantal DRCs for the beneficial effects of a drug, we can also construct similar curves for the dose-dependent ADRs of drugs.

Drug Selectivity

Selectivity refers to the ability of a drug to bind preferentially to one receptor over another. If the dose or concentration needed to bind to one receptor is significantly less than that needed to bind to any other receptor, the drug is considered selective. Concentration-binding curves and DRCs provide information useful in making this determination.

As discussed earlier, concentration-binding curves provide information about the affinity of a drug for a receptor but not the efficacy. DRCs provide us information about efficacy and also give us a relative sense of potency provided we can control for ADME processes. In the drug discovery process, affinity and selectivity are very important considerations for antagonists. Efficacy and selectivity are important considerations for agonists. Potency of a drug is typically not an issue unless the dose is either incredibly small or incredibly large and administration of such a dose is problematic.

Figure 14.10 helps to illustrate the point about affinity and selectivity. Consider for this example the development of antibiotic drugs. The drug targets are often times enzymes that the bacteria need for survival. Many times, the host cell has a similar, but not identical, enzyme. The intent is to design a drug that binds to and inhibits the bacterial form of the enzyme at a concentration that does not inhibit the human form. That is, we want the drug to be selective for the bacterial enzyme. In Figure 14.10, the dose of drug A needed to inhibit the bacterial enzyme will also inhibit greater than 50% of the host enzyme. The difference in their K_d values, a measure of affinity, is approximately three times. In contrast, drug B requires a concentration that is approximately 100 times greater to inhibit the host enzyme versus the bacterial enzyme. Therefore, drug B is more selective for the bacterial enzyme than the host enzyme compared to drug A. Note that drug A is more potent at inhibiting the enzyme than drug B.

Therapeutic Index

The ultimate adverse side effect of a drug is lethality or death. In animals, we characterize this as the LD_{50}, the *median lethal dose*, the dose of the drug that kills 50% of the animals tested during a set period after an acute exposure. Ideally, the LD_{50} of a drug should be much larger than its ED_{50} because this would make the drug safer to use. The LD_{50} values may vary for the same drug given by different routes of administration because of differences in

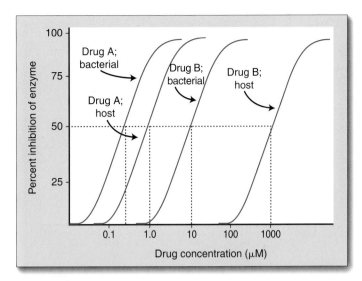

Figure 14.10. A concentration–response curve comparing the ability of two drugs to inhibit the bacterial and host forms of an enzyme. The concentration needed to inhibit 50% of the host form of the enzyme (K_i) for drug A is three times greater than the K_i for the bacterial form of the enzyme. Drug B, however, has a K_i value for the host enzyme that is 10 times higher than the K_i for the bacterial form of the enzyme. Therefore, while drug A is more potent than drug B, drug B has greater selectivity for the bacterial form of the enzyme.

absorption and bioavailability from different administration sites.

The pharmacological therapeutic index (TI), also called the *therapeutic ratio*, of a drug is defined as

$$TI = \frac{LD_{50}}{ED_{50}} \qquad (Eq.\ 14.2)$$

A large TI implies that a drug is safe. For example, a drug with a TI of 25 is safer than a drug with a TI of 8.

Because the LD_{50} cannot be determined in human subjects, clinicians instead define the TD_{50}, the median toxic dose, as the dose that produces a defined toxic effect in 50% of individuals. In this case the clinical therapeutic index is given by

$$TI = \frac{TD_{50}}{ED_{50}} \qquad (Eq.\ 14.3)$$

Here again the TI is a measure of the safety of the drug. A clinical TI of 5 means that the dose that produces a particular toxic effect (such as liver damage) in 50% of individuals is five times higher than the effective dose in 50% of individuals. We will use TI to mean the clinical TI for the remainder of the chapter.

Figure 14.11 illustrates the effective (therapeutic) and toxic dose–response relationships of drug X with a TI of 10. Drug X has considerable separation between these two DRCs, indicating that it has good safety. A general rule of thumb is that drugs with a TI less than 2 will show significant toxicity in some patients when used clinically at therapeutic doses. Thus, such drugs should be used only if the risk–benefit analysis for a particular patient is favorable. The selectivity of a drug is very important in determining its safety profile.

A drug can have many toxic effects of different degrees of severity. Relatively mild side effects such as nausea, gastrointestinal upset, or headaches may occur at low doses whereas more serious toxic effects such as liver or kidney damage may occur at higher doses. Therefore, a

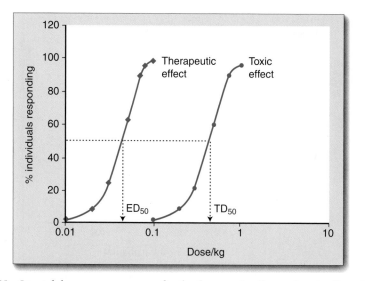

Figure 14.11. Quantal dose–response curves for the therapeutic effect and toxic effect of drug X. The ratio TD_{50}/ED_{50} gives the therapeutic index (TI) of the drug. Drug X has a TI = 10. Note that very little toxicity will be seen at a dose that gives therapeutic effect in greater than 90% of individuals.

drug has different TD_{50} and TI values for each of its toxic effects.

Certain Safety Factor

The TI is not always a good measure of the safety of a drug because it compares only the midpoints of efficacy and toxicity DRCs.

These curves could have significant overlap, so that some patients might experience toxicity without significant therapeutic benefit even though the average patient is effectively treated.

This problem is apparent in the DRCs shown in Figure 14.12 for drug Y. Although the TI of drug Y is the same as that of drug

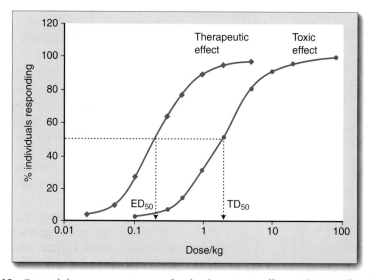

Figure 14.12. Quantal dose–response curves for the therapeutic effect and toxic effect of drug Y. The ratio TD_{50}/ED_{50} gives the TI of the drug. Drug Y has a TI = 10. Note that significant toxicity will be seen at a dose that gives therapeutic effect in greater than 90% of individuals.

X in Figure 14.11, drug Y is obviously not as safe as drug X. The reason for this is that we would need potentially toxic doses of drug Y to obtain desired effectiveness in some patients. Thus, TI alone is not useful for true determination of drug safety because it does not give any information about the slopes of the DRCs for therapeutic and toxic effects. If the therapeutic DRC is relatively flat, there may be significant overlap between the two curves even if TD_{50} and ED_{50} of a drug are quite different.

Ideally, we would like a drug that is effective in all individuals at a dose that does not produce toxic effects in any individual. This concept is characterized by a parameter called the certain safety factor (CSF) as follows:

$$CSF = \frac{TD_1}{ED_{99}} \qquad (Eq.\ 14.4)$$

Here, TD_1 represents the *minimally toxic dose*, the dose that is toxic to only 1% of individuals, whereas ED_{99} represents the *maximally effective dose*, the dose that is effective in 99% of individuals. The percentages used here—1% and 99%—are just illustrations. In practice, one can establish the desired population percentage acceptable for both toxicity and effectiveness.

The CSF is a measure of the overlap of the high end of the therapeutic DRC with the low end of the toxic DRC. A drug with a CSF of 1 can be dosed effectively to 99% of individuals while being toxic in only 1% of individuals. A higher CSF means that there is virtually no overlap between the two DRCs, and a maximally effective dose can be used with little chance of toxicity.

Risk Versus Benefit

A drug is usually considered safe if serious side effects or toxicity are unlikely when the drug is used at its *recommended* dosage in the *average* patient. This does not mean that there are no ADRs; it only means that the risk–benefit ratio of the drug is acceptable in most patients.

The TI and CSF are often used to predict the probability of toxicity in patients. When side effects or toxicity are likely, patients are given low doses to begin with and the dose is slowly boosted while monitoring the patient for ADRs. A drug that is safe in most patients may be toxic in a patient with a specific disease, impaired physiological function, or genetic predisposition.

Key Concepts

- Drug action at receptors or enzymes can be depicted as graphical dose–response relationships.
- The biological response to a drug forms a plateau at high drug concentrations because receptors are fully occupied.
- Graded DRCs compare efficacy, potency, and toxicity of different drugs. They also reveal whether a drug is a full or partial agonist, or a competitive or noncompetitive antagonist.
- Quantal dose–response relationships are useful in illustrating the variability of drug response in a population.
- The safety of a drug can be illustrated by dose–toxic response relationships.
- The clinical therapeutic index of a drug is a ratio of the median toxic dose to the median effective dose.
- Dose–response and dose–toxic response curves are used together to define the risk–benefit of a drug and to select an appropriate dose.

Review Questions

1. Explain the important features of a concentration–response curve for a full and partial agonist. What are the similarities of this curve and a curve of enzyme activity? How do these curves change when the concentration is plotted on a logarithmic scale?
2. How does the concentration–response curve for an agonist change in the presence of competitive and noncompetitive antagonists?
3. How does the concentration–response curve for a substrate change in the presence of competitive and noncompetitive inhibitors?
4. What are the differences between a concentration–response relationship and a dose–response relationship? Why is the latter more useful in therapeutic application?
5. Explain the difference between potency and efficacy of a drug. How is this revealed in a dose–response curve?
6. What is meant by a selective drug? How can one determine selectivity from a dose–response curve?
7. Clarify the difference between the pharmacological therapeutic index and the clinical therapeutic index. Why is the latter more relevant to drug therapy?
8. Discuss why the certain safety factor is more appropriate in the choice of a drug dose than the clinical therapeutic index.

CASE STUDY 14.1

Competing for β-receptors

A pharmacist and a first year pharmacy student intern were participating in a brown bag event where people are encouraged to gather up all their prescription and over-the-counter medicines and take them to a pharmacist for review. One particular patient was taking extended release tablets of albuterol (VoSpire ER®, 4 mg, twice a day) for asthma and propranolol (60 mg twice a day) for high blood pressure. He also had albuterol as an inhaler (Ventolin® HFA: 90 μg/inhalation) that he uses when he has trouble breathing, which has been becoming more frequent recently.

The pharmacist thought the patient's medication therapy could be managed better and asked the patient if she could contact his physician to discuss alternatives.

The pharmacist asked the student to look up information on the patient's drugs and they would discuss what options may be available. The student found the following information:

- β_1 receptors are located in the heart and when blocked can decrease heart rate and when activated can increase heart rate.
- β_2 receptors are located on bronchial smooth muscle and when activated can cause bronchodilation and when blocked can cause bronchoconstriction.

Drug	α value	K_D or K_i Values (nM)	
		β_1	β_2
Propranolol	0	2.7	0.8
Metoprolol	0	45	2300
Pindolol	0.5	4.0	8.9
Isoproterenol	1	200	224
Albuterol	1	7500	2400

1. Using the above data, draw concentration-binding curves for propranolol and metoprolol for each receptor. Assume the slope of each curve is identical.
2. Which drug is more potent? Can you make a case that either drug is selective for a receptor subtype?
3. Using the above data, draw concentration response curves for pindolol, isoproterenol, and albuterol for each receptor. Assume the slope of each curve is identical.
4. Which drug is more potent? Which drug has the greatest efficacy? Can you make a case that any of the drugs is selective for a receptor subtype?
5. Which drug is most likely to cause bronchodilation without changing heart rate?
6. Which drug is most likely to decrease heart rate without altering lung function?
7. In the case of the above patient, explain why albuterol in the inhaler form is relieving his breathing troubles even though it is the same drug as he is taking orally.
8. What would happen if he took an extra dose of VoSpire ER® each day?
9. Could pindolol be used to treat both his high blood pressure and his asthma?
10. The pharmacist recommended switching from propranolol to metoprolol. What is the basis for this recommendation?

Additional Readings

Brunton L, Lazo J, Parker K (eds). Goodman & Gilman's The Pharmacological Basis of Therapeutics, 11th ed. McGraw-Hill Professional, 2005.

Golan D, Tashjian A, Armstrong E. Principles of Pharmacology, Pathophysiological Basis of Drug Therapy, 2nd ed. Lippincott Williams & Wilkins, 2008.

Harvey RA, Champe PC, Finkel R, Cubeddu L. Lippincott's Illustrated Reviews: Pharmacology, 4th ed. Lippincott Williams & Wilkins, 2008.

Katzung BG (ed). Basic and Clinical Pharmacology, 11th ed. McGraw-Hill/Appleton & Lange, 2009.

PART V

Drug Therapy

There does not exist a category of science to which one can give the name applied science. There are science and the applications of science, bound together as fruit and the tree which bears it.
—Louis Pasteur

Chapter 15 Therapeutic Variability

Chapter 16 Drug Interactions

Chapter 17 Pharmacogenomics

Therapeutic Variability

Earlier chapters have discussed what the body does to the drug (absorption, distribution, metabolism, and excretion [ADME] and pharmacokinetics) and what the drug does to the body (drug action and pharmacodynamics). In these previous chapters, we have focused on the disposition and action of drugs in normal, relatively healthy individuals, suggesting that most patients process the drug in the same manner and that the drug works similarly in all individuals. In fact, the standard dose and dosing frequency of most drugs are based on the drug's behavior in an average patient population: approximately 18 to 65 years of age, weighing about 70 kg (150 lb), with normal body functions.

However, patient attributes can affect the nature and degree of pharmacological response significantly. Not everyone responds to the same dose of a given drug in exactly the same manner at all times; variability in response to drug therapy is the rule rather than the exception for most medications. Even at the recommended standard doses of a drug, the *intensity* of the response is often different among patients because of individual differences in pharmacokinetics or pharmacodynamics. Even the *nature* of the response may vary in some patients,

resulting in effects (such as drug allergy) not seen in the average patient. Alteration of physiological and pathological conditions in patients further complicates this picture.

Even the most successful drugs provide optimal benefits to only a fraction of patients. Variability in patient response to drug therapy must be taken into account to adapt drug treatment to individual patient needs.

Types of Therapeutic Variability

Therapeutic variability may be *interpatient,* i.e., between different people, or *intrapatient,* in which the drug response changes for a given person at different times. Many interwoven and overlapping factors contribute to variability. Scientists are reaching the conclusion that genetic variability among individuals is the primary underlying cause of altered response to drugs; we shall discuss genetic factors in detail in Chapter 17. Drug interaction, in which one drug influences the behavior of another, also contributes to therapeutic variability; this too, is the subject of a separate chapter (Chapter 16).

This chapter deals with common and generally predictable factors contributing to therapeutic variability, such as

- Pharmacokinetic factors that produce differing concentrations of the drug at the target receptor.
- Pharmacodynamic factors that cause different pharmacological responses to the same drug concentration.
- Immunological factors that result in allergic response.

Other nondrug-related factors such as the personality, beliefs, and attitudes of both patient and clinician have been occasionally linked to therapeutic variability. We will not explore these in this book.

Many different factors contribute to therapeutic variability, and the same factor may cause pharmacokinetic as well as pharmacodynamic variability. Some common causes of variability can be anticipated by proper evaluation of a patient. In other cases, variability is unexpected and can result in therapeutic failure or toxicity.

Pharmacokinetic Variability

Pharmacokinetic variability refers to variability in delivery of drug to or removal of drug from sites of action involved in efficacy and/or toxicity. The obvious result of this is a change in the intensity of drug effect because either too much or too little drug reaches the site of action, and side effects because of higher than normal drug concentrations. Pharmacokinetic variability is particularly problematic for drugs with a narrow therapeutic range or *therapeutic window* (or low therapeutic index) because small differences may result in therapeutic failure or toxicity, as illustrated in Figure 15.1.

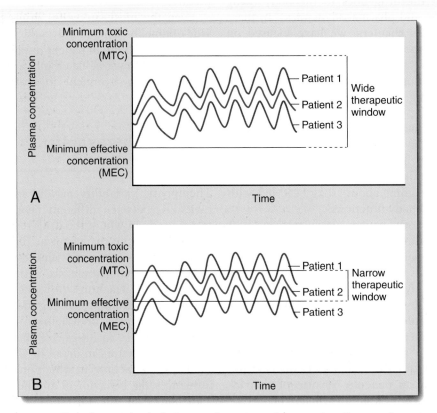

Figure 15.1.   Effect of interindividual pharmacokinetic variability on the efficacy and toxicity of a drug with a wide (**A**) and narrow (**B**) therapeutic window, after multiple dosing in three patients.

A patient who does not fit the "average" patient mold can show differences in absorption, distribution, metabolism, and excretion of drugs. Much of this can be anticipated, and appropriate changes in the dose or dosing schedule made before the initiation of drug therapy.

Pharmacokinetic variability may also be attributable to genetic effects, arising from alterations in certain proteins such as drug-metabolizing enzymes, and drug transporters that mediate drug uptake into and efflux from intracellular sites. Such genetic effects are often unpredictable, although new research is allowing clinicians to identify patients with an abnormal ADME profile for a certain drug. The relationship between genetic characteristics, drug effects, and toxicity is called *pharmacogenetics;* we shall discuss this in greater detail in Chapter 17.

Discussed below are some common sources of pharmacokinetic variability.

Body Weight and Composition

The magnitude of the pharmacological effect depends on the concentration of drug reaching the site of action, which in turn depends on the drug dose and pharmacokinetics. The recommended standard dose of most drugs is typically based on a 70-kg adult male. If we assume ADME processes are functioning normally in an individual, then drug concentration at the site of action depends on dose and volume of distribution V_d. For a given dose, the greater the V_d, the lower the concentration in all tissues, including the site of action. This means that a given dose of drug gives lower tissue concentrations in large individuals compared with smaller individuals. Thus, overweight individuals may need a higher than standard dose to achieve adequate tissue concentrations, whereas small individuals may need a lower than standard dose. Many drug products are available

in multiple strengths (e.g., 10-, 20-, and 30-mg tablets) to allow dose adjustments in individual cases.

Although larger individuals generally require a higher dose to achieve therapeutic plasma or tissue concentrations, the difficulty lies in defining what large and small mean when referring to patients. A simple approach is to adjust doses based on body weight as follows:

$$\text{Dose required} = \frac{\text{Average dose}}{70 \text{ kg}} \times \text{weight of indvidual (kg)}$$

(Eq. 15.1)

Dose adjustments based on Eqn. 15.1 do not work for people who are extremely lean or obese because it does not account for dramatically altered body composition such as body fat and body water. Recall that V_d of drugs depends on drug lipophilicity. Thus, in an obese individual, a lipophilic drug may have an unusually large V_d, whereas the V_d of a hydrophilic drug may not be changed as dramatically. Consequently, doses for lipophilic and hydrophilic drugs may have to be adjusted by different factors in obese patients. In such cases, body surface area rather than body weight is often used to adjust dosage.

Age

Many drugs behave differently in children and the elderly compared with the average adult. Some of this difference is caused by variation in body size and composition, as discussed earlier. However, even when body size is taken into account, additional factors are responsible for increased sensitivity of the very young and the very old to drugs.

Special populations—the very young (infants and pediatrics) and the very old (geriatrics)—are usually excluded in clinical testing of drugs, and their response to drugs is generally unknown when a drug is first marketed. This is changing, however, and more and more drugs are now being tested in geriatric and pediatric populations to identify appropriate doses and dosing schedules.

Infants and Children. Infants constitute a very special subgroup of patients in which drugs must be used with extreme care. In addition to a much smaller body weight, there are significant physiological differences between infants and the average adult. The most important of these are

- Increased permeability of all tissues, including the skin and blood–brain barrier
- Proportionately greater volume of body water, and a consequently higher V_d for certain drugs
- Lower rate of blood flow to most organs
- Decreased biotransformation as a result of underdeveloped metabolic enzymes
- Decreased renal clearance attributable to reduced glomerular filtration rate.

Consequently, use of any drug in an infant must be carefully considered and the dose adjusted appropriately. At an age of about 1 year, metabolic and excretion functions are better developed, and the risk of using drugs in young children is less than in infants. At about 12 years of age, adult doses are often used. However, compensation for a lower body weight and altered body composition must always be considered when using all drugs in children.

Elderly. Many organ systems show a normal decline in function with age in the elderly population. Muscle mass decreases, whereas percentage of body fat rises. Absorption efficiency is usually only slightly reduced, but there are significant decreases in efficiency of metabolism and excretion of drugs. Hepatic effects include

- Decreased hepatic mass
- Decreased hepatic blood flow
- Decreased enzyme activity.

Renal effects consist of

- Reduced number of nephrons
- Reduced number of functioning glomeruli
- Decreased renal blood flow.

The result is that plasma and tissue concentrations in the elderly are often higher than expected, and sensitivity to the drug is increased.

Sex-Related Differences

Until the 1990s, health researchers used male subjects to determine safety and efficacy of new drugs and treatments. Reasons for this were concerns about the potentially confounding effects of women's hormonal changes on treatment, the desire to protect a potential fetus, and fear of liability if a fetus was harmfully exposed. As a result, women of child-bearing age were systematically excluded from clinical trials. Treatment interventions, toxicity, and safety data were studied in men and then applied or assumed to be the same in women.

Sex. The discovery of differences between male and female response to disease and treatments has changed the landscape of new drug development. Women are now included in clinical trials unless the risk is unacceptable.

Sex-related differences in body weight and composition account for some pharmacokinetic variability. Women generally have a lower body weight and a higher proportion of body fat, and may therefore require a different drug dose. There is evidence that metabolic rates may also be different (usually lower) in women compared with men, requiring dosage adjustment. The issue of sex in drug safety becomes particularly important in women of childbearing age, and in pregnant and lactating women.

Pregnancy and Lactation. Many drugs administered to a mother during pregnancy and lactation may adversely influence the embryo, fetus, and infant. The placenta allows transport of many drugs from mother to embryo or fetus by passive diffusion, and drug concentrations in the embryo and in fetal circulation are often the same as those in the mother's circulation. Embryonic and fetal cells are highly sensitive to drugs, and severe toxic effects are seen when these are exposed to drugs. The type and extent of toxicity depend on the stage of embryonic or fetal development when exposure occurred.

The embryonic stage is the time between fertilization and the eighth week of pregnancy. Because major organ structures are being formed during this period, a major toxicity is teratogenicity, the ability of a drug to cause damage to a developing fetus, resulting in congenital malformation of various structures. Serious malformations result in a miscarriage. The fetal stage of development occurs after differentiation of major organ structures; here, toxic effects of drugs can be seen on already formed organ systems.

Many drugs, particularly lipophilic drugs, distribute readily into the breast milk of the mother during lactation. Infants in their first 3 months of life do not have fully developed enzyme systems for biotransformation and renal excretion of drugs. Thus, toxic levels may accumulate in nursing infants, resulting in a variety of effects depending on the drug.

Health and Disease

The overall health of the patient is critical in determining how a drug behaves and works in the body. Drugs are often used in patients whose organ systems are not functioning normally; particularly important are organs involved in drug elimination—the liver and kidney. Patients with impaired hepatic or renal function do not eliminate drugs readily, resulting in higher plasma levels and resultant potential toxicity. A change in dose or dosing frequency is often necessary in such patients.

Impaired circulation (resulting in lower blood flow rates to organs) seen in cardiovascular disease can affect all aspects of drug pharmacokinetics. Other factors such as body temperature, hydration or dehydration, and acidosis or alkalosis may also change the pharmacokinetics of some drugs. The dosage regimen for patients with disease often needs to be individualized on the basis of assessment of hepatic, renal, and cardiovascular function.

The nutritional status of a patient can influence drug pharmacokinetics. Malnutrition, vitamin deficiencies, or decreased protein synthesis may result in altered plasma protein and metabolic enzyme levels.

Pharmacodynamic Variability

Pharmacodynamic variability refers to variable drug effects despite equivalent drug delivery to the sites of action. It may reflect differences in the structure and function of target receptors or in the broad pathophysiological context in which a drug interacts with its target. The existence of pharmacodynamic variability means lack of a relationship between drug response and plasma concentration, and pharmacokinetic–pharmacodynamic correlations are not useful in these situations.

Sex-Related Differences

Physiological differences between men and women may result in altered pharmacodynamics of some drugs in women compared with men. For example, differences have been shown between men and women in both perception of and response to pain. Emerging scientific evidence points to sex-related pharmacological differences in opioid-receptor binding and in responses to certain opioid pain medications. These differences suggest the importance of developing sex-specific strategies for pain relief and highlight the need for further investigation of sex-related pain treatment.

Idiosyncrasy

A few individuals respond to drugs in a highly unusual and unpredictable manner, giving a response quantitatively much different than in the average patient. For example, some patients may have an intense response to a very small dose of the drug, whereas others may not respond to very high doses. The response may also be qualitatively different in some situations, with new pharmacological effects being observed. Such responses, referred to as drug idiosyncrasy or *idiosyncratic response*, are infrequent and believed to result from a genetically determined metabolic or enzyme deficiency that is not expressed under normal situations (e.g., hemolytic anemia occurring in patients with glucose-6-phosphate dehydrogenase deficiency after receiving an oxidant drug). These responses show a dose–response relationship, but not the same one shown by the average patient.

Circadian Rhythms

A circadian rhythm is the regular recurrence of a biological process or activity in cycles of about 24 hours. These cycles are set by a biological clock that seems to respond to recurring daylight and darkness. This clock, which lies in the brain, regulates organs such as the liver, kidneys, and blood vessels by controlling circadian clocks within them; consequently, a daily reproducible pattern of

peaks and troughs is seen in many physiological variables. The acknowledgment of circadian rhythms is philosophically different from the concept of homeostasis, which assumes that most physiological processes are in a state of equilibrium and do not change significantly with time.

It is now generally understood that there are circadian rhythms in many receptors, in signaling pathways, and in activity of enzymes. If these are targets of a drug, then pharmacodynamics of the drug can also be different at different times. There are a number of hormones that are primarily secreted in the morning, such as cortisol, catecholamines, plasma renin, aldosterone, and angiotensin. In contrast, other substances peak at the end of the day or at night, e.g., gastric acid, growth hormone, prolactin, melatonin, follicle-stimulating hormone, luteinizing hormone, and adrenocorticotropic hormone.

There are consequences to the circadian changes in these hormones, and many common diseases show significant circadian variation in onset or exacerbation of symptoms. Asthma symptoms generally worsen during the night; in fact, estimates are that symptoms of asthma occur 50 to 100 times more often at night than during the day. Many circadian-dependent factors may contribute to the worsening of nocturnal asthma. For example, researchers have reported that cortisol (an anti-inflammatory ligand) levels were lowest in the middle of the night, and histamine (a mediator of bronchoconstriction) peaked at a level that coincided with the greatest degree of bronchoconstriction at 4 AM.

Because of its effect on physiological processes, circadian rhythm can affect all aspects of drug disposition and action and is one of the factors responsible for intraindividual variability of medications depending on time of administration. Many drugs display normal, reproducible daily variations in pharmacokinetics and pharmacodynamics. Circadian effects on drug pharmacokinetics have been related to time-dependent changes in the following processes and parameters:

- Gastrointestinal motility and intestinal absorption rates
- Intestinal enzyme activity
- Gastric acid secretion
- Hepatic drug metabolism activity and enzyme concentration
- Glomerular filtration rate
- Blood flow rate
- Urine pH.

The narrower the therapeutic window for a specific drug, the more important the implication of circadian variation in plasma levels. Although most drug doses and dosing schedules have not yet taken into account such diurnal variation in drug action and disposition, mounting evidence suggests these factors must be considered in drug therapy.

For example, rhythmic changes in cell division may explain circadian variation in the sensitivity to the toxic effects of chemotherapy. Many anticancer agents are most cytotoxic to normal tissues that are actively dividing during specific phases of the cell division cycle. Studies indicate the timing of cancer chemotherapy may be of practical importance in improving the therapeutic index of common cancer treatments. Corticosteroids and interferons are less toxic and no less effective when given, respectively, on awakening and just before sleep.

Drug Tolerance

Tolerance may be defined as either (1) the loss of effect over time to the same dose of a drug or (2) the need for more of a drug over time to get the same effect. Tolerance, at first, appears counterintuitive because addition of more of an activating ligand lessens the elicited response.

Recall, however, that receptor number and receptor sensitivity are dynamic and that signaling can adjust based on the conditions of ligand availability. Given that drugs often times act as a replacement for endogenous ligands or alter the response to endogenous ligands, it is possible that drugs may change receptor activity. Tolerance, therefore, is a normal response reflecting the body's ability to adapt to the presence of a drug.

Tolerance may be pharmacokinetic in origin, but is most often related to drug pharmacodynamics. Pharmacokinetic tolerance develops when a drug induces its own metabolism and thus decreases concentration of drug at the site of action. Pharmacodynamic tolerance arises as a result of adaptive changes in receptor sensitivity in response to repeated exposure to a particular drug. The result is usually a decrease or loss of sensitivity to the drug, resulting in a decreased response. Adaptive changes may be related to receptor downregulation, cellular adaptation, or *tachyphylaxis* (a rapidly decreasing response to a drug after administration of a few doses).

Receptor Regulation by Drugs. In Chapter 12, Ligands and Receptors, we learned that when receptors are exposed to a persistent concentration of a ligand, the tissue adjusts by decreasing the number of receptors by *receptor downregulation*. The same phenomenon can occur with drugs. For example, continuous administration of an agonist drug can result in the development of tolerance, so that the usual dose of drug produces a progressively smaller effect and larger doses are needed to achieve the same effect.

In contrast, if there is a decrease in ligand stimulation of receptors, the body compensates by increasing receptor density; this is known as *receptor upregulation*. This can occur after continuous treatment with an antagonist that blocks receptors from being stimulated by their ligands. The homeostatic response by the body is an increased rate of receptor synthesis. A *rebound effect* is often seen on abruptly discontinuing the antagonist because of the large number of receptors now available to bind to endogenous ligands or other agonists.

Drug Resistance

Drug resistance is defined as insensitivity or decreased sensitivity of cells to drugs that ordinarily cause growth inhibition (such as antitumor drugs) or cell death (such as antimicrobial drugs). It occurs despite administration of doses equal to or higher than those usually recommended but within limits of safety, and despite adequate absorption from the administration site.

Drug resistance may be classified as *intrinsic resistance*, in which the cell or organism is inherently insensitive to the drug and predisposed to respond poorly to it, or *acquired resistance*, in which organisms or cells initially respond to the drug, but eventually some or all fail to respond because of an acquired resistant property.

Intrinsic Resistance. Intrinsic or primary resistance may occur as a result of systemic or cellular factors:

- *Systemic factors:* factors causing low drug concentration in the organism or tumor such as decreased absorption, increased elimination, or decreased distribution to the site of action because of functional membrane barriers (e.g., blood–brain barrier limits effective therapy of bacterial infections in the brain).
- *Cellular factors:* factors that affect ability of the drug to reach and interact with the drug target receptor or enzyme. Such factors include low intracellular levels of drug (owing to efflux proteins), low affinity of receptor for drug, absence of a particular receptor, or lack

of activation of a prodrug to an active metabolite in the cell.

Acquired Resistance. Acquired resistance is usually related to genetic changes that alter the sensitivity of the target to a single drug (or to a chemically similar group of drugs) through a variety of mechanisms. Acquired resistance is an inheritable trait. It may be the result of induction by the drug of DNA mutations in some cells in the population. Alternatively, it may arise as a result of a drug selectively affecting the genetically susceptible cells within a population while not affecting a small number of resistant cells in the population. In both cases, the drug will be initially effective, but will become progressively less effective as acquired resistance develops.

Once a cell has developed acquired resistance, i.e., is altered such that it is partially or completely resistant to a drug, there is a selective advantage for its survival in a drug-containing environment. Selection is the process by which drug-resistant organisms or cells are enriched in a cell population. Consequently, with continued presence of drug, eventually only drug-resistant organisms or cells will survive, resulting in a resistant population.

Cross-resistance arises when cells become resistant to drugs that are chemically related or have the same mechanism of action. Therefore, it is possible that resistance develops to a drug that was never given to a patient because the drug is so similar either chemically or mechanistically to the original drug the patient had received and developed tolerance. More problematic is *multiple drug resistance*, or multidrug resistance, in which cells become resistant to drugs with different chemical structures and mechanisms of action.

Multidrug resistance (MDR) occurs when cells become resistant to a broad range of structurally and functionally unrelated drugs after exposure to a single cytotoxic agent. This type of resistance is a serious problem in chemotherapy and in antiviral and antimicrobial therapy.

A number of different mechanisms can cause development of MDR, including increased drug efflux from the cell by ATP-dependent transporters, decreased drug uptake into the cell, or activation of biotransformation enzymes. However, MDR has most often been linked to the overexpression of P-glycoprotein (P-gp), a 170-kilodalton ATP-dependent membrane transporter that acts as a drug efflux pump.

Clinical observation has shown that MDR may develop after a course of chemotherapy (acquired resistance) or may be present on diagnosis (intrinsic resistance). MDR in chemotherapy has been associated with overexpression of P-gp transporters that act as efflux pumps to remove cytotoxic compounds from tumor cells, thereby preventing drugs from reaching therapeutic concentrations in the cell. The cytotoxic drugs most frequently associated with MDR are hydrophobic, amphipathic natural products, such as the taxanes (paclitaxel, docetaxel), vinca alkaloids (vinorelbine, vincristine, vinblastine), anthracyclines (doxorubicin, daunorubicin, epirubicin), epipodophyllotoxins (etoposide, teniposide), topotecan, dactinomycin, and mitomycin C.

Expression of P-gp is usually highest in tumors that are derived from tissues that normally express P-gp, such as epithelial cells of the colon, kidney, adrenal, pancreas, and liver. Such tumors may show resistance to some antitumor drugs even before chemotherapy is initiated. In other tumors, the expression of P-gp may be low at the beginning of treatment but increase after exposure to the drugs, resulting in the development of MDR.

Inhibiting P-gp as a way of reversing MDR has been extensively studied. Many P-gp inhibitors, both competitive and noncompetitive, have been identified, with the objective of administering the inhibitor along with the antitumor drug. However, clinical results have been disappointing. The inhibitors are either too toxic themselves, have a relatively low affinity for the transporter, or have other undesirable drug interactions.

Several clinical approaches have been implemented to avoid or minimize resistance.

- Use of high doses to achieve adequate intracellular concentrations to inhibit or kill the intended organism or cell. Because subtherapeutic concentrations encourage development of resistance, this approach reduces the probability that drug-resistant populations will develop.
- Combination therapy with two or more drugs with different mechanisms of action. The probability that DNA changes will emerge in the same cell resulting in resistance to both drugs is small. Thus, this approach reduces the probability of selection of a population of resistant cells.
- Cells resistant to one drug often exhibit increased sensitivity to another drug that acts by a different mechanism. Thus, knowledge of the mechanism of resistance to a drug can provide an approach to specifically target drug-resistant organisms or cells.

Immunological Variability

Drug allergy is a variability in drug response among individuals that is related to an immunological reaction and is seen only after a second or subsequent exposure of the patient to the drug. The effects are qualitatively different from the normal pharmacological effects of the drug. Allergic reactions to drugs do not show the usual dose–response relationships; even a small, subtherapeutic dose may be sufficient to cause allergy.

Drug Allergy

An allergic reaction is an adverse response to a drug as a result of a previous exposure to the same drug. Drug allergy is different from drug toxicity or idiosyncrasy in that it is not dose-dependent and not drug-specific. Thus, even therapeutic doses can cause an allergic reaction in some patients. Symptoms of drug allergy are similar for all drugs that cause an allergic response, and are not related to usual pharmacological effects of the drug.

Many macromolecules (such as foreign proteins) are viewed as antigens by the body, and their presence triggers formation of antibodies. Thus, many biopharmaceutical protein drugs have the potential of initiating antibody formation. However, small molecule drugs can also indirectly cause sensitization. This indirect effect occurs if the drug (or its metabolite) binds covalently to an endogenous protein (*hapten*), creating an antigen complex with specificity for the drug part of the complex. A subsequent exposure to the same drug then triggers an antigen–antibody response in the body, a chain reaction that is always the same regardless of drug.

The most important cause of drug-related immediate hypersensitivity reactions are associated with antibiotics. Other common drugs that cause such reactions are insulin, enzymes (streptokinase and chymopapain), heterologous antisera (equine antitoxins and antilymphocyte globulin), murine monoclonal antibodies, protamine, and heparin.

The first contact of the drug with a potentially allergic patient is called sensitization. On subsequent contacts, the body produces large amounts of histamine, an autacoid that causes potentially serious effects such as a skin rash, breathing difficulty, decrease in blood pressure and, ultimately, shock. This exaggerated immune response to a foreign agent such as an antigen or drug is called hypersensitivity. Symptoms may occur within seconds or minutes after the second drug exposure (*immediate hypersensitivity*) or may begin gradually with maximum effect in days or weeks after the second exposure (*delayed hypersensitivity*). The most serious manifestation of such an allergic reaction is called *anaphylaxis* or *anaphylactic shock*—a severe and life-threatening allergic reaction. Structurally similar drugs with the same determinant group (group recognized by the antibody) can show *cross-sensitivity*, in that an allergic response to the second drug is shown even without previous contact with it.

The predisposition of a patient to be allergic to a particular drug is partly genetic, but may be related to other factors such as duration of treatment or route of administration. Allergic reactions often occur without warning and cannot be predicted.

Penicillin Allergy

Penicillin antibiotics are one of the most common causes of medication allergies. Penicillins are a family of antibiotics called β-lactams and include benzylpenicillin, penicillin V and penicillin G, amoxicillin, ampicillin, dicloxacillin, and nafcillin. These drugs are generally used to eradicate many common bacterial infections such as skin, ear, sinus, and upper respiratory infections.

Common allergic reactions to penicillin include rashes, hives, itchy eyes, and swollen lips, tongue, or face. Serious and occasionally fatal hypersensitivity (anaphylaxis) has been reported in patients on penicillin therapy. The anaphylactic reaction can develop within an hour of taking penicillin. Symptoms include difficulty breathing, hives, wheezing, dizziness, loss of consciousness, rapid or weak pulse, skin turning blue, diarrhea, nausea, and vomiting. Although anaphylaxis is more frequent after parenteral therapy, it also occurs in patients receiving oral penicillin.

Allergic reactions are more likely to occur in individuals with a history of penicillin hypersensitivity or a history of sensitivity to multiple allergens. Some people who are allergic to penicillin show cross-sensitivity to other closely related antibiotics, particularly other β-lactams. Drugs in this category include cephalosporins (e.g., cephalexin, cefprozil, and cefuroxime), carbapenems (e.g., imipenem), monobactams (e.g., aztreonam), and carbacephems.

The prevalence of penicillin hypersensitivity in the general population is not known. Before any penicillin therapy is initiated in a patient, it is important to make a careful inquiry concerning previous hypersensitivity reactions to penicillin, cephalosporins, or other antibiotics. Approximately 10% of hospitalized patients report a history of allergy to penicillin, and for this reason, many of these patients receive alternative antimicrobial drugs. The most reliable method for evaluating penicillin allergy is by skin testing to both major and minor determinants of penicillin.

If an allergic reaction occurs, the penicillin product should be discontinued immediately. Emergency treatment of penicillin allergy includes injections of epinephrine or intravenous administration of antihistamines and corticosteroids. Oxygen, intravenous steroids, and airway management, including intubation, are also administered as indicated.

Drug Compliance

Compliance is the willingness and ability to follow a prescribed course of drug treatment. Medication noncompliance or nonadherence, i.e., the failure to take drugs on time in the doses and manner prescribed, is as dangerous and costly as many illnesses.

Noncompliance can be classified as either complete nonadherence (missing dosages) or partial adherence (prescribed dose is not completely administered) to a therapeutic regimen. Whether compliance is absent or partial, the outcome is a reduction of pharmacological effect or emergence of drug resistance. Some causes for noncompliance include:

- The patient is taking many medications (polypharmacy) on a complex dosing schedule and is unable to keep track of them.
- The cost of medications may cause the patient to miss doses or take reduced doses.
- Side effects may discourage the patient from taking the drug.
- The patient may lack understanding of a drug's benefits.

Although an obvious cause of therapeutic variability, noncompliance must be taken into account and strategies developed to encourage adherence to a dosing regimen.

Individualization of Therapy

The standard drug therapy, i.e., drug, dose, and dosing frequency, for a particular disease or condition is merely the starting point of treatment. Before the standard drug or dose is used, the patient needs to be assessed for factors discussed in this chapter to see whether this approach is suitable. Even if a patient is started on standard therapy, monitoring of response (efficacy, adverse effects) is necessary as therapy continues. For drugs with a narrow therapeutic window and in certain sensitive patients, blood levels may need to be monitored to ensure they are within the therapeutic range. The dose or the drug may have to be changed to individualize therapy to each patient. Figure 15.2 summarizes factors causing therapeutic variability and actions to be taken in these situations.

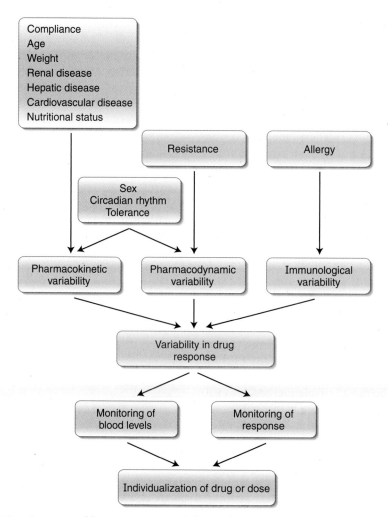

Figure 15.2.   Summary of factors causing variability in drug response.

Key Concepts

- The standard dose of a drug is based on response of a majority of average patients.
- The effect of a particular dose of a particular drug is never the same in all persons, or even in the same person at different times. The standard drug or dose may need to be modified for the needs of a particular individual.

- Pharmacokinetic variability arises because of differences in ADME of the drug in patients.
- Pharmacodynamic variability is caused by differences in target receptors or in pathophysiology of the patient.
- Circadian rhythms are an important source of pharmacokinetic and pharmacodynamic variability.

- Drug tolerance and drug resistance can limit the therapeutic utility of a drug in some patients.
- Immunological variability, e.g., drug allergy, can cause serious adverse reactions in certain patients.

- Poor drug compliance is an important component of interindividual therapeutic variability.

Review Questions

1. Why do patients respond differently to the same dose of a drug?
2. Why is pharmacokinetic variability particularly problematic for drugs with a narrow therapeutic range?
3. What factors can cause pharmacodynamic variability among patients?
4. What factors can cause variability in the same patient at different times?
5. Differentiate among drug toxicity, drug idiosyncrasy, and drug allergy.
6. Differentiate between drug tolerance and drug resistance. List the clinical approaches to minimizing drug resistance.
7. Differentiate between cross-resistance and multiple-drug resistance.
8. What is an allergic reaction to a drug? How does an allergic response differ from other responses seen after administering a drug?
9. What are the clinical approaches to ensuring that each patient is given the right dose of the right drug?

CASE STUDY 15.1

Better Dosing Through Chemistry

Identifying the correct dose to use in patients with increased body size is not often a straightforward process. The physiologic changes in obesity and the physicochemical properties of the drug can influence the volume of distribution of medications, potentially leading to sub- or supratherapeutic concentrations. As a result, increasing the dose or dosing on a mg/kg basis is not always appropriate in obese patients.

Consider the following three drugs:

Gentamicin is an aminoglycoside antibiotic.
- It is a polar molecule used to treat soft-tissue infections.
- It is administered intravenously.

- It distributes primarily into the intravascular space and only moderately into the interstitial space.

Propofol is an anesthetic.
- It is a very lipophilic molecule used to induce sleep.
- It is administered intravenously.
- It rapidly distributes into adipose tissue.

Enoxaparin is an anticoagulant.
- It is a large polar molecule (low-molecular-weight heparin) used to prevent blood clots from forming in veins and arteries (thromboprophylaxis).
- It is administered subcutaneously.
- It distributes primarily into the intravascular space.

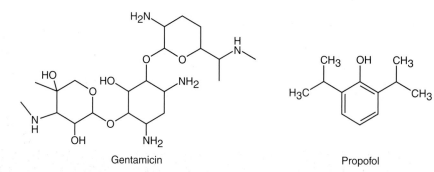

Gentamicin   Propofol

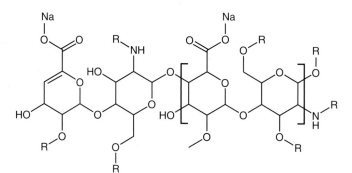

n=1 to 21, R= hydrogen or sodium sulfate salt or methoxy group
Enoxaparin

1. Briefly explain how the volume of distribution is determined for a drug.
2. In a normal population (nonobese), which of the three drugs given above would you predict to have the largest V_d?
3. What physicochemical property of the drug cited in the previous question is responsible for a high V_d?

   Standard dosing for gentamicin is 4 mg/kg. Clinical studies indicate there are problems when using the standard dose of gentamicin in obese patients. As a result, the following adjustments are used to determine the dosing weight of an obese patient.

   Dosing weight = (DWCF × [ABW – IBW]) + IBW

   where DWCF is the dosing weight correction factor = 0.4 for gentamicin,

   ABW = actual body weight, and IBW is the ideal body weight given by

   IBW = 50 kg + (2.3 × [height in inches – 60])

4. What is the appropriate dose of gentamicin for a 300-lb man who is 5'5' tall?
5. Based on the physicochemical properties of gentamicin and the physiological changes associated with obesity, explain why the dose of gentamicin is adjusted in this manner.
6. Propofol does not require a DWCF and is best dosed on an mg/kg basis. Based on the physicochemical properties of propofol and the physiological changes associated with obesity, explain why the dose of propofol is adjusted in this manner.
7. The physicochemical properties of gentamicin and enoxaparin are similar. Yet, the dose of enoxaparin for obese and nonobese adults is the

same, 40 mg. A pharmacist states that the therapeutic index for enoxaparin is larger than the therapeutic indices for gentamicin and thiopental. Explain why or why not this statement applies in this case.

8. If one dose of a drug is effective in 95% of the population, does this support the concept that the drug has a steep dose response curve? Explain why or why not.

Additional Readings

Brunton L, Lazo J, Parker K (eds). Goodman & Gilman's The Pharmacological Basis of Therapeutics, 11th ed. McGraw-Hill Professional, 2005.

Levine RR, Walsh CT, Schwartz-Bloom RD. Pharmacology: Drug Actions and Reactions, 7th ed. CRC Press-Parthenon Publishers, 2005.

Pacifici GM, Pelkonen O. Interindividual Variability in Human Drug Metabolism, 1st ed. Taylor and Francis, 2001.

Rowland M, Tozer TN. Clinical Pharmacokinetics: Concepts and Applications, 4th ed. Lippincott Williams & Wilkins, 2011.

CHAPTER 16

Drug Interactions

During development of a new drug, each compound is tested extensively for pharmacokinetic, pharmacodynamic, and pharmaceutical properties to evaluate its safety and efficacy. An acceptable drug product is one that produces the desired therapeutic effect in the recommended dosing range without serious adverse events. However, while each approved drug may be safe and effective on its own, this cannot be said definitively when drugs are used together.

In clinical practice, several drugs are often given to a patient concurrently (*polypharmacy*), either to treat multiple medical conditions or to use multiple approaches in treating a single disease. Whenever two or more drugs are coadministered there is a possibility of some type of interaction between them, i.e., a situation in which the action of one drug is altered by the use of another drug. Unexpected drug interactions can cause severe adverse drug reactions (ADRs) in patients and may result in death. Drug interactions also contribute to therapeutic variability among patients and are particularly common in the elderly owing to age-associated changes in pharmacokinetics and pharmacodynamics. The use of multiple drugs also increases the chance of a drug interaction; once a person takes four or more drugs at one time, the risk of a drug interaction occurring increases exponentially. The health care community is becoming increasingly aware of the role of drug interactions in loss of therapeutic effectiveness and increase in side effects.

Many drug interactions can be predicted based on known mechanisms and pathways and, as a result, can be prevented by making appropriate changes in dose or by choosing an alternative drug. Interestingly, drug interactions can sometimes be exploited to enhance a drug's therapeutic effectiveness. A second drug is sometimes prescribed intentionally to modify effects of the first. Such an approach might be used to increase efficacy or reduce side effects of the primary drug. Thus, drug interactions are not necessarily to be always avoided; they just need to be anticipated and dealt with.

Interactions between foods and drugs are also possible because many physiological and biochemical pathways in the body (such as those for absorption, metabolism, excretion, and transport) are shared by nutrients and drugs. The action of a drug may be altered by a food or nutrient, or vice versa. It is important to know whether safety or efficacy of a drug will be affected by coadministration with certain kinds of foods.

Drug–Drug Interactions

Interactions between drugs may be conveniently classified as

- Pharmaceutical drug interactions
- Pharmacokinetic drug interactions
- Pharmacodynamic drug interactions

Pharmaceutical interactions occur when two drugs react chemically or physically during administration or absorption so that the amount of drug available for absorption (of one or both drugs) is altered. *Pharmacokinetic interactions* arise when one drug changes the absorption, distribution, metabolism, or excretion (ADME) behavior of another drug. Finally, *pharmacodynamic interactions* develop when one drug increases or decreases the pharmacological effect of another.

Pharmaceutical Drug Interactions

Interactions that interfere with drug absorption as a result of chemical or physical reactions between drugs are called pharmaceutical drug interactions. Most of these occur during release or absorption after drug administration, such as in the stomach when two oral drugs are given concurrently. The main result of a pharmaceutical interaction is to reduce the concentration of drug available for absorption. This decreases the concentration gradient for absorption, thereby reducing the amount of drug absorbed and, therefore, its bioavailability. The more common causes of pharmaceutical interactions are discussed here.

Chelation

Chelating agents are compounds that can bind to a metal ion to form a salt or complex that is poorly absorbed; several drugs have chelating properties. Metal ions such as Ca^{2+}, Mg^{2+}, Al^{3+}, and Fe^{3+} are present in antacids, many nutritional supplements (vitamins and minerals), and foods (milk and other dairy products). When coadministered with metal ion-containing products, chelating drugs can combine with metal ions in the gastrointestinal (GI) tract to form complexes that are poorly absorbed.

A classic example of a chelation interaction occurs with orally administered tetracycline and fluoroquinolone (e.g., ciprofloxacin) antibiotics (Fig. 16.1).

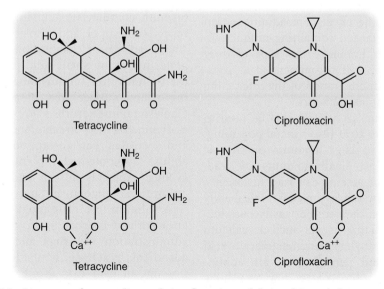

Figure 16.1. Structures of tetracycline and ciprofloxacin, and their calcium chelates.

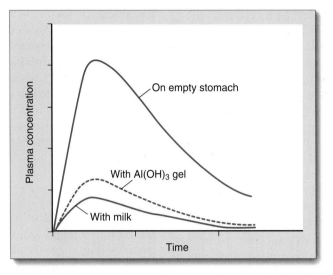

Figure 16.2. Plasma concentration–time curves for tetracycline showing the effect of coadministration with an antacid product (Al[OH]₃ gel) or with calcium-containing food (milk), compared with administration on an empty stomach. Plasma levels are significantly lower when tetracycline is administered with a product containing metal ions.

The chelation reaction involves an electron donor (usually N, S, or O) forming a bond with the metal ion to form a 5- or 6-membered ring system. In the case of tetracyclines and fluoroquinolones, the newly formed drug–metal complex is insoluble, resulting in reduced bioavailability. Figure 16.2 shows a typical plasma concentration-time curve for tetracycline depicting the effect of coadministration with a metal ion-containing product. To prevent or minimize this type of drug interaction, it is recommended to separate the administration of the interacting drugs by at least 2 hours.

Chelating agents can also be used as antidotes to treat heavy metal poisoning. Ingestion of large amounts or chronic exposure to small amounts of lead, mercury, or arsenic can lead to toxicity. Because these heavy metals bind readily to proteins, they are not easily excreted. Polar chelating agents such as calcium disodium ethylenediaminetetraacetic acid (EDTA) and penicillamine are administered in order to form a water-soluble complex that is renally eliminated.

Adsorption

Adsorption interactions are nonspecific and arise when molecules of a drug physically bind to the surface of another solid that acts as an adsorbent, reducing the concentration of drug available for absorption. Examples of adsorbents are antacids, antidiarrheal products (kaolin, bismuth subsalicylate), and ion exchange resins (colestipol and cholestyramine). These adsorbent medications disintegrate into many small solid particles in the GI tract after administration, providing a large surface area for adsorption. Cholestyramine adsorbs many drugs such as dicumarol, methotrexate, and digitoxin and decreases their absorption, bioavailability, and potential for enterohepatic cycling. Antacids adsorb and decrease absorption of digoxin and iron.

A solution to a drug interaction with an adsorbent is, once again, to separate administration of drugs and potential adsorbents by at least 2 hours. The adsorption mechanism can also be exploited for a beneficial use; adsorbents such as activated charcoal are used orally as antidotes to treat various types of poisoning or overdoses.

Alteration of Gastric pH

Antacids, anticholinergic drugs, histamine (H$_2$) blockers, and proton-pump inhibitors are used to decrease stomach acidity and increase stomach pH. This alteration of gastric pH can influence the ionization of other coadministered weak acid and weak base drugs and change the ratio of their ionized to un-ionized forms in the GI tract. This change could, in turn, influence dissolution, absorption rate, and bioavailability of the drug after oral administration.

For example, absorption of iron salts, ketoconazole, or ampicillin administered in ester form requires a low gastric pH for adequate dissolution. If omeprazole, a proton-pump inhibitor that increases stomach pH, is coadministered with these drugs, it can interfere with their absorption.

Incompatibilities

Some drug products such as intravenous (IV) solutions are mixed together before administration for convenience, but may be incompatible with each other when combined. These incompatibilities can be considered a type of pharmaceutical interaction. For example, phenytoin precipitates in the IV bag as an insoluble salt when added to dextrose solutions, and is consequently unavailable to control seizures. Amphotericin precipitates if it is administered in saline and can cause serious complications. Gentamicin is incompatible with most β-lactams in IV fluids, resulting in loss of antibiotic effect.

Pharmacokinetic Drug Interactions

Most drug interactions are pharmacokinetic in nature, involving an alteration of absorption, distribution, metabolism, or excretion of one drug by another. Although many pharmacokinetic interactions have been studied, documented, and can be anticipated, unexpected interactions arise frequently. From a pharmacokinetic standpoint, the major effect of such a drug–drug interaction results in unusually high or unusually low plasma or tissue levels of one or all interacting drugs.

Interactions Involving Absorption

In contrast to pharmaceutical drug interactions, which mainly change concentration of drug available for absorption, pharmacokinetic interactions affecting absorption can change the absorption process itself. Some common causes of such interactions are discussed here.

Changes in GI Motility. The small intestine is the major site of absorption for orally administered drugs; very little drug is absorbed from the stomach. Therefore, the longer a drug remains in the stomach, i.e., the longer its *gastric emptying time*, the slower it is absorbed. Conversely, the shorter the gastric emptying time, the faster a drug can be absorbed. Drugs such as phenytoin and morphine inhibit gastric emptying and increase gastric emptying time. Other agents such as metoclopramide, erythromycin, and reserpine speed up gastric emptying and decrease gastric emptying time. Therefore, drugs that alter gastric emptying can affect the absorption rate of other concurrently administered drugs. Some drugs, particularly anticholinergics and laxatives, affect the small intestines by changing its *motility*, i.e., they change peristaltic activity that moves intestinal contents down the tract. This will also affect residence time in the GI tract and potentially influence bioavailability and absorption rate.

Alterations in GI residence time by one drug can influence absorption of another oral drug administered to the patient. In general, drugs that decrease GI motility (e.g., anticholinergics) reduce the rate but not the extent of absorption of concurrently administered drugs; reduction in rate may cause delay in achieving desired blood levels. The extent of absorption also may be reduced in some cases. An example is reduction in GI motility caused by the antihistamine chlorpheniramine. When the drug levodopa (used in Parkinson's disease) is coadministered with chlorpheniramine, there is a decrease in levodopa absorption. The reduction in GI motility allows greater degradation of levodopa in the GI tract, decreasing the amount available for absorption.

Medications that increase GI motility considerably (such as laxatives) may reduce both extent and rate of absorption of other drugs, resulting in lower blood levels and poor bioavailability. This occurs because the drug spends an insufficient time in the small intestines to be completely absorbed.

Alteration of Intestinal Flora. Some oral antibiotics reduce the bacterial flora in the large intestines. These bacteria are responsible for metabolism of certain drugs (e.g., digoxin) and deconjugation of other drugs (e.g., oral contraceptives) that enter the large intestines during enterohepatic recycling. In the case of digoxin, concomitant administration with antibiotics (such as erythromycin or tetracycline) may result in higher blood levels than expected. When oral contraceptives and antibiotics are given together, a lack of deconjugation interrupts the enterohepatic recycling process and decreases reabsorption from the small intestine back into the circulation, lowering blood levels below the therapeutic range. Figure 16.3 depicts the enterohepatic cycling process.

Saturation of Carrier-Mediated Absorption. A few drugs rely on active transporters in the intestinal wall for their absorption. If another substrate for this

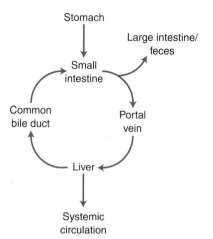

Figure 16.3. Enterohepatic cycle. Digoxin and conjugated oral contraceptives are secreted into the bile duct and delivered to the small intestine. Normal flora in the intestine may metabolize digoxin allowing the more polar metabolite to be excreted in the feces. Normal flora may also deconjugate oral contraceptives to yield the more lipophilic parent compound allowing it to be reabsorbed in the intestine. Destruction of the normal flora with antibiotics can cause increased plasma levels of digoxin and reduced plasma levels of oral contraceptives.

transporter is also present in the intestinal contents, competition may arise, reducing absorption of one or both substrates.

Interactions Involving Distribution

The main interaction affecting distribution is displacement of one drug from plasma protein binding by another. The result is that the drugs displace one another from the protein, increasing free drug concentrations in plasma. How much displacement is seen depends on relative affinities of the drugs for the protein. Increase in free drug concentrations in plasma means more drug is available to distribute into tissues, increasing the volume of distribution (V_d). A higher free drug concentration in plasma also means elimination (metabolism and excretion) rates of the displaced drug will increase, resulting in an increase in renal and hepatic clearances. This will serve to rapidly decrease plasma concentration of free drug, counteracting the increase caused by the displacement of drug from plasma proteins. Therefore, if the patient has normal liver and kidney functions, and if the drugs do not have narrow therapeutic ranges, the transitory increase in plasma concentrations of free drug is not usually clinically important.

Interactions Involving Excretion

Renal excretion of a drug can be affected by a coadministered drug for many different reasons. The second drug can alter any of the contributing processes of renal clearance, such as reabsorption, tubular secretion, glomerular filtration rate, or renal blood flow.

Modification of Urinary pH. The effects of urine pH on tubular reabsorption of weak acids and bases have been discussed in Chapter 9. Compounds that lower urinary pH (such as ammonium chloride) can increase excretion rate of basic drugs and decrease excretion rate of acidic drugs. Compounds that elevate urinary pH (such as sodium bicarbonate) have the opposite effect. For example, excretion of antihistamines and amphetamines (weak bases) is decreased by sodium bicarbonate and increased by ammonium chloride. Conversely, excretion of weak acids such as aspirin and phenobarbital is decreased by ammonium chloride and increased by sodium bicarbonate. Such modifications in urinary pH may be intentionally used to increase excretion rates of drugs after an overdose.

Regular administration of antacids has also been shown to increase urine pH and decrease excretion rates of basic drugs, which are less ionized at high pH. The result is higher blood levels of these drugs, with potential toxic effects.

Alteration of Tubular Secretion. Tubular secretion from plasma into urine is an active transport process involving specific transporters for weak acids and weak bases. Thus, one weak acid (or base) can compete with another for these transporters, thereby reducing tubular secretion rate, decreasing renal clearance, and consequently increasing plasma concentrations. For example, weak bases such as acetylcholine, histamine, morphine, and atropine compete with each other for tubular transporters and can reduce each other's excretion.

A classic example for such an interaction is with the drug probenecid, a weak acid that blocks tubular secretion of other weak acids. Therefore, probenecid can reduce renal clearance of many drugs such as penicillins, cephalosporins, and sulfonamides. In fact, probenecid is administered concurrently with some antibiotics when high antibiotic levels in plasma and tissue are required.

Interactions Involving Biotransformation

The majority of serious drug–drug interactions are caused by interference of metabolism of one drug by another because of inhibition or induction of metabolic enzymes. In general, drugs with a low extraction ratio are more affected by these interactions than drugs with a high extraction ratio. Moreover, interactions involving biotransformation have more serious consequences for drugs with a narrow therapeutic range.

We have learned that oxidation by CYP450 is the most common pathway for phase I metabolism of many drugs. Thus, it is no surprise that most biotransformation interactions involve inhibition or induction of CYP450 isozymes. There are six subfamilies responsible for metabolism of a majority of drugs. Of these six subfamilies, the CYP3A family is responsible for metabolizing approximately 55% of all drugs and CYP2D6 family another 30% of all drugs, making these two enzyme families the most commonly implicated in metabolism-related drug interactions.

Enzyme Induction. Most enzyme induction situations arise when a substance increases the cellular biosynthesis of enzymes that metabolize another drug. When the level of metabolic enzymes is increased by induction, possible effects include:

- Decreased duration of action of the drug owing to increase in its rate of biotransformation.
- Loss of therapeutic effect of the drug because plasma concentrations are lower than the minimum effective concentration.
- Increased concentration of metabolites of the drug, which is important if a metabolite has therapeutic or toxic effects.

Barbiturates and other drugs such as carbamazepine, rifampin, and phenytoin are known to induce hepatic enzymes and increase drug biotransformation. For example, phenobarbital increases metabolism of warfarin and thereby decreases warfarin's anticoagulant activity. The dose of warfarin is usually increased to compensate for this. However, if phenobarbital is subsequently discontinued, the warfarin dose has to be reduced to avoid toxic effects. A few drugs (ethanol, carbamazepine) induce their own metabolism after repeated administration (*auto-induction* or *self-induction*); this may result in development of tolerance.

The process of induction is relatively slow and requires chronic administration of the drug that causes induction. The mechanism for induction involves the drug binding to a nuclear receptor to activate transcription of enzymes. The process of protein synthesis is relatively slow and the full effect is typically realized 10 to 21 days after continuous administration of the drug. As a result of this process, the effects of enzyme induction may not be displayed until weeks after therapy has begun. Likewise, the offset of induction is also delayed. Discontinuing the drug will remove the stimulus for increased enzyme synthesis but enzyme levels will return to normal only after the excess proteins have been destroyed by normal cellular processes, typically this process may take several days or weeks.

Enzyme Inhibition. Enzyme inhibition is, by far, the mechanism most often responsible for life-threatening drug interactions. If biotransformation of a drug is impeded as a result of inhibition of an enzyme predominantly responsible for its metabolism, possible effects include:

- High plasma levels, resulting in increased pharmacological activity. This may or may not be a problem depending on the therapeutic window for the drug. If plasma levels rise above maximum safe concentration (MSC), increased toxicity may also be seen.
- In cases when biotransformation of a prodrug is impeded, less of the active drug will be formed, presumably resulting in lower therapeutic effectiveness.
- If the major metabolic pathway of a drug is impeded, secondary pathways may come into play, resulting in higher concentrations of usually uncommon metabolites. If these metabolites are toxic, a new pattern of side effects may be observed.

The mechanism for enzyme inhibition in cases of drug interactions follows the same concepts discussed earlier regarding competitive inhibition of enzymes and receptors. Inhibitors act by binding to the enzyme at the active site and prevent other drugs from binding and thereby getting metabolized. Drugs may be classified as either inhibitors or substrates. This designation is based in part on the drug's affinity for the enzyme (K_i or K_m value) as compared to its concentration in the body and whether the drug is converted to a product. An inhibitor binds to the enzyme but is not converted to a product (i.e., is not metabolized). In order for it to produce this effect, the affinity and the concentration of the inhibitor must be great enough to outcompete other drugs (substrates) for binding. In some instances, a drug is classified as an inhibitor and a substrate for the same enzyme. In these cases, the drug is still likely outcompeting other drugs for the enzyme and metabolism occurs but is a relatively slow reaction that continues to make the enzyme unavailable for binding to other drugs and substrates.

Confusion often times occurs when trying to predict what will happen when two drugs that are classified as substrates for the same enzyme are administered together. In most cases, this does not present a problem or potential drug interaction. While both drugs are theoretically competing for the same enzyme, it is likely that either (1) the concentration of each drug is below the K_m values and therefore, not saturating the enzyme or (2) the metabolic reaction is fast enough that over the course of hours, there is no perceptible change in the metabolic rate. In other words, for drugs classified as substrates (and not inhibitors) there is enough enzyme present and drug concentrations are low enough (relative to their K_m values) that neither drug impedes the metabolism of the other. Keep in mind, a number of other factors can play a role in determining whether two substrates may interact, such as timing of the peak plasma levels, distribution of the drugs, presence of endogenous substrates, presence of alternate metabolic or excretion pathways, and whether the change in metabolism produces a significant adverse effect.

There are a few cases where two substrates can interact to cause a drug interaction. For example, methanol is a toxic substance that is metabolized by the enzyme alcohol dehydrogenase. The product of this reaction causes blindness and death. A common treatment for methanol poisoning is ethanol. Ethanol is also a substrate for alcohol dehydrogenase. When given at doses that cause intoxication, ethanol saturates the enzyme and prevents methanol from being metabolized to its toxic metabolite. Ethanol, in effect, can act like an inhibitor when its concentration is high enough to (1) outcompete methanol for the enzyme and (2) saturate all of the available enzymes.

The timing or the onset of interactions involving enzyme inhibition differs from that of enzyme induction. Inhibition occurs when the drug is present in a high enough concentration. Thus, the onset for inhibition-related drug interactions occurs within the first few doses of the drug and is terminated when the drug is cleared from the body. The onset and offset, therefore, are readily predictable.

Many drugs inhibit hepatic CYP450 enzyme systems and cause potential drug interactions. For example, fluoxetine inhibits the enzyme CYP2D6 and thus elevates the blood levels of drugs metabolized by this pathway such as metoprolol, simvastatin, and tramadol. Table 16.1 shows some important inducers and inhibitors of CYP3A4, the enzyme involved in metabolism of the majority of drugs.

TABLE 16.1. Some Important Inhibitors and Inducers of CYP3A	
CYP3A Inhibitors	CYP3A Inducers
Ketoconazole	Carbamazepine
Itraconazole	Rifampin
Fluconazole	Rifabutin
Cimetidine	Ritonavir
Clarithromycin	St. John's wort
Erythromycin	
Troleandomycin	
Grapefruit juice	

Pharmacodynamic Drug Interactions

Pharmacodynamic drug interactions arise when one drug alters tissue sensitivity or responsiveness to another drug, resulting in additive or opposing effects. We have considered the principles behind these types of interactions in Chapter 13. Pharmacodynamic interactions may be classified as additive, synergistic, or antagonistic.

Additive

Additivity, or summation, is the most common type of pharmacodynamic drug interaction and occurs when two drugs act on the same receptor or effector system. The effect is additive in the sense that it is predictable and would be similar to that seen if the dose of one drug was simply increased. A simple mathematical formula to express this effect is $1 + 1 = 2$. An example of a drug regimen with additive interactions is the use of a combination of inhalation anesthetics. Using the half maximal dose (ED_{50}) of two inhalation anesthetics produces a maximal effect with fewer adverse effects because they act by the same mechanism to produce anesthesia but act at different sites to produce adverse effects. A common drug interaction not often intended is when two central nervous system (CNS) depressants such as ethanol and certain antihistamines are used together and produce excessive sedation.

Synergistic

Synergism is seen when the combined effect of two drugs is greater than the sum of their individual effects, and requires that the two drugs act at different sites in the same signaling pathway or effector system. A simple mathematical formula to express this effect is $1 + 1 = 3$. The use of nitroglycerin with sildenafil (Viagra®) is a well-documented synergistic drug interaction. Nitroglycerin causes vasodilation by activating a pathway to increase synthesis and release of the second messenger cyclic guanosine monophosphate (cGMP). Sildenafil also causes vasodilation by inhibiting the enzyme that destroys cGMP. The interaction increases the levels of cGMP through two different mechanisms and causes a profound decrease in blood pressure.

Potentiation is similar to synergism in that the effect is greater than the sum of its parts. The difference is that one drug has no effect on its own but can significantly enhance the effect of another. Potentiation can be expressed mathematically as $1 + 0 = 2$. For example, benzodiazepines such as diazepam (Valium®) have a very high therapeutic index and are considered nonlethal on overdose. When typical or well-tolerated doses of benzodizapines and ethanol are taken together, however, the combination can be severely toxic or even lethal.

Antagonistic

Antagonism, or inhibition, occurs when one drug (the antagonist or inhibitor) diminishes or prevents the action of another (usually the agonist or substrate). Antagonism can be further classified as competitive, noncompetitive, functional, or chemical; these were discussed in detail in Chapter 13. An antagonistic drug interaction may occur, for example, when the β-blocker propranolol (used to treat hypertension) prevents the effects of β-agonist albuterol (used to treat asthma).

Food–Drug Interactions

Many foods and beverages contain substances capable of interacting with drugs because they often share the same ADME pathways. The most common of these interactions are summarized here.

Administration with Meals

Dosing drugs during a meal is often recommended to reduce gastric irritation and for convenience of remembering a dosing schedule. However, food may change absorption of drugs by slowing gastric emptying, binding with the drug, decreasing access to absorptive sites on the intestinal mucosa, altering pH of gastric contents, or changing dissolution rate. Food reduces rate or extent of absorption of many antibiotics and of drugs such as alendronate, captopril, and didanosine. These drugs should be taken on an empty stomach. Absorption of some lipophilic drugs (e.g., theophylline) is improved when they are taken with a high-fat meal; the fat presumably accelerates dissolution rate of the drug by providing a lipid medium and by slowing gastric emptying time, increases the time the drug is in contact with the lipid medium (GI residence time).

Alcohol

Alcohol has so many pharmacokinetic and pharmacodynamic interactions with drugs that simultaneous intake of alcohol and any drug is strongly discouraged.

Alcohol is a CNS depressant and can have additive or synergistic pharmacological interactions when taken with other CNS depressant drugs. Alcohol also causes vasodilation and can result in hypotension when taken with vasodilator drugs.

Alcohol is oxidized by mixed-function oxidase (MFO) enzymes and competes with drugs for metabolism with this enzyme system. Chronic alcohol consumption can also induce certain MFO enzymes, resulting in production of higher concentrations of toxic metabolites of certain drugs. An example is metabolism of acetaminophen, which produces higher levels of a toxic metabolite when alcohol is consumed by the patient. Alcohol also depletes glutathione supply in the liver, decreasing glutathione conjugation of drugs and their metabolites.

Grapefruit Juice

Drugs that undergo oxidative metabolism by CYP450 enzymes in the intestinal wall or liver (particularly by CYP3A4) have the potential for an interaction with grapefruit juice. Grapefruit juice contains various bioflavonoids and furanocoumarins, which may bind to the CYP3A4, impairing first-pass metabolism either by inactivation or inhibition of the enzyme. Grapefruit juice thus improves oral bioavailability of several important medications by inhibiting CYP3A4 in the enterocytes of the intestinal wall, which are responsible for presystemic metabolism of many drugs. Extensive consumption of grapefruit juice may inhibit hepatic CYP450 as well, further increasing bioavailability. Drugs affected by this interaction include calcium-channel blockers (i.e., felodipine) and HIV-protease inhibitors (i.e., saquinavir). One glass of grapefruit juice or half a grapefruit can significantly increase blood levels of these drugs, resulting in increased therapeutic effect or increased toxicity.

However, grapefruit juice can also inhibit absorption of other drugs, including vinblastine, cyclosporine, digoxin, and fexofenadine. A study performed in cellular models shows that grapefruit juice activates P-glycoprotein (P-gp)–mediated efflux pumps in intestinal epithelial cells. This effect partially counteracts the CYP3A4 inhibitory effects of grapefruit juice, reducing the absorption and bioavailability of susceptible drugs from the small intestines. The consequences are lower blood levels and reduced therapeutic efficacy. The combination of effects of grapefruit juice on CYP3A4 and P-gp may explain why the effect of grapefruit juice on drug absorption is unpredictable and highly variable.

Other Food Ingredients

Tyramine is a natural component of foods and beverages such as cheese, alcoholic drinks, yeast extracts, and pickled herring. It is normally metabolized by the enzyme monoamine oxidase (MAO) in the liver. Drugs that inhibit MAO (such as the antidepressants phenelzine and tranylcypromine) will reduce metabolism of tyramine, resulting in tyramine accumulation, which causes a subsequent release of norepinephrine from adrenergic neurons. This can cause a hypertensive crisis in patients as a result of a sudden elevation in blood pressure.

Dietary sources of vitamin K, such as spinach or broccoli, may increase the dosage requirement for warfarin by pharmacodynamic antagonism of its effect. Patients should be counseled to maintain a consistent diet during warfarin therapy.

Sometimes, eating certain foods may minimize a drug's side effects. For example, many antibiotics destroy not only infectious organisms, but also the natural intestinal bacteria that maintain critical balances. These imbalances can result in diarrhea and vaginal yeast infections. Research has shown that eating foods that contain active *Lactobacillus acidophilus* bacteria (found in most yogurts) can help eliminate these GI-related side effects.

Some other common drug–food interactions are listed in Table 16.2.

Drug–Herbal Interactions

Changes in dietary habits favoring diets rich in fruits and vegetables, and a significant rise in the consumption of dietary supplements and herbal products, have substantially increased human exposure to *phytochemicals*, chemical substances found in plants or plant-derived products. It is, therefore, not surprising that herbal remedies and other nutritional supplements can interact with each other and with prescription drugs. Phytochemicals have the potential to both elevate and inhibit CYP450 activity. Such effects are more likely to occur in the intestine, in which high concentrations of phytochemicals are achieved. Alteration in CYP450 activity will influence, in particular, the fate of drugs that are subject to extensive presystemic and first-pass metabolism. Moreover, it is increasingly apparent that phytochemicals can also influence the pharmacological activity of drugs by modifying their cellular uptake through interaction with drug transporters. Thus, phytochemicals have the potential to alter the effectiveness of prescription and nonprescription drugs,

TABLE 16.2. Some Common Drug–Food Interactions	
Drugs	*Effect(s) of Food*
Acetaminophen, aspirin, digoxin	Delayed absorption
	Reduced absorption
ACE inhibitors (captopril and moexipril)	Significant decrease in plasma concentration
Fluoroquinolones (ciprofloxacin, levofloxacin, ofloxacin, trovafloxacin), tetracycline	Decreased absorption with antacids (especially magnesium and aluminum) and iron supplements
Didanosine (ddl)	Food, especially acidic foods or juices, significantly decreases absorption
Saquinavir, griseofulvin, itraconazole, lovastatin, spironolactone	Food, especially high-fat meals, improves absorption
Famotidine	Delayed absorption
	Reduced absorption
Ketoconazole	Acidic foods and drinks significantly increase absorption
Iron, levodopa, penicillins (most), tetracycline, erythromycin	High-carbohydrate meals decrease absorption

ACE, angiotensin-converting enzyme.

TABLE 16.3. Some Interactions Between Drugs and Herbal Products that have been Reported in the Literature and that Pose a Potential Risk

Drug	Herbal Product	Potential Adverse Drug Interactions
Alprazolam	Kava	Synergistic CNS activity of alprazolam
Digoxin	Licorice	Significantly elevated plasma digoxin concentration
	Hawthorn	Increased cardiac toxicity
	Ginseng	Significantly elevated plasma digoxin concentration
	St. John's wort	Reduced plasma digoxin concentration
Lithium	Broom, buchu, dandelion, juniper	Increased plasma concentration of lithium
Estrogen	Herbal tea	Increased estrogen plasma levels
Paroxetine and other SSRIs	St. John's wort	Confusion, nausea, weakness, and fatigue
Phenelzine	Ginseng (Siberian)	Insomnia, headaches, irritability, and visual hallucinations
Spironolactone	Licorice	Hypokalemia and muscle weakness
Theophylline	St. John's wort	Increased plasma theophylline concentration
Warfarin	Ginkgo biloba, garlic, feverfew, and cayenne	Increased risk of bleeding or bruising
	Ginseng (Siberian)	Decreased anticoagulant activity
	Licorice	Increased risk of bleeding
	Alfalfa	Decreased anticoagulant activity
	Vitamin E (doses of 200 IU/d)	Increased anticoagulant activity and increased platelet aggregation inhibition, increased risk of bleeding
	Ginger	Increased anticoagulant activity, prolonged bleeding

CNS, central nervous system; SSRIs, selective serotonin reuptake inhibitors.

either impairing or exaggerating their pharmacological activity.

For example, ingestion of St. John's wort has resulted in several clinically significant interactions with drugs metabolized by CYP1A2 or CYP3 A, including indinavir (Crixivan) and cyclosporine (Sandimmune and Neoral). An interaction with digoxin (Lanoxin) has also been reported, which may be mediated by interference with a P-gp efflux pump. These interactions are believed to be related to induction of the CYP isozyme or the drug efflux transporter, and have caused decreased plasma levels of drugs. In the case of cyclosporine, subtherapeutic levels resulted in transplant organ rejection. Warnings about St. John's wort drug interactions have been extended to oral contraceptives, because there is a possibility of breakthrough bleeding and potential for loss of contraceptive effect.

Table 16.3 lists some interactions between drugs and herbal products that have been reported in the literature and that pose a potential risk. Many more drug–herbal interactions probably exist but have not yet been reported.

Dealing with Interactions

Hundreds of drug interactions have been reported in the pharmaceutical and medical literature and the prevalence has increased because of an aging population and a rise in the number of prescriptions being dispensed. As noted earlier, drug interactions range from inconsequential in some patients to serious and life-threatening in other patients, while other interactions are intentionally provoked to enhance treatment or reduce side effects. The ability to identify, assess, and manage potential drug interactions is becoming a more important function of the pharmacist. A number of databases, compendia, and software programs is available to aid in identifying and managing drug interactions. However, these resources are unable to account for all variables that may contribute to a clinically relevant drug interaction, i.e., one that will result in some adverse event. The determination of clinical significance is

TABLE 16.4. Most Serious Drug Interactions in the Elderly

Drug 1	Drug 2	Adverse Effect	Mechanism
Warfarin (anticoagulant)	NSAIDs (e.g., naproxen, ibuprofen)	Serious GI bleeding	NSAIDs destroy protective lining of stomach and decrease platelet aggregation
Warfarin (anticoagulant)	Macrolide antibiotics (e.g., erythromycin, azithromycin)	Increased effects of warfarin, with potential for bleeding	Macrolides inhibit the metabolism of warfarin. Warfarin action may also be prolonged owing to reduction in intestinal flora by macrolides, causing a decrease in production of vitamin K for clotting factor production
Warfarin (anticoagulant)	Quinolone antibiotics (e.g., ciprofloxacin, ofloxacin, and norfloxacin)	Increased effects of warfarin, with potential for bleeding	Exact mechanism is unknown. Probable causes are reduction in intestinal flora and decreased warfarin clearance
Warfarin (anticoagulant)	Phenytoin	Increased effects of warfarin and phenytoin	Currently unknown, but probably a genetic basis involving liver metabolism of warfarin and phenytoin
ACE inhibitors (e.g., captopril, enalapril)	Potassium supplements	Elevated serum potassium levels	ACE inhibition results in lower aldosterone production and decreased potassium excretion
ACE inhibitors (e.g., captopril, enalapril)	Spironolactone	Elevated serum potassium levels	Unknown, possibly an additive effect
Digoxin	Amiodarone	Digoxin toxicity	Exact mechanism unknown. Amiodarone may decrease digoxin clearance, resulting in prolonged digoxin activity. May also be an additive effect on sinus node of heart
Digoxin	Verapamil	Digoxin toxicity	Synergistic effect of slowing impulse conduction and muscle contractility leading to bradycardia and possible heart block
Theophyllines (e.g., theophylline, aminophylline, and oxtriphylline)	Quinolones (e.g., ciprofloxacin, ofloxacin, and norfloxacin)	Theophylline toxicity	Inhibition of hepatic metabolism of theophylline by aminophylline and quinolones

GI, gastrointestinal; NSAIDs, nonsteroidal anti-inflammatory drugs; ACE, angiotensin-converting enzyme.

a decision that requires skills (collecting patient information and analyzing drug information) and judgment.

The first consideration in prescribing a new drug to a patient is to determine what medications (prescription, over-the-counter, and herbal) the patient is already taking and what if any disease state may be a contributing factor. If an interaction is a potential problem, several options or approaches are possible. A different drug that does not interact with currently used therapy can be chosen. If use of an alternative agent is not possible, existing therapy may need to be modified (either with a different drug, different dose, different dosage form, or route of administration) to allow for use of the newly prescribed agent. Often times, the drug interaction is known and anticipated, but the mag-

nitude of the effect is unpredictable. In these cases, the patient is monitored and changes are made later as needed.

Clinicians have identified a set of drug interactions that is particularly problematic in long-term care settings. Each of these drug interactions involves medications that are commonly used chronically in the elderly, and each has the potential to cause significant harm if not managed appropriately. They are listed in Table 16.4. Drugs on the list are those that are used frequently in older adults in the long-term care setting, and have a potential for adverse consequences if used together. Because of individual variability, not every patient who takes these medications together will experience an adverse reaction. However, these combinations have the potential to produce serious side effects.

Key Concepts

- Polypharmacy can result in drug interactions that cause serious side effects in patients.
- Coadministered drugs can alter each other's pharmaceutical, pharmacokinetic, or pharmacodynamic properties.
- Common pharmaceutical interactions involve reduction in the amount of drug available for absorption, usually from the GI tract.
- Pharmacokinetic interactions involve one of the ADME processes; alterations of elimination (metabolism or excretion) of one

drug by another are the most common interactions.
- Pharmacodynamic interactions are a result of additivity, potentiation, or antagonism of one drug by another.
- Food and nutritional supplements can interact with drugs and either enhance or reduce their effectiveness, or cause adverse reactions.
- Herbal and nonprescription medications can interact with many prescription drugs, and should be considered in evaluation of drug interactions.

Review Questions

1. Why are drug interactions most often encountered in the elderly?
2. Explain which pharmaceutical drug interactions can increase, and which can decrease, the absorption rate or bioavailability of drugs.
3. How do interactions involving distribution occur? Why are these clinically significant for only a few types of drugs?

4. What types of drugs modify urine pH, and why can this alter excretion of other drugs?
5. Discuss the consequences of enzyme induction and inhibition on plasma levels of interacting drugs.
6. Explain how administration with meals can increase or decrease the bioavailability of certain drugs.
7. How does coadministration of grapefruit juice alter plasma levels of certain drugs?
8. Which types of drug interactions can be minimized by separating administration of interacting drugs by 1 to 2 hours? What types of interactions will not be avoided by this approach?
9. What are some common clinical approaches to minimizing drug interactions in patients?

Drug interactions can be a pain

A 23-year-old female was playing basketball during her lunch break when she severely twisted her ankle. Upon examination a few hours later, the physician noted redness and swelling and gave her a dose of Celecoxib (Celebrex®) to be taken immediately and wrote a prescription for a 5-day supply of Celebrex® to treat the pain and inflammation.

Two days later, she was not getting adequate relief of her pain and inflammation. She also began to experience symptoms of a urinary tract infection.

The physician told her to double the dose of the Celebrex® and gave her a prescription for Septra® DS (sulfamethoxazole 800 mg/trimethoprim 160 mg) to treat her infection.

Her patient profile also notes she is allergic to penicillin and has been taking Dilantin® (phenytoin, 100 mg tid) for the last 6 years to treat seizures associated with head trauma received in a car accident.

Use the following chart to identify potential drug interactions.

Drug	2C8	2C9	2C19	2D6	3A4
Celecoxib (Celebrex®)		⊙			
Phenytoin (Dilantin®)		⊙	⊙		↑
Sulfamethoxazole		↓			
Trimethoprim	↓				
Zolpidem (Ambien®)					⊙

⊙ = substrate for isozyme; ↑ = inducer of isozyme; ↓ = inhibitor of isozyme.

1. Is there a drug interaction that may explain why celecoxib was not effective at the initial dose?
2. Identify other reasons that may explain why celecoxib may not be effective when using the standard dose in a patient.
3. With the addition of Septra DS, what potential drug interactions may develop?
4. Describe the mechanism and the timing of these interactions.
5. In this particular case, the interaction between Septra DS and celecoxib resulted in a clinically significant interaction but the interaction between Septra DS and phenytoin was not clinically significant. What factors may account for this?
6. What changes can be made to avoid the interaction and still treat the patient effectively?
7. Zolpidem is a fast onset, short-acting hypnotic used to initiate sleep. What will the patient experience if she took the drug while taking all of the above drugs?
8. Describe the mechanism and the timing of the interaction involving zolpidem.
9. Do you think the interaction involving zolpidem will be clinically significant? If so, what changes can be made to avoid the interaction?

Additional Readings

Baxter K. Stockley's Drug Interactions, 9th ed. Pharmaceutical Press, 2010.

Hansten PD, Horn JR. Drug Interactions Analysis and Management. Facts and Comparison, 2010.

McCabe BJ, Wolfe JJ, Frankel EH. Handbook of Food–Drug Interactions. CRC Press, 2003.

Rodrigues AD. Drug–Drug Interactions, 1st ed. Marcel Dekker, 2001.

Tatro DS. Drug Interaction Facts 2011. Facts and Comparisons, 2010.

Pharmacogenomics

Different patients often respond quite differently to the same dose of a given drug; variability in response to drug therapy is the rule, not the exception. Chapter 15, Therapeutic Variability, discussed common physiological and environmental factors that cause differing drug effects among patients. However, even when these factors are taken into account, there remains a large variability in individual drug response.

Interindividual variability in response to drugs complicates new drug discovery and approval. How does one weigh the benefit-to-risk ratio of a drug, taking into account the entire population that might use it? Such questions often result in potentially beneficial drugs never coming to market because of toxicity in a subgroup of subjects, or in the withdrawal of useful drugs from the market when serious adverse events are seen in a small percentage of patients. If the origin of variability in drug response could be identified and compensated for, all drugs could be safe and effective in the correctly chosen patient.

Environment, diet, age, lifestyle, and state of health can influence how an individual reacts to a drug, but the response also has a genetic component that can make a drug therapeutic in one patient, ineffective in a second, and toxic in a third.

The existence of large population differences with smaller intrapatient variability is consistent with inheritance as a determinant of drug response. Understanding an individual's genetic makeup is believed to be the key to designing and using drugs with greater efficacy and safety.

Genetic factors are also very important in determining health and illness. Many diseases, whether infectious diseases, cardiovascular disease, or cancer, have a genetic component. Genetic research will enable us to identify the genes that cause disease and the individuals who are at risk, and will suggest therapeutic approaches. Analyzing genetic variations will also allow selection of patients who might be helped by a treatment, and those who may show resistance or adverse reactions.

To understand the influence of genetic factors on disease and drug therapy, let us first briefly review how genes control the expression of proteins.

Review of Genetics

Chromosomes

Our genetic material is located primarily in structures called chromosomes contained in the nucleus. Humans have 23 pairs of chromosomes for a total of 46. One pair (chromosome pair 23) is made up of the sex chromosomes—females have two X chromosomes whereas males have an X and a Y chromosome. The other 22 pairs of chromosomes (1 through 22) are called *autosomes.*

Each chromosome contains a single DNA molecule, composed of two polynucleotide strands that wind about each other into a double helix, often compared with a spiral ladder. The sides of the ladder are composed of two sugar-phosphate backbones, and each rung of the ladder consists of two paired bases, one from each strand. The helix is stabilized by van der Waals forces, hydrogen bonds between the base pairs, and hydrophobic interactions between the bases and surrounding water. The hydrogen bonding between base pairs is such that the most energetically stable DNA configuration is achieved when adenine (A) pairs with thymine (T) and guanine (G) pairs with cytosine(C); A–T and G–C are called *complementary base pairs.* Each human chromosome can contain as many as 300 million base pairs.

Genes

A gene is a precise sequence of DNA on a chromosome that encodes information for a particular characteristic or function. Different sequences of base pairs contain different coded messages. The coded information is contained in triplets or *codons,* such as ATG. Almost all genes have one primary function: they code for proteins. The process of *transcription* converts DNA to mRNA, and *translation* converts the mRNA to a functional protein. The *genetic code* is the correspondence between the codons in DNA and the amino acids that are ultimately assembled into protein. It is the precise sequence of these codons that results in the synthesis of different proteins.

Less than 10% of human DNA is believed to contain functional genes.

Between genes are other DNA sections called *regulatory regions* that control gene activity. There are also long stretches of noncoding DNA that has no apparent function.

Each gene is found at a specific location or *locus* on a chromosome. A gene can have two alternative forms, or alleles, one copy from each parent on each chromosome pair. If both chromosomes have the same allele occupying the same locus on the two chromosomes, the individual or cell is referred to as homozygous for this allele; if the alleles at the two loci are different, the condition is referred to as heterozygous for both alleles. Alleles are often responsible for alternative traits, and some alleles are dominant over the other in the pair.

The majority of genes are the same for all humans. In fact, even chimpanzees are more than 98% genetically similar to humans. Individual gene sequences in people may differ to the extent of about 1 in 1,000 base pairs, which at first seems to be too small to account for all the differences we see in humans. However, these small differences can result in significant differences in the protein they code for, and an infinite number of DNA sequence variations. In the broadest sense, human genetic variation refers to the differences in DNA sequence among individuals.

The Human Genome

A *genome* is all the genetic information of an organism. The human genome consists of about 30,000 known genes, a small number considering the complexity of humans. This means that other factors such as the environment play an important role in human biology. The *genotype* refers to the genetic makeup or genome of an individual; it can pertain to all genes or to a specific gene. By contrast, the *phenotype* results from interaction between the genotype and the environment. It is the outward expression, appearance or behavior shown by a cell, an individual, or an organism under a particular set of environmental conditions.

Gene Expression

The genetic code or genotype does not control all biological functions. Some of the differences among species and among individuals are also a result of differences in *gene expression* rather than dissimilar genes because not all genes are expressed all the time. In its simplest terms, gene expression is the manifestation of the genotype of an organism into the phenotype, involving execution of the instructions held in the genes into a final, functioning protein.

One can think of the genome as a book of recipes and gene expression as the selection of recipes for a meal. Very different meals can result depending on which recipes from the same book are used at a particular time. A small difference in timing and level of gene expression could account for many interindividual differences. Variability in *mRNA* expression patterns rather than in the DNA itself may help find the cause of some diseases and of variable response to drugs. Thus, an understanding of gene expression may be as useful as knowing the DNA sequence in understanding diseases and approaches to drug therapy.

Changes in protein structure can occur as a result of differences in DNA transcription into mRNA or translation of the mRNA into protein. The gene transcript (mRNA) can be spliced in different ways before translation into protein. After translation, many proteins are chemically changed through posttranslational modification, mainly through the addition of carbohydrate and phosphate groups. Such modification plays a vital role in modulating the function of many proteins but is not directly coded by genes. As a consequence, the information from a single gene can encode as many as 50 different protein species.

Genetic Variation and Disease

Genomic research has provided a vast amount of information linking gene structure, function, and activity with disease.

Types of Genetic Variation

Mutation

One type of genetic variation is a mutation, a permanent change or structural alteration in the DNA. Mutations are a result of random chance events or can be caused by external factors, including environmental insults such as radiation and mutagenic chemicals.

Mutation refers to a genome variation that is present in less than 1% of the population and is usually harmful. However, some mutations may have no physiological or biochemical effect if they occur in the noncoding part of DNA. Occasionally, a mutation can be beneficial and improve the organism's chance of survival, contributing to adaptation and evolution of a population over time. Such beneficial mutations usually become polymorphisms if they persist in the gene pool, as discussed a little later.

A *germline mutation* or *hereditary* mutation is an inheritable change in the DNA that occurred in a germ cell (a cell that will become an egg or a sperm) or the zygote at the single-cell stage. Such a mutation is incorporated into every cell of the body of the resulting offspring. Germline mutations play an important role in many genetic diseases. They are also involved in certain types of cancer (e.g., eye tumor retinoblastoma and Wilms tumor, a childhood malignancy of the kidney).

By contrast, an *acquired mutation* is a change in a gene or chromosome that occurs in a single cell after conception. This change is then transmitted to all cells descended from the altered cell, giving rise to a clone of cells marked by the mutation. Acquired mutations occur in general body cells as opposed to germ

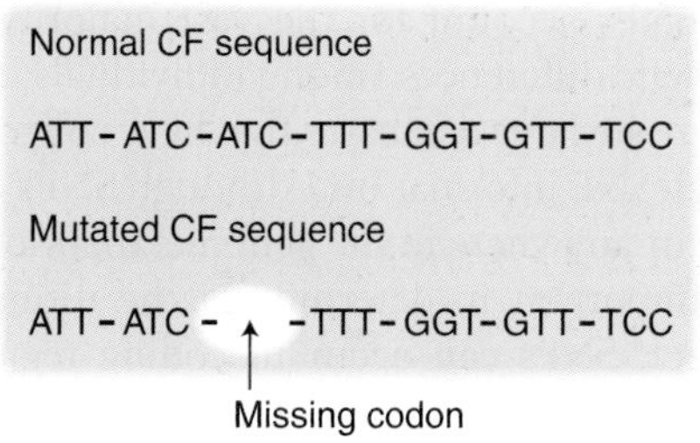

Normal CF sequence

ATT - ATC - ATC - TTT - GGT - GTT - TCC

Mutated CF sequence

ATT - ATC - ↑ - TTT - GGT - GTT - TCC

Missing codon

Figure 17.1. Example of a mutation causing cystic fibrosis (CF). A codon (ATC) that codes for the amino acid phenylalanine has been deleted in the mutated CF gene, resulting in an abnormal CF protein that does not have phenylalanine in this position. Individuals with the abnormal protein develop CF.

cells, and are not passed on to descendants. Many diseases arise as a result of acquired mutations; for instance, the great majority of people who get breast cancer or colon cancer have not inherited such altered genes. Inherited forms of cancer represent only perhaps 5% or 10% of all cancers. This is true even for families that have several members with cancer; certain cancers are so common that some clusters are bound to happen purely by chance. Cases that are diagnosed at older ages, in particular, are more likely to be caused by acquired mutations.

Many mutated genes make physiologically important proteins that do not function correctly and are, therefore, directly responsible for disease. For example, a change in a single amino acid in the normal hemoglobin protein causes sickle cell anemia. Figure 17.1 illustrates a mutation that causes cystic fibrosis (CF). By searching for mutations, scientists can identify and understand the molecular genetic basis for disease. A flaw in virtually any gene may potentially result in a disease, or in an altered response to a drug.

Genetic Polymorphism

Another kind of genetic variation is a polymorphism, a variation in the DNA that occurs with an appreciable frequency in the population and is too common to be

caused merely by a new mutation. In general, polymorphisms have a frequency of at least 1% in the general population. Polymorphisms that occur at a lower frequency are called mutations or genetic variants.

Polymorphisms probably begin as germline mutations but become common in a certain patient population because of inheritance. Polymorphisms are generally more benign than mutations, and many polymorphisms persist in the gene pool because they confer a survival advantage to the individuals in certain environments. However, the same polymorphism may result in another detrimental trait.

An example is the gene for sickle cell disease, in which a mutation occurred thousands of years ago. The altered gene was passed on to offspring and became common in malarious areas because it gave individuals a selective advantage against malaria. However, the altered gene is also responsible for making abnormal hemoglobin, so children who inherit an altered gene from both parents have sickle cell anemia. Children who inherit only one altered gene have no symptoms of the disease, but can pass on the genetic predisposition trait to their offspring.

Polymorphisms are particularly important in certain ethnic groups and races. Glucose-6-phosphate dehydrogenase (G6PD) is an enzyme normally present in red blood cells that protects these cells from oxidative stress. G6PD deficiency is a sex-linked polymorphism that affects 400 million people worldwide; about 10% of black men and fewer black women have G6PD deficiency. Inheriting the G6PD deficiency gene is believed to also protect against malaria. However, the polymorphism causes life-threatening hemolytic anemia, in which red blood cells burst. This anemia develops only under specific conditions—eating fava beans, inhaling certain types of pollen, contracting certain infections, or taking certain drugs. Some drugs that potentiate hemolytic anemia in people with G6PD deficiency are chloroquine, pamaquine and primaquine, aspirin, probenecid, and vitamin K.

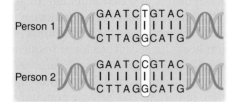

Figure 17.2 Illustration of a single-nucleotide polymorphism in a DNA sequence. In this case, a T in the general population (person 1) has been replaced with a C in a small subgroup of the population (person 2).

Single-Nucleotide Polymorphism. The most common form of genetic polymorphism is a single-nucleotide polymorphism (*SNP*), a change of one base pair at a specific point in the DNA molecule. This occurs when a single nucleotide, such as an A, replaces one of the other three nucleotides—C, G, or T. An example of an SNP is the alteration of the DNA segment AAGGTTA to ATGGTTA, where the second "A" in the first segment is replaced with a "T." Figure 17.2 illustrates the concept of an SNP. Other less common sources of genetic variation are duplications or deletions in a single base pair or in multiple base pairs in the DNA.

SNPs account for the vast majority of genetic differences among individuals, and there are large databases that have collected such SNP information. Although SNPs can occur anywhere in the genome, their locus is important in determining the ultimate effect. SNPs can occur in coding regions of DNA (cSNPs), in regulatory regions of DNA (rSNPs), or most commonly, in noncoding regions, in which case they are referred to as *anonymous* SNPs.

SNPs that occur in the noncoding region, thought to be the most common type of SNPs, have no known effect on gene function. Even among cSNPs, *synonymous* SNPs do not change the amino acid sequence of the encoded protein and are not expected to have any functional consequences. Only *nonsynonymous* SNPs, those that result in a code for a different amino acid, have the potential of influencing propensity to disease or drug response. The magnitude of their effect will depend on how much the two amino acids differ and how this difference changes protein structure, folding, and active site configuration. There are an estimated 200,000 cSNPs present in the human genome.

Figure 17.3 shows one approach for locating disease-susceptibility genes in individuals using SNP association studies.

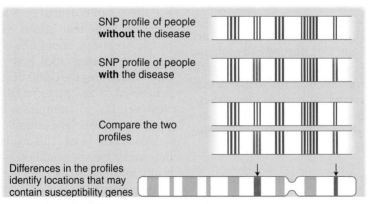

Figure 17.3 Association studies for locating disease susceptibility genes in individuals using single-nucleotide polymorphisms (SNPs). The process involves looking at particular genes or variations in two groups (e.g., affected patients and control subjects) to establish an association with a phenotype by finding significant genetic variations in the two groups.

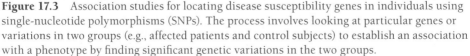

Monogenic Diseases

Human genetics first focused on the identification of genes that cause monogenic diseases or *single-gene disorders*, those caused by a defect in just one gene. Scientists currently believe single-gene mutations cause approximately 6,000 inherited diseases. These conditions include a number of lung and blood disorders, such as CF, Huntington's disease, sickle cell anemia, and hemophilia. Although not common, as a group these monogenic disorders still affect millions of people worldwide. The precise molecular defects that result in more than 100 of these disorders have now been characterized. The study of monogenic disorders has led to important advances in early diagnosis, understanding the disease process, and finding potential cures.

Most monogenic diseases, with very few exceptions, occur regardless of the environment; if an individual inherits a mutation that causes the disease, it will manifest itself regardless of the person's lifestyle and living conditions.

Monogenic diseases can be classified as X-linked, autosomal recessive, or autosomal dominant. The defective version of the gene responsible for the disease is known as a mutant allele or a disease allele. X-linked diseases are monogenic disorders that are linked to defective genes on the X chromosome (the sex chromosome). X-linked alleles can be dominant or recessive. Only a few disorders (e.g., X-linked hypophosphatemia) have a dominant inheritance pattern. Examples of X-linked recessive disorders are hemophilia A and Duchenne muscular dystrophy. Autosomal disorders are those caused by defects in chromosomes 1 through 22. Autosomal recessive diseases (e.g., CF and sickle cell anemia) require an individual to have two disease alleles. Autosomal dominant diseases (e.g., Huntington's disease) can be manifest when there is only one disease allele.

Table 17.1 lists some common monogenic disorders.

Polygenic Diseases

Attention is now turning to more common polygenic diseases or complex diseases, those that arise as a result of defects in several genes. Such diseases or disorders are often a result of a combination of genetic flaws in alleles of multiple genes. Polygenic disorders include common conditions that affect many millions of people, such as asthma, heart disease, adult-onset diabetes, migraine, and Alzheimer's disease. Depression and other mental illnesses are also believed to be the result of alterations in several genes at once. These diseases do not show the clear patterns of inheritance seen in monogenic diseases because genotype does not necessarily translate into phenotype. However, complex diseases still tend to cluster in families, but not in

TABLE 17.1. Some Common Monogenic Disorders, the Chromosome Where the Mutation is Located, and the Type Of Mutation		
Disorder	Mutation	Chromosome
Color blindness	P	X
Cystic fibrosis	P	7
Down syndrome	C	21 (extra chromosome)
Hemophilia	P	X
Klinefelter syndrome	C	X (extra chromosome)
Spina bifida	P	1

P, point mutation, or any insertion or deletion entirely inside one gene; C, whole chromosome extra, missing, or both.

the predictable manner shown by monogenic diseases.

Many common polygenic diseases are a result of a complex interaction between a combination of flawed susceptibility genes and external environmental factors (such as a person's diet, air pollutants, tobacco smoke, and exposure to allergens). Susceptibility genes contribute to an individual's risk of developing a specific disease, but usually are not enough to cause the disease. Different alleles of a gene may be associated with different degrees of susceptibility or risk. The *APOE* gene on chromosome 19 is one example of a disease susceptibility gene. An individual who has two copies of one variant allele of *APOE* is more likely to develop Alzheimer's disease at an earlier age than an individual with a different *APOE* genotype. Infectious diseases reveal even more complexity, because manifestation of the disease involves the genome of the individual, the genome of the infectious invader, and environmental influences on both.

The relative importance of genetics versus environment as determinants of disease varies across a broad spectrum. In some diseases, external factors appear to be more important, whereas in others intrinsic predispositions prevail. Susceptibility genes may influence the age of onset of a disease, contribute to its rate of progression, or help to protect against it. Understanding the rules of their inheritance and their roles in disease is a complicated challenge. Researchers believe genetic factors account for much of the susceptibility of an individual to a disease; environmental factors may determine whether the disease actually manifests itself. For example, if two individuals with the same genetic susceptibility to a particular disease grow up in two entirely different environments, one that contributes to disease and one that does not, only the individual in the disease-contributing environment will manifest the disease. Thus, early knowledge about disease susceptibility may make it possible to control environmental and lifestyle factors to prevent disease, or to initiate prophylactic or early treatment.

Figure 17.4 illustrates the difference between monogenic and polygenic diseases.

Linkage

Scientists have found that long blocks of DNA have traveled from one generation to the next with little genetic shuffling. Along any given stretch of chromosome, the genetic variation within these blocks comes in only four or five patterns in different people. These DNA segments often contain one or more genes that make important proteins, many gene regulatory segments, and many fragments with no known function.

Linkage refers to the tendency for DNA segments that are located close to each other on the same chromosome to be inherited together. One of the segments may be the gene of interest, whereas the other is a *marker*–a segment of DNA with an identifiable physical location on a chromosome whose inheritance can be followed. A marker can be a gene or a section of DNA with no known function. The closer together two segments are on a chromosome, the lower the probability that they will be separated during DNA repair or replication processes, and hence the greater the probability that they will be inherited together.

Thus, the marker is typically unrelated to the phenotype of interest, but is nonetheless useful for predicting the phenotype owing to the marker's proximity to the gene that is functionally producing the phenotype. Markers are often used as indirect ways of tracking the inheritance patterns of genes that have not yet been identified, but whose approximate locations are known. Because SNPs occur frequently throughout the genome and tend to be relatively stable genetically, they serve

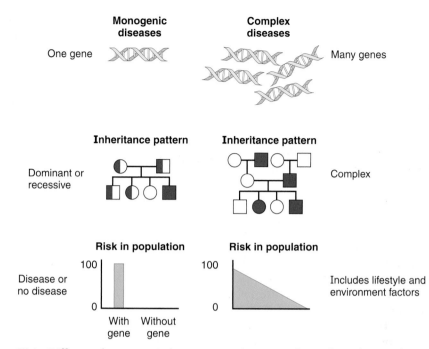

Figure 17.4 Difference between simple monogenic diseases and complex polygenic diseases. Monogenic diseases arise owing to a defect in one gene and have a fairly predictable inheritance pattern. Polygenic diseases develop as a result of defects in several genes, any combination of which can be inherited, giving rise to a complex inheritance pattern. Monogenic diseases show a clear relationship between genotype and phenotype; a person either has the disease or does not. The correlation between genotype and phenotype is complex in polygenic diseases, and is further complicated by the influence of one or more lifestyle and environmental factors. Persons may have different degrees of susceptibility or risk for the disease, and the exact degree of risk cannot be determined with any certainty.

as excellent biological markers to track disease-linked genes.

Genetic Variation and Response to Drugs

Some genetic variations are responsible for the disease itself, as we have just discussed. Other types of genetic variations, although not involved in the disease process, can influence the pharmacokinetic behavior or pharmacodynamic response to a drug in an individual. Genetic variation refers not only to gene alterations leading to protein structure modifications but also to gene regulation that results in the synthesis of different amounts of protein. A drug's behavior in the body is a result of complex interactions with a variety of endogenous cellular proteins such as receptors, metabolizing enzymes, transporters, and binding and carrier proteins. Small but important genetic polymorphisms among individuals can result in differences in structure or amount of these proteins among individuals, leading to dramatic differences in the way each person responds to a drug.

Pharmacogenetics and Pharmacogenomics

The field of pharmacogenetics, which is about 40 years old, is the study of genetically determined variability in the response of individuals to drugs. Much of the research in this area has focused on genetic variations affecting hepatic metabolizing enzymes, particularly the CYP450 family. Pharmacogenetics attempts to identify those individuals within the population who are susceptible to possible alterations in drug metabolism so that this may be taken into account during development of a therapeutic regimen. The ability to identify hereditary differences in metabolism allows drugs to be prescribed in a more efficacious and safe manner to begin with, without having to adjust dosage after observing an undesired patient response. Many pharmacogenetic studies have explained drug idiosyncrasy, which is the abnormal response to a drug in a few patients, resulting in serious toxicity. Most idiosyncratic reactions are now known to arise because of genetic variation in metabolizing enzymes.

Although the field of pharmacogenetics began with a focus on drug metabolism, it now encompasses the entire spectrum of drug disposition, including a growing list of transporters that influence drug absorption, distribution, and excretion.

Pharmacogenomics is the study of the effect of an individual's genetic inheritance, their genome, on the body's response to drugs. It is a broader study of multiple genes and their alleles, of the entirety of expressed and nonexpressed genes in any given physiological state and how they affect all aspects of pharmacokinetics and pharmacodynamics. Although the terms pharmacogenetics and pharmacogenomics are often used interchangeably and are synonymous for all practical purposes, pharmacogenomics uses a genome-wide approach while pharmacogenetics generally focuses on specific interindividual differences.

Consequences of Genetic Variation

The pharmacokinetic behavior of a drug and the pharmacodynamic response of an individual are directly related to drug–protein interactions and, to a lesser extent, to interactions of the drug with other biomolecules. Thus, a more complete understanding of genetic variability in drug therapy may be gained by looking directly at polymorphisms in cellular proteins. Interindividual differences in drug response may be caused by sequence variants in genes encoding drug-metabolizing enzymes, drug transporters, or drug targets.

Drug-Metabolizing Enzymes

Genetic polymorphisms in drug-metabolizing enzymes give rise to distinct population subgroups that differ in their ability to carry out certain biotransformation reactions. These differences can lead to changes in enzyme levels or enzyme activity in particular groups of people. Structurally altered enzymes can exhibit either an increased or decreased Michaelis constant K_m or maximum velocity V_{max}, or both. There are more than 30 families of drug-metabolizing enzymes in humans, almost all with polymorphic variants. Many of these polymorphisms translate into functional changes in the enzymes encoded, although all variations in enzyme structure may not lead to clinically significant differences in metabolizing ability.

Gene amplification leads to increased expression of the mRNA for an enzyme and subsequently a greater amount of the enzyme. This can result in a patient population resistant to the drug because the drug is eliminated very rapidly. Gene deletion leads to a deficiency in enzyme activity either because the enzyme is not made at all or an incomplete or nonfunctional one is made. This gives rise to a patient population that is a slow metabolizer of a particular drug. In this situation, plasma drug concentrations can quickly reach toxic levels even at standard therapeutic doses. Figure 17.5 shows a typical frequency distribution of normal metabolizers and slow metabolizers of a drug.

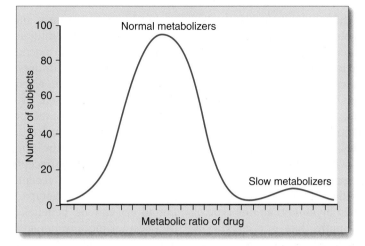

Figure 17.5. A typical bimodal graph showing the frequency distribution of normal metabolizers and slow metabolizers of a drug. The *X*-axis is the metabolic ratio, defined as the ratio between parent drug concentration and metabolite concentration in plasma. The higher the ratio (slow metabolizers) the greater the probability of adverse drug reactions. A small percentage of the population is slow metabolizers of the drug in this example. Trimodal graphs, showing three different metabolic subgroups, are also seen for some drugs.

CYP Enzymes. Much work has been done with the CYP450 family of enzymes, which is responsible for the biotransformation of most drugs. There appears to be a relatively high incidence of polymorphism in the six most common CYP drug-metabolizing enzymes (CYP1A2, CYP3A4, CYP2A6, CYP2C9, CYP2C19, and CYP2D6). For example, approximately 90 SNP variants of CYP2D6, 10 of which have been shown to be clinically important, have been found. This enzyme is responsible for biotransformation of more than 50 different drugs, including antidepressants (amitriptyline, fluoxetine, paroxetine), antipsychotics (risperidone, haloperidol), and opioid analgesics (morphine, codeine). The CYP2D6 metabolism of the antihypertensive drug debrisoquine is used as an index of CYP2D6 activity. This drug has been used in population studies to classify individuals as "poor metabolizers," "intermediate metabolizers," "extensive metabolizers," or "ultra-rapid metabolizers" of CYP2D6 substrates. Approximately 1% to 10% of people in various ethnic groups are poor metabolizers of drugs that are substrates for CYP2D6.

Other Enzymes. Other enzyme systems are affected by SNPs as well. For example, SNPs are responsible for a number of variants of the enzyme N-acetyl-transferase-2, which plays a role in the phase II acetylation of several drugs, including isoniazid. In particular, a rapid-metabolizing and a slow-metabolizing variant can be distinguished, the corresponding individuals being known as "rapid acetylators" and "slow acetylators," respectively. Rapid acetylators require high doses of the drugs concerned whereas slow acetylators need smaller doses. This is because the drug persists longer and in higher concentrations in the cells of patients with the slow-metabolizing variant of the enzyme. It was observed that therapeutic failure rates for pulmonary tuberculosis treated with isoniazid were higher in rapid acetylators than in slow acetylators, presumably because the duration of action of isoniazid was shorter.

Clinical Implications. One way to identify slow metabolizers of a particular drug is to monitor blood levels after dosing.

Unusually high drug levels may be a sign of slow metabolism as a result of an enzyme defect. However, drug level monitoring is expensive and inconvenient, and high drug levels may be caused by other physiological problems as well.

Genotyping of individuals to identify genetic polymorphisms of drug-metabolizing enzymes is a more direct approach and may be widely available some day. Using such genotype information may not be self-evident, however. Many drugs are metabolized by more than one type of reaction, and more than one enzyme is involved. In addition, each enzyme may have several possible polymorphisms, not all of which may be clinically important. Thus, identification of an individual with a polymorphism in a particular enzyme may shed little light on how to plan drug therapy.

In general, clinically significant genetic polymorphisms of drug metabolism occur when the metabolic pathway subject to polymorphism is a major route of elimination for the drug, if the drug has a narrow therapeutic range, or if the drug is a prodrug that must be metabolized to produce pharmacologically active metabolites.

Many pharmaceutical companies are trying to get around the issue of slow metabolizers in a different way. For example, because of the high incidence of CYP2D6 polymorphism, pharmaceutical companies are designing drugs with structures that do not involve CYP2D6 for biotransformation.

Drug Targets

Pharmacodynamic effects can lead to interindividual differences in drug effect despite the presence of appropriate concentrations of drug at the intended site of action. Here, effects of the drug are modulated by variations in how the target molecule, or another downstream element of the target molecule's signal transduction pathway, responds to the drug. In contrast to the wealth of information available on the genetic polymorphism of metabolizing enzymes, the importance of polymorphism in influencing receptor structure and the pharmacodynamics of a drug is yet to be well understood.

Mutations in receptor genes can make receptors *hyporesponsive* or *hyperresponsive*. A hyporesponsive receptor is one less susceptible than normal to up- or down-regulation, whereas the opposite is true for a hyperresponsive receptor. However, not all mutations in receptor genes are problematic in drug therapy. In fact, some mutations can be beneficial by making the receptor more responsive to the drug, whereas others may not significantly influence drug–receptor interactions at all.

For example, asthmatic patients with a certain genotype of the β_2-adrenergic receptor do not respond to the most commonly prescribed inhaled drug, albuterol. The gene in this case carries the information for the β_2-adrenergic receptor at which the drug acts. If the base present at position 16 of this gene is adenine, albuterol is able to exert its effect. If, on the other hand, guanine is present at this position, the receptor fails to perform its function and the drug is inactive.

Tumors often express unusual combinations of genes and proteins compared with normal cells. For example, individuals with a mutation in *BRCA1* or *BRCA2* genes express a different pattern of mRNA and proteins are responsible for regulating the cell cycle and cell proliferation. The classification of cancer tumors on the basis of their mutation or genetic variation may be very valuable as a diagnostic tool and may help to select the best therapy.

Genotyping of infectious agents such as bacteria and viruses is also expected to be useful in selecting the best therapy. Many infectious agents mutate and become resistant to certain antimicrobial or antiviral drugs. For example, the HIV-AIDS virus in a patient can be genotyped to determine whether it is resistant to certain drugs. Selection of the appropriate drugs for the patient can make therapy more successful and less expensive.

There are also several cases of genetic variability in signal transduction or other downstream proteins influencing drug response. An example is angiotensin-converting enzyme (ACE) inhibitors, which block conversion of angiotensin I to angiotensin II and prevent breakdown of bradykinin. Polymorphism in the G protein-coupled receptor of bradykinin results in cough, one of the side effects of ACE inhibitors. Thus, although the polymorphism is not directly in the protein that is the target of ACE inhibitors, it influences the overall response of these drugs.

Transporters

Many transport proteins are involved in the absorption, distribution, and excretion of drugs so that their genetic variation will contribute to variability in drug disposition among individuals. Transport proteins may also be implicated in pharmacodynamics if they are themselves drug targets. Because many drug transporters are still unknown and the functions of many transporters have not been fully defined, much work needs to be done before we can understand the impact of transporter polymorphisms on drug disposition and response.

Among the most extensively studied transporters involved in drug disposition is P-glycoprotein encoded by the human *ABCB1* gene (also called *MDR1*) on chromosome 7. It is believed a polymorphism of the multidrug-resistant efflux protein MDR1 can explain the differences in oral absorption and target organ accumulation of several drugs. For example, a variation in the *MDR1* gene results in low expression of the transporter and, consequently, high plasma levels of digoxin after oral dosing.

The serotonin transporter, which is the target of serotonin reuptake inhibitor drugs, is another transporter known to show genetic variation that is related to drug response. Studies have documented an association between genotype and antidepressant response.

Clinical Applications of Pharmacogenomics

Even the most successful drugs provide optimal benefits to only a fraction of patients; some patients show no benefit, whereas others experience unacceptable toxicity. For example, studies have shown up to 30% of patients do not respond to 3-hydroxy-3-methylglutaryl coenzyme A (HMG-CoA) reductase inhibitors (statins such as atorvastatin), up to 35% do not respond to β-blockers (e.g., propranolol), and as many as 50% do not respond to tricyclic antidepressants (e.g., desipramine).

Even for patients who are helped by a particular drug, optimal doses can vary widely among individuals. For example, the daily therapeutic dose varies 20-fold for warfarin, and 40-fold for propranolol. The variability in dose and response is very apparent for the common cholesterol-lowering drug simvastatin. It lowers LDL (low-density lipoprotein) levels in patients by an average of 41% at the recommended 40-mg dose, 47% at an 80-mg dose, and 53% at a 160-mg dose. However, even at the highest dose of 160 mg, about 5% of patients show only a 10% to 20% reduction and 6% of patients show no LDL lowering at all. These numbers illustrate the interindividual variability in drug response, even for very successful and relatively safe drugs.

Many aspects of interindividual variability in drug efficacy and toxicity can be traced back to genetic variability. One of the goals of pharmacogenomics is to identify the precise subgroup of patients that will benefit from a particular drug. The reverse situation—trying to identify those at risk for toxicity from a certain drug—is also important. Screening tests to identify the presence or absence of critical genes are being developed, and will help to identify the optimal drug for a given patient. Figure 17.6 shows one way that pharmacogenomics will influence future drug therapy.

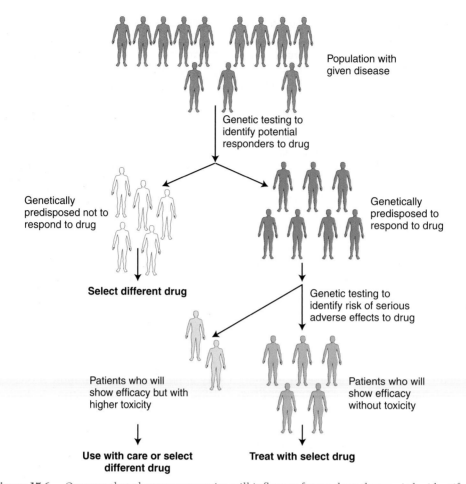

Population with given disease

Genetic testing to identify potential responders to drug

Genetically predisposed not to respond to drug

Genetically predisposed to respond to drug

Select different drug

Genetic testing to identify risk of serious adverse effects to drug

Patients who will show efficacy but with higher toxicity

Patients who will show efficacy without toxicity

Use with care or select different drug

Treat with select drug

Figure 17.6.   One way that pharmacogenomics will influence future drug therapy is by identifying the right drug therapy for the right patient.

For example, it is estimated in various studies that only 20% to 40% of Alzheimer's patients benefit from the drug tacrine. Researchers have discovered that patients with the gene subtype *ApoE4* are less likely to benefit from the drug. Such knowledge helps to target the use of tacrine, facilitates valid data analysis of clinical trials of Alzheimer's therapies, and will promote investigation of new therapies specifically for *ApoE4* carriers.

The anticipated benefits of pharmacogenomics on future drug therapy are numerous:

- *Advanced screening for disease:* Knowing one's disease susceptibility will allow a person to make lifestyle and environmental changes at an early age to avoid or lessen the severity of a genetic disease. Prior knowledge of a patient's disease susceptibility will allow physicians to monitor and initiate therapy at the appropriate stage of the disease.
- *Targeted drugs:* Pharmaceutical companies will be able to design drugs based on the proteins, enzymes, and RNA associated with diseases, facilitating therapies better targeted to specific diseases with maximum therapeutic effects and minimal damage to healthy cells.
- *Choice of drug:* Instead of the standard trial-and-error method of matching patients with the right drugs, physicians

will be able to analyze a patient's genetic profile and prescribe the best available drug therapy from the beginning. This will speed recovery time, decrease likelihood of adverse effects, and increase safety.

- *Choice of dose:* The current practice of basing doses on patient weight and age will be replaced with doses based on a person's genetics—how an individual's pharmacokinetics handles a drug. This will maximize efficacy and safety.

- *Designing "universal" drugs:* Some scientists believe that pharmacogenomics could be used to design drugs that are intentionally not affected by, or bypass, common polymorphisms among individuals. Such drugs could be given safely to all patients and ensure both efficacy and safety.

Figure 17.7 illustrates the approach to discovering targeted drugs using pharmacogenomic and genetic information.

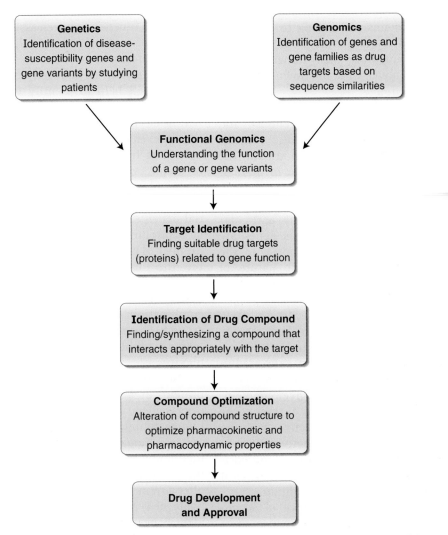

Figure 17.7. Use of genetic and genomic strategies in new drug discovery. It will be useful to combine genetic and genomic strategies and to focus on identification of targets that will lead to new and effective drugs. Genomics and genetics complement each other by providing focus and speed to target identification.

Proteomics

The elucidation of the human genome and numerous pathogen genomes will have a profound impact on our understanding of human disease and its treatment. The Human Genome Project has given scientists the structure and sequences of thousands of genes that encode for hitherto unknown proteins. About 30,000 genes could well translate into one million proteins. In most cases, gene sequence reveals little about the protein structure or its role in disease. Although many of these proteins will belong to well-characterized families with predictable biological functions, many others will be entirely novel with unknown structure and function.

The term proteome refers to all the proteins expressed by a genome, and proteomics is the systematic identification of proteins in the body and the determination of their role in biological functions. Although an individual's genome remains unchanged to a large extent, the proteins in any particular cell change dramatically as genes are turned on and off in response to the environment. The dynamic nature of the proteome has led to the term *functional proteome* to describe all the proteins produced by a specific cell at a particular time. Although there may be more than 100,000 proteins in humans, only a fraction of these are expressed in any given cell type. Only certain genes in a cell are active at any given moment, and as cells mature, many of their genes become permanently inactive. It is the pattern of active and inactive genes in a cell and its resulting protein composition that determines what kind of cell it is and what it can and cannot do.

To discover the relevance of a protein to a disease process, scientists must catalog where, when, and to what extent a protein is expressed, and how these parameters are altered in the disease state. If all the proteins present in a cell at any one time were known, it would indicate which genes were currently expressed and producing these proteins. If this cataloging process were repeated at various stages in a cell's life cycle, it would yield a biochemical timeline of the particular physiological process of interest.

Many human diseases occur because of irregularities in protein interactions that can be related directly to alterations in protein structure. However, not all proteins are going to be involved in producing disease. The true value of genome sequence information will only be realized after a function has been assigned for each of the encoded proteins; this is the task of proteomics.

Ultimately, it is believed that proteomics will help to identify new disease markers and drug targets, which will then help to design compounds that prevent, diagnose, and treat disease. The future of biotechnology and medicine will be impacted greatly by proteomics, but there is still much to do before patients can realize the potential benefits. Genome sequencing was a large but finite problem; there are a fixed number of genes in the human genome. But the human proteome involves or impacts hundreds of tissues, thousands of diseases, hundreds of cell types all in combination, and it all changes by the second. This makes sequencing the proteome a problem of much greater complexity.

Most drugs work by interacting with proteins in some way, but all the known drugs affect only about 300 to 500 human proteins. That leaves more than 100,000 human proteins with unknown functions, waiting for drugs that might interact with them. These novel proteins offer a tremendous opportunity to investigate new pathways for disease and to identify new molecular targets to address unmet therapeutic needs. If one could make chemical compounds that interfere with the synthesis of the protein, the resulting changes in the organism would help to understand the protein's role. The chemical compound structure could then be appropriately fine-tuned to yield a drug.

Promise of Pharmacogenomics

The statement "no single drug fits all patients" is the new maxim in drug therapy. The emerging challenge for the pharmaceutical sciences is to understand why individuals respond differently to drug therapy, and then to design drugs taking this variability into account. Many pharmaceutical companies have begun to direct their research activities toward achieving individualized medicine; the approach is now toward finding the "right" patient population for a given drug.

In the near future, genetic analysis may help us to get to individualized medicine: the right drug for the right patient at the right time. By understanding the molecular basis of individual variation in drug response, we will be able to focus on the patient as an individual and identify the drug and dose most suited for the patient at that time. We also know environmental factors will play an important role in the success of the therapy. The complete understanding of the environmental and molecular basis of drug response will be a long, complicated but exciting process.

Key Concepts

- Genetic variation arises as a result of mutations or polymorphisms. Mutations are relatively rare, whereas a polymorphism is a genetic variation present in at least 1% of the population.
- Single-nucleotide polymorphisms (SNPs) are the most common type of polymorphism and arise from an alteration of one base pair in a gene.
- Monogenic disorders occur because of a genetic defect in one gene. Most monogenic diseases manifest themselves regardless of the individual's lifestyle or environment.
- Polygenic or complex disorders are the most prevalent illnesses and arise because of a complex interaction of defects in several susceptibility genes and the individual's environment and lifestyle.
- Genetic variation can influence an individual's response to drugs by affecting drug pharmacokinetics or pharmacodynamics.
- Polymorphisms of drug-metabolizing enzymes can give rise to distinct subgroups (slow, intermediate, and fast metabolizers) in the population.
- Variations in drug targets (receptors, enzymes) or their signal transduction pathways can affect drug pharmacodynamics.
- Genetic variability of transporters can influence absorption, distribution, metabolism, or elimination, or pharmacodynamics, of a drug.
- Pharmacogenomics will have a large impact in improving drug therapy outcomes for patients, and in developing new drugs with better safety and efficacy profiles.
- Proteomics, the characterization of the structure and function of all the proteins in the body, promises to be the next major advance in this area.

Review Questions

1. Describe three causes of mutations in DNA. How is a germline mutation different from a somatic mutation?
2. Describe the major types of genetic variation, including mutations and single-nucleotide polymorphisms.
3. How are mutations different from genetic polymorphisms? What is meant by a single-nucleotide polymorphism (SNP)?
4. Do all mutations and genetic polymorphisms lead to disease? Why not?
5. Elaborate on the effect of genetic variability on drug-metabolizing enzymes, drug transporters, and drug targets.
6. Why are polygenic disorders more complex than monogenic disorders?
7. How does the environment influence the probability of getting a disease? What is meant by susceptibility genes?
8. How can SNPs influence the metabolism, transport, and action of a drug?
9. Why are SNPs in *CYP* genes particularly relevant in variability of drug response among individuals?
10. What are the benefits of a pharmacogenomic approach to drug research and therapy?
11. Why is the proteome as important as or more important than the genome for understanding disease and for the discovery and development of new drugs?

CASE STUDIES

Drug metabolism: It's hereditary

Over 100 allelic variants of *CYP2D6* have been reported, some of which can lead to altered enzyme activity. A commonly accepted classification system designates individuals homozygous for two wild-type *CYP2D6* alleles as CYP2D6*1/*1, and refers to such persons as extensive metabolizers (EMs). The majority of the population is classified as EMs and smaller proportions are classified as poor metabolizers (PM), intermediate metabolizers (IM), and ultra metabolizers (UM).

Case Study 17.1

Tamoxifen is a standard endocrine therapy for the prevention and treatment of estrogen receptor (ER)-positive breast cancer. It acts as an antagonist at ERα in breast tissue to inhibit the growth of ER-positive and estrogen-sensitive breast cancer cells.

Tamoxifen is administered orally as the citrate salt and undergoes extensive metabolism by the following pathways.

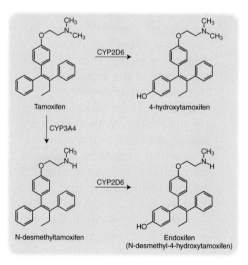

The plasma concentrations of endoxifen are 6- to 12-fold higher than 4-hydroxy-tamoxifen in patients receiving chronic tamoxifen therapy. Endoxifen and 4-hydroxy-tamoxifen are equipotent and have a 10-fold higher affinity for ERα than tamoxifen.

1. Describe the genotype for each of the above phenotypes—PM, IM, and UM.
2. It has been noted that when tamoxifen is used in women with a certain CYP2D6 phenotype, they tend to have higher relapse rates and shorter disease-free survival times than women with other CYP2D6 phenotypes. Which phenotype tends to render a less successful outcome and why?
3. A characteristic adverse effect of tamoxifen therapy is moderate to severe hot flashes. Women with the PM phenotype, however, experience tamoxifen-induced hot flashes to a far lesser extent. Why may this be the case?
4. It was noted that women taking certain antidepressants (fluoxetine, paroxetine) would not experience hot flashes when taking tamoxifen. Co-prescribing these antidepressants with tamoxifen became a common practice. What is one potential mechanism by which fluoxetine may decrease tamoxifen-induced hot flashes?

5. Would this combination of fluoxetine with tamoxifen have any effect on the efficacy of tamoxifen?

Case Study 17.2

Metoprolol is a selective β₁-receptor blocker and is a substrate for CYP2D6. Metoprolol is used in the treatment of hypertension and the dose is titrated over time to achieve the desired effect.

1. How would the different phenotypes of CYP2D6-mediated metabolism affect the dosing of metoprolol?
2. A case can be made that genotyping for CYP2D6 alleles may be necessary prior to use of tamoxifen but not prior to use of metoprolol. Explain why that may be true.
3. Consider the addition of a drug that inhibits CYP2D6 in a patient currently taking metoprolol. Which phenotype, the extensive metabolizer or the poor metabolizer, will more likely experience a clinically significant drug interaction?
4. What are the consequences of using codeine in a patient with a CYP2D6 ultra-rapid metabolizer phenotype?
5. Explain how a patient with the CYP2D6*1/*1 genotype (extensive metabolizer) can be changed to an ultra-rapid metabolizer phenotype for codeine by the addition of clarithromycin.

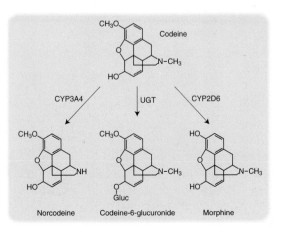

Additional Readings

McLeod HL (ed). Pharmacogenomics: Applications to Patient Care, 2nd ed. American College of Clinical Pharmacy, 2009.

Weber W. Pharmacogenetics, 2nd ed. Oxford University Press, 2008.

Wong S, Linder MW, Valdes R (eds). Pharmacogenomics and Proteomics: Enabling the Practice of Personalized Medicine. AACC Press, 2006.

Zdanowicz M. Concepts in Pharmacogenomics. ASHP, 2010.

PART VI

Special Topics

The important thing in science is not so much to obtain new facts as to discover new ways of thinking about them.
—Sir William Bragg

Chapter 18 Biopharmaceutical Drugs

Chapter 19 Drug Discovery and Approval

Biopharmaceutical Drugs

Most drugs on the market are small molecules that are typically manufactured through chemical synthesis. Most of our discussion in this book has focused on the behavior of these "conventional" drugs. However, an increasing number of new therapeutic agents are macromolecules (e.g., proteins and antibodies) and the trend is expected to continue. Most of these drugs are large, complex molecules or mixtures of molecules that cannot be easily extracted from natural sources or manufactured by conventional chemical synthesis. They may be variously called biotech drugs, biologics, biologicals, biopharmaceuticals, etc., although each of these terms has a slightly different meaning.

Biopharmaceuticals are defined as substances produced in living systems by biotechnology and used for therapeutic purposes or in vivo diagnostics. Because of the way they are made, these agents are often called *biotech drugs* and include therapeutic peptides and proteins, antibodies, oligonucleotides and nucleic acid derivatives, and DNA preparations. Biopharmaceuticals are part of a broader category of therapeutic agents called biologics (or biologicals), defined as any therapeutic agent manufactured in living systems such as microorganisms, or plant and animal cells. Biologics not only include biopharmaceuticals, but

also blood and blood components, vaccines, and other biomolecules extracted directly from natural (nonengineered) sources.

Most of our discussion of biopharmaceuticals in this chapter will focus on therapeutic proteins and antibodies. We will also touch upon nucleic acid derivatives and gene therapy, because these newer therapeutic approaches, although still in their infancy, show great promise.

Biotechnology and Genetic Engineering

Most biopharmaceutical drugs are made using biotechnology, a general term for processes that use living organisms or parts of living organisms to make or modify products for human use. During natural biosynthesis of proteins in our body's cells, several complex enzymes ensure that proteins are made and folded correctly into their active three-dimensional structure. These interactions are optimal in a very narrow range of conditions present naturally in the organism that makes the protein. These strictly controlled processes make it next to impossible to duplicate protein production by chemical synthesis. Instead, proteins must be produced

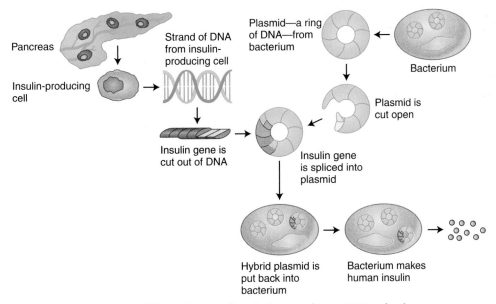

Figure 18.1. An overview of the production of insulin by recombinant DNA technology.

in and isolated from laboratory animals, microorganisms or special cultures of animal or plant cells.

The rapid growth of biotechnology has been primarily due to our ability to manipulate an organism's genes. Genetic engineering, or recombinant DNA (rDNA) technology, is the process of moving genetic information from one chromosome to another or from one organism to another. It includes a group of techniques for locating the desired gene, isolating it, and then moving it into the genome of another cell or organism to achieve the desired goal. It is this integration of natural sciences and engineering sciences that allows the use of organisms, cells, or their parts to make therapeutic biopharmaceutical products on a large scale. The terms biotechnology, genetic engineering, and rDNA technology are often used interchangeably. An overview of how rDNA technology is used to produce human insulin is shown in Figure 18.1.

Before the advent of genetic engineering, biopharmaceutical drug supplies were limited because proteins had to be obtained from natural sources. For instance, insulin was collected from slaughtered pigs and human growth hormone was obtained from human cadavers. With genetic engineering, the gene for a protein drug of interest can be transferred into an appropriate "host" organism that can produce large amounts of the protein. A number of therapeutic proteins and protein-based drugs are now readily available commercially as a result of progress in biotechnology and genetic engineering. A detailed discussion of biotechnology is outside the scope of this book.

Advantages of the Biopharmaceutical Approach

The targets for most conventional drugs are proteins; in particular receptor proteins present at the surface of cells, or catalytic proteins (enzymes). The goal is to either increase or decrease the inherent activity of the protein, and thus alter a physiological process that is causing disease or illness. Because these proteins are diverse and found at many different cellular locations, each new drug has to be developed from scratch. In addition, interference with the activity of the protein at an unintended location can cause side effects. The drugs are also not completely selective, so may bind to similar, non-target, proteins, also resulting in side effects.

Rather than using a small molecule to alter protein function, the protein itself could be the drug. Therapeutic proteins and peptides represent a class of biopharmaceutical drugs that allow management of diseases not treated adequately with conventional drugs. rDNA and cell culture can now be used to produce these therapeutic proteins, which are then administered to the patient.

Some diseases are caused when defective genes do not produce the correct protein, or enough of the protein, that the body requires. Examples are insulin for the treatment of diabetes and clotting factors in hemophilia. Other diseases are caused when the production of certain proteins is unusually high. For example, in about 25% of cases of breast cancer, the presence of a certain receptor protein (HER2) on the surface of tumor cells is greatly increased. As a result, the cells are more receptive to growth signals and keep on dividing. We can use an antibody (a type of protein) to block these receptors and prevent them from receiving growth signals and thus slow tumor growth. In addition, antibody-receptor binding stimulates certain immune cells to kill the tumor cell. Therefore, using therapeutic proteins or antibodies as drugs represents a more specific and direct form of therapy.

An even more direct approach is to alter the production of the protein in the body. One could design biopharmaceutical drugs targeted against the messenger RNA (mRNA) molecules that encode the proteins. This approach is referred to as nucleic acid-based therapeutics.

Ultimately, gene therapy could be used to introduce the correct copy of a gene to replace a defective or absent one. All these therapeutic approaches are illustrated in Figure 18.2.

Types of Biopharmaceutical Drugs

Therapeutic Proteins

Therapeutic proteins represent a class of drugs that allow management of diseases not treated adequately with conventional small molecule drugs. Proteins can be used in therapy in two ways. In one application, large amounts of a particular protein drug may be given to suppress a process that contributes to the disease or trauma. For example, fibrinolytics (clot-destroying biotech drugs such as Activase® and Retavase®) are used in facilitative therapy for the treatment of heart attacks. When administered in large doses, their natural biological function can be used to dissolve blood clots.

Another application is in replacement therapy; the therapeutic protein replaces or supplements a protein that is deficient or defective in a patient. For example, insulin is used as replacement therapy to compensate for the lower levels of insulin made by the pancreas of diabetic patients. Selected examples of therapeutic protein drugs on the market are shown in Table 18.1.

Structure of Proteins

Peptides and proteins are made up of amino acid building blocks. The distinction between a peptide and a protein is often based on size, and is somewhat arbitrary and variable. A peptide is a compound with two or more amino acids covalently bonded by a peptide bond. A protein is a functional polypeptide with at least 50 amino acids and a distinctive three-dimensional conformation. Many polypeptide drugs can be made synthetically and are therefore not strictly classified as biotech drugs, although they may share some of the characteristics of biopharmaceuticals. Other small polypeptides cannot yet be made synthetically, and have to be manufactured by recombinant

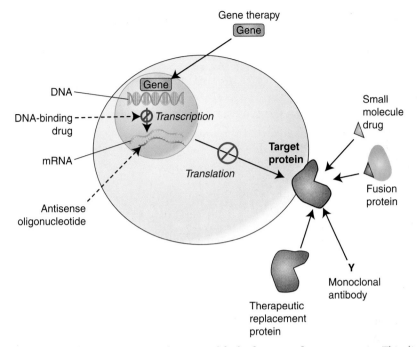

Figure 18.2. Various therapeutic approaches to modify the function of a target protein. This diagram shows a cell surface protein target, but the target could be intracellular. A small molecule drug can bind to the protein. The protein can be replaced if it is in short supply. A monoclonal antibody can bind to the protein in a very specific manner and alter its function. A fusion protein (therapeutic protein with an antibody fragment) can help to target the replacement protein. An antisense drug can prevent the translation process for making the protein. A DNA binding drug can alter the transcription process. Gene therapy can alter the genome to adjust protein synthesis.

TABLE 18.1. Examples of Marketed Therapeutic Protein Drugs			
Brand Name	*Active Drug*	*Class*	*Indication*
Procrit®	Epoetin alfa	Erythropoietin	Anemia (chemotherapy)
Aranesp®	Darbepoetin alfa	Erythropoietin	Anemia (chemotherapy)
Humatrope®	Somatotropin	Human growth hormone	Growth hormone deficiency
Follistim®	Follicle stimulating hormone	Follicle stimulating hormone	Ovulatory dysfunction
Remicade®	TNF alpha	Tumor necrosis factor	
Neupogen®	Filgrastim	Granulocyte colony stimulating factor	Bone marrow transplant
Avonex®	Interferon beta-1a	β-Interferon	Multiple sclerosis
Humulin®	Human recombinant insulin	Insulin	Diabetes
Activase®	Recombinant alteplase	Tissue plasminogen activator	Acute myocardial infarction

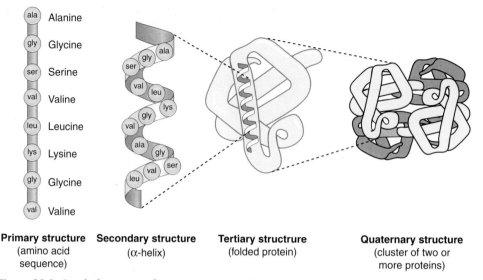

Figure 18.3. Level of structure of proteins. Amino acids linked by peptide bonds form the chain of the primary structure. Secondary structure results from interactions (mainly hydrogen bonding) between the side chains of the amino acid residues in the chain. The side chains of the amino acids interact further via hydrogen bonds or disulfide bonds to fold the protein into its three-dimensional tertiary structure that is compatible with the environment. The quaternary structure arises as a result of association of two or more protein molecules to form a complex.

methods. For our purposes, the term *protein* will used to include all polypeptide made by biotechnology.

For example, nafarelin acetate (Synarel®), a synthetic analog of the natural gonadotropin-releasing hormone (GnRH), is a decapeptide (molecular weight 1,322) and is not strictly a biotech drug. It is used to treat endometriosis or uterine fibroids in women. Nesiritide (Natrecor®), the recombinant form of the 32 amino acid human B-type natriuretic peptide (molecular weight 3,464), is a biotech drug, used to treat acute congestive heart failure.

The secondary and tertiary structure of proteins is important to their function. The 3D structure depends on diverse, often weak, interactions between amino acids. Often, a number of proteins form functional complexes with quaternary structures; only when arranged in this way can they perform their intended functions. The level of structure of proteins is shown in Figure 18.3. Many, but not all, endogenous proteins also undergo posttranslational modifications in which a carbohydrate is attached to the protein (glycosylation) to give a glycoprotein (Fig. 18.4). Correct glycosylation is very important for the physicochemical and

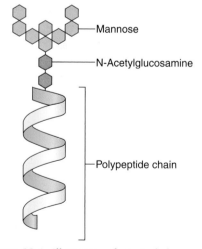

Figure 18.4. Illustration of a typical glycoprotein, with a carbohydrate (mannose) covalently bonded to the protein by N-acetylglucosamine

TABLE 18.2. Physicochemical and Biological Properties That Are Changed When a Protein Undergoes Glycosylation or Other Posttranslational Modification	
Physicochemical Properties	*Biological Properties*
Solubility	Immunogenicity
Protein folding behavior	Affinity for, and binding to, target
Stability of 3D conformation	Interaction with other proteins
Susceptibility to hydrolysis	Plasma half-life
Susceptibility to denaturation	Localization

biological behavior of a therapeutic protein drug, as listed in Table 18.2.

Manufacture of Therapeutic Proteins

Protein drugs are generally made by large-scale cultivation of genetically engineered "host" cells; rapidly growing cells with artificially inserted genes that encode the protein being made. These cells are grown in large fermenters, lysed at the appropriate time, and the protein of interest isolated and purified. The selection of the host organism for production is a technical and economic decision. The isolation and purification of the protein in its intact form is also an immense technical challenge.

Small molecule drugs with known chemical structures can be synthesized exactly in the laboratory, and their structure and purity can be confirmed with great precision and accuracy. On the other hand, biotechnological production is more technically demanding and consequently more expensive than simple chemical synthesis. Relatively small changes in the temperature, salt content or pH during manufacture can alter the structure of the final protein. Manufacturing variability can cause unanticipated changes in the folding and therefore the efficacy and safety profile of the protein.

After manufacture, characterization of the concentration and purity of biopharmaceutical drugs is difficult, because the analytical tools for biologics are 10 to 100 times less sensitive than for conventional drugs. Therefore, very extensive and stringent tests have to be put into place during manufacture of biopharmaceuticals to ensure that the final drug is what was intended. In other words, the process conditions during manufacture will determine the identity and purity of the drug. Post-manufacture testing is not reliable enough to guarantee quality.

Bacterial Hosts. Many bacteria, such as *Escherichia coli*, can readily acquire new genes by taking up DNA molecules such as plasmids from their surroundings. Large amounts of bacterial cells can be grown easily in commercial-sized fermenters to give useful quantities of therapeutic proteins. This has made it possible to produce virtually unlimited amounts of many human proteins in vitro.

However, bacterial hosts present some disadvantages. There is a possibility of the presence of pyrogenic (fever causing) and endotoxin (immunogenic) contaminants from bacterial cell membranes in the final product. In addition, the exact human protein may not be produced because bacteria do not perform post-translational modifications such as glycosylation or phosphorylation.

Bacterial hosts are particularly suited to producing smaller proteins (less than about 30 kD), or those that do not require post-translational modification, such as insulin or growth hormone. An inexpensive, easy-to-grow culture of genetically engineered bacteria such as the common *E. coli* can manufacture these protein drugs.

Yeast Cell Hosts

Yeasts have been used to express recombinant proteins to overcome the shortcoming of bacterial expression systems. The most obvious advantage in yeast over bacteria is the capability of processing diverse posttranslational modifications required to produce "authentic" and bioactive mammalian proteins. In addition, yeast expression systems have the following advantages: high level of protein secretion, rapid growth rate, ease of large-scale production, ease of genetic manipulation, lower cost compared with animal expression systems, lack of endotoxins, lytic viruses, and no known pathogenic relationship with man. Yeasts are also capable of expressing larger proteins, greater than 50 kD.

Saccharomyces cerevisiae, a common and safe yeast used in baking and brewing, was the first to be used for the production of recombinant proteins such as interferon and hepatitis surface antigen. But *S. cerevisiae* often causes super-high glycosylation in expressing glycosylated proteins, so other yeast hosts have been identified that offer the characteristics well suited to the expression of a particular protein. *Pichia pastoris* is a yeast that has been extensively used for this purpose. Even when posttranslational modification patterns generated by yeasts are different than those desired, they can sometimes be changed by altering experimental conditions or other genetic engineering techniques.

Mammalian Cell Hosts

Proteins that are difficult to express, or those that require "complete authenticity" to human proteins, can only be produced using host cells of higher organisms such as mammals. However, prediction and consistency of glycosylation in the manufacture of therapeutic proteins is an issue with mammalian hosts as well.

Genetically engineered Chinese hamster ovary (CHO) cells have been used extensively for production of many biotech drugs. These cells can perform the posttranslational processing necessary for the secretion of a biologically active recombinant protein. In addition, CHO cells have a very low susceptibility to contamination by human viruses, usually a potentially serious problem in the manufacture of recombinant products. However, because CHO cells are not of human origin, proteins produced in CHO are often glycosylated differently compared with their native human counterparts, and further genetic engineering is needed to produce the correct protein.

Unfortunately, mammalian hosts are difficult and expensive to grow and transfect, and the cultures have lower cell densities and slower growth rates, resulting in smaller yields of protein. Mammalian cells also carry the risk of containing oncogenes or viral DNA, so recombinant protein products derived from them must be tested more extensively.

Transgenic Animal Hosts. Cloned genes can also be expressed in vivo if introduced into the germline of an animal. An animal that is genetically engineered by insertion of a foreign gene into its genome is called a transgenic organism, and the introduced engineered gene is a *transgene*. The protein encoded by the transgene is secreted into the animal's milk, eggs, or blood, and then collected and purified. Livestock such as cattle, sheep, goats, chickens, rabbits, and pigs have been modified in this way to potentially produce several useful proteins and drugs. A new term, *pharming*, is now being used, a combination of the words *farming* and *pharmaceuticals*, to describe the combination of methods of agriculture with advanced biotechnology. Another term for this technology is *molecular farming*. Cloning methods have dramatically improved farming technology; when one suitable transgenic animal has been raised, an unlimited number of genetically identical animals can be produced rapidly.

Milk production by mammals has been the target for production of therapeutic

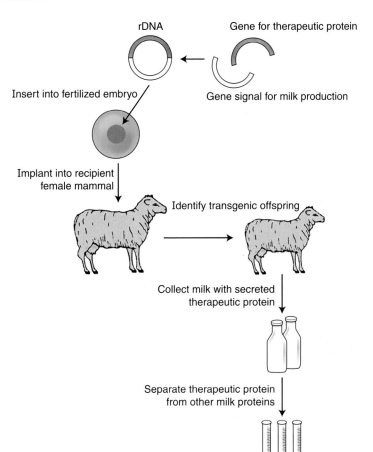

rDNA   Gene for therapeutic protein

Insert into fertilized embryo   Gene signal for milk production

Implant into recipient
female mammal

Identify transgenic offspring

Collect milk with secreted
therapeutic protein

Separate therapeutic protein
from other milk proteins

Figure 18.5. Process for the development of a transgenic animal that secretes a therapeutic protein into milk.

proteins, illustrated in Figure 18.5. The gene for the therapeutic protein is coupled with a DNA signal directing milk production in the mammary gland. This rDNA is injected into a fertilized animal embryo (cow, sheep, goat, or mouse). The embryos are then implanted into recipient females where, hopefully, they survive and are born normally. Female offspring of these animals may also continue to produce the desired protein.

Transgenic animals are now being used for the production of therapeutic proteins that require complex posttranslational modifications or are needed in large quantities. The isolation of the protein is much easier from transgenic animals than from cellular hosts. However, because of the long time periods involved in the development of a mature animal, obtaining biopharmaceuticals from transgenic animals is currently very expensive.

ATryn®, a recombinant form of human antithrombin, also known as ATIII, is at the forefront of transgenic technology for the production of biotherapeutics. It is the first transgenically produced therapeutic protein to be approved by the Food and Drug Administration (FDA). Antithrombin is an anticoagulant and anti-inflammatory plasma protein that is currently obtained from human blood supply, and has been difficult to express using conventional recombinant protein production methods. ATryn is produced in the milk of genetically engineered goats. Its amino acid sequence is identical to that of human plasma-derived antithrombin. The glycosylation profile of ATryn is different from plasma-derived antithrombin, which actually results in an increased heparin affinity and efficacy.

Transgenic Plant Hosts. Plant biotechnology was developed to improve agricultural products but is now being studied to manufacture biopharmaceuticals, including vaccines, for human health. Like transgenic animals, transgenic plants may be engineered to produce the therapeutic protein of choice. Plants and plant cells are easier and cheaper to grow on a large scale, and human pathogens do not replicate in plants, making the final product safer. A variety of plants are being examined, such as corn, soybean, canola, alfalfa, and tobacco.

One approach is to use bioreactors plant cell systems rather than the crops themselves. Genetically engineered plant cells, such as carrot and tobacco cells, can be grown on an industrial scale in a closed and controlled environment. The closed system provides stable, optimized conditions, with manufacturing capabilities for the entire range of proteins, including antibodies, complex enzymes, and plant-derived pharmaceuticals.

There are some obstacles with transgenic plant-based biopharmaceutical production. One is low product yield, i.e., the low concentration of drug in plant tissues, such as a leaf or a seed. Research efforts continue on increasing these yields. Another is the slightly different glycosylation process in plants compared with mammals. Plant glycans can be immunogenic to humans. Genetic manipulation to modify glycosylation processes in plants is being studied to better mimic glycosylation in humans. Finally, the impact of pharmaceutical plants on the environment and potential cross-contamination with food crops has also been an issue, but is minimized in bioreactors.

To date, no transgenic plant-based drug has been approved by the FDA. One therapeutic agent, taliglucerase alfa, has been successful in Phase III clinical trials; it is a plant cell expressed recombinant glucocerebrosidase enzyme for the treatment of Gaucher disease.

Therapeutic Antibodies

Antibodies are immunoglobulins (Igs), a type of glycoprotein synthesized and secreted by B cells (also called B lymphocytes) of the immune system. They recognize foreign structures (antigens) present on the surface of bacteria, viruses or tumor cells, and mark these for attack by the immune system. Unfortunately, the immune system is often unable to mount an antibody response large enough to remove the infected or injured cells, which leads to disease.

Almost all cells display a range of surface antigens. Some are found on a variety of cell types whereas others, called unique surface antigens (USAs), are specific to a given cell type. Antibodies produced against USAs bind selectively to the surface of only these cells. In effect, these antibodies are "magic bullets" capable of selectively targeting a specific cell type such as cancer cells, virally infected cells, or microbial cells at an infection site.

Therapeutic antibodies are precisely targeted biopharmaceuticals that recognize and bind to a cell surface antigen and then trigger a biological response. The therapeutic antibody may itself be the drug, or may be a carrier to target a potent drug to specific cells. After binding to the target antigen, the therapeutic antibody may perform one of several functions: activate cell membrane receptors and change the cell's function, block the growth of a tumor, recruit the body's immune system to attack the cell, or sensitize a cancer cell to chemotherapy.

Antibody Structure

Igs are heavy plasma proteins usually with added sugar chains. The basic unit of each

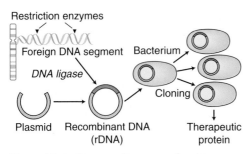

Figure 18.6. The overall process of making a recombinant DNA therapeutic protein.

antibody is a monomer, a Y-shaped molecule with two identical heavy glycoprotein chains and two identical light glycoprotein chains connected to each other by disulfide bonds (Fig. 18.6). The amino acid sequence at the tips of the Y of both heavy and light chains varies greatly among different antibodies and constitutes the *antigen-binding regions*. Each antibody has two identical antigen-binding sites that provide specificity for binding to a particular antigen.

Heavy chains can exist as five different types (γ, δ, α, μ, and ε); these types are used to define the different Ig classes (IgG, IgD, IgA, IgM, and IgE, respectively). Each heavy chain has a *constant region*, the same for all Igs of the same class, and a *variable region* that differs among Igs made by different B cells, but is the same for all Igs of the same B cell. Light chains exist in two types, γ and κ, and all antibodies have one or the other type. Each light chain has one *constant region* and one *variable region*.

Once the heavy and light chains are assembled, however, the areas or domains of the antibody become more important than the individual chains. Each half of the forked end of the Y-shaped molecule is called a Fab (fragment, antigen binding) region, containing the antigen-binding ends of one light chain and one heavy chain. When an antibody is enzymatically cleaved, it yields two Fab fragments and one Fc fragment (fragment crystallizable), the stem of the Y with constant regions of the heavy chains. The Fab region has great diversity so that antibodies can be made to recognize any and every antigen the body encounters, whereas the constant Fc region defines the class of antibody (IgG, for example). The Fc portion also provides for a long half-life of antibodies in the bloodstream, an important factor in the efficacy of therapeutic antibodies.

Polyclonal Antibodies. When an antigen is injected into a mouse or a human, some B cells start producing antibodies that bind to that antigen. Each B cell produces only one kind of antibody, but different B cells produce structurally different antibodies that bind to different parts of the antigen. This mixture of antibodies is known as a polyclonal antibody. Although the mixture contains Igs of different structures, each antibody in the mixture is specific to the same antigen. This specificity of antibodies makes them attractive as therapeutic agents.

Monoclonal Antibodies. The conventional method of making an antibody was to inject laboratory animals (e.g., mice) with an antigen and to collect antibodies from the blood serum (antibody-containing serum is called *antiserum*). The problems with this method are that the antiserum contains undesired substances, and a very small amount of usable antibody can be recovered. Another important disadvantage is that these antibodies are polyclonal, derived from many kinds of B cells.

A monoclonal antibody (MAb) is an antibody with uniform structure and specificity derived from a single clone of cells. MAbs are produced in the laboratory by cells created through the fusion of an antibody-producing cell (such as a B lymphocyte), with an immortal rapidly multiplying tumor cell, to produce a hybrid cell (hybridoma) that expresses properties of both cells. The hybridoma cells are identical because they derive from a single cell, and multiply rapidly, creating a clone that produces large quantities of the

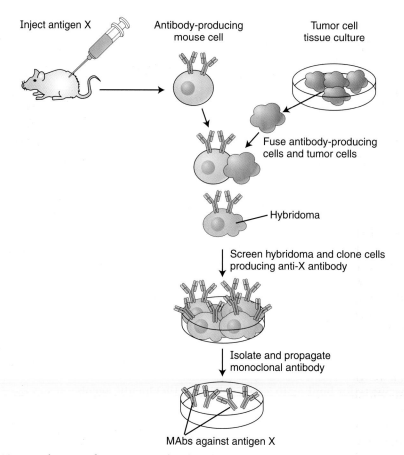

Inject antigen X   Antibody-producing   Tumor cell
                        mouse cell   tissue culture

Fuse antibody-producing
cells and tumor cells

Hybridoma

Screen hybridoma and clone cells
producing anti-X antibody

Isolate and propagate
monoclonal antibody

MAbs against antigen X

Figure 18.7. A schematic of murine monoclonal antibody (MAb) production using hybridomas.

antibody. This application of rDNA technology, illustrated in Figure 18.7, allows the production of large amounts of identical, pure antibodies. The stem -*mab* is used as a suffix to name monoclonal antibodies as well as their fragments. The nomenclature of some early MAbs does not follow the newer naming conventions.

Chimeric, Humanized, and Human Antibodies. The main difficulty of using an animal such as a mouse to make antibodies is that mouse (or *murine*) antibodies are considered foreign by the human immune system, which mounts an immune response against them by producing human anti-mouse antibodies (HAMA). The first consequence of a HAMA response is that the therapeutic antibody is cleared rapidly from the body, reducing its half-life.

Second, the HAMA response, essentially an allergic reaction to the murine antibodies, can result in mild side effects such as a rash, to more serious and life-threatening responses such as renal failure. HAMA can also set the stage for a future allergic reaction if the patient is given a subsequent treatment containing mouse antibodies. These drawbacks limited the use of therapeutic murine antibodies, although a few murine antibody drugs still exist; their names end in the suffix -*omab*.

The HAMA problem was reduced by introducing human sequences into the murine antibody. Depending on the proportion of human sequences in the final molecule, the resulting product is called either a chimeric antibody (approximately 65% human sequences; names end in -*ximab*) or a humanized antibody (greater

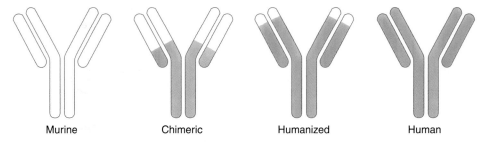

| Murine | Chimeric | Humanized | Human |

Figure 18.8. Differences among murine, chimeric, humanized, and human monoclonal antibodies.

than 90% human sequences, names end in -*zumab*). The presence of the human sequences helps reduce the immune response to the therapeutic antibody. However, humanized antibodies often bind antigen more weakly than murine antibodies, resulting in lower efficacy.

Fully human antibodies have also recently been developed (names end in the suffix -*umab*), and are a rapidly growing class of biopharmaceutical drugs. One approach is to make use of transgenic mice in which mouse antibody gene expression is suppressed and replaced with human antibody gene expression. These mice have the ability to make fully human monoclonal antibodies, avoiding the need to humanize murine monoclonal antibodies. The human genes in these transgenic mice are stable and are passed on to offspring of the mice.

Figure 18.8 illustrates the differences among murine, chimeric, humanized, and human monoclonal antibodies.

Fusion Proteins. Fusion proteins are made by joining two or more genes that originally code for separate proteins. Translation of this fusion gene results in a single polypeptide with functional properties derived from both of the original proteins. rDNA technology has facilitated the development of fusion proteins (recombinant fusion proteins) that contain antibody domains fused to therapeutic proteins. The purpose of creating fusion proteins as therapeutic agents is to impart properties from each of the "parent" proteins to the resulting chimeric protein; chimeric and humanized MAbs may be classified as fusion proteins. An example of a fusion protein is the drug etanercept (Enbrel®) for rheumatoid arthritis, an autoimmune disease. It is a fusion protein of the human TNF (tumor necrosis factor) receptor attached to the Fc portion of human IgG. Enbrel works by acting as a specific TNF inhibitor; it binds to TNFα and decreases its role in disorders involving excess inflammation in human.

Antibody Fragments. Monoclonal antibodies, due to their large size, have difficulty penetrating into their target tissues and organs. This has spurred the development of antibody fragments, especially Fab fragments. Such fragments, because of their smaller molecular size, are capable of more readily penetrating tissues, organs, or tumors and should therefore show increased efficacy. The smaller FAbs may also allow access to binding sites on enzymes that MAbs cannot access. Also, the removal of the Fc portion may reduce immunogenic potential. Antigen-binding Fab fragments can be made by direct proteolytic cleavage of intact antibodies, or by genetic engineering.

An example of a FAb therapeutic is ranibizumab (Lucentis®). It is much smaller than the parent murine antibody molecule, or its humanized MAb bevacizumab (Avastin®). This gives it higher affinity to its target, VEGF-A (vascular endothelial growth factor A), in the eye. Both ranibizumab and bevacizumab are used to reverse loss of vision by macular degeneration.

TABLE 18.3. Examples of Marketed Therapeutic MAbs, Antibody Fragments, and Fusion Proteins

Brand Name	Monoclonal Antibody	Indication
Murine		
Orthoclone OKT-3®	Muromonab-CD3	Organ transplant rejection
Zevalin®	Ibritumomab	Non-Hodgkin's leukemia
Bexxar®	Tositumomab	Non-Hodgkin's leukemia
Chimeric		
Erbitux®	Cetuximab	Metastatic colorectal cancer
Remicade®	Infliximab	Rheumatoid arthritis, Crohn's
ReoPro®	Abciximab	Clotting after angioplasty
Humanized		
Avastin®	Bevacizumab	Metastatic colorectal cancer
Herceptin®	Trastuzumab	Breast cancer
Lucentis®	Ranibizumab	Wet macular degeneration
Synagis®	Palivizumab	Compromised respiratory function
Human		
Humira®	Adalimumab	Rheumatoid arthritis
Vectibix®	Panitumumab	Colorectal cancer
Fusion Protein		
Enbrel®	Etanercept	Rheumatoid arthritis

Table 18.3 lists some examples of currently marketed MAbs, antibody fragments, and fusion proteins.

Antibody-Drug Conjugates. Antibody-drug conjugates (also called immunoconjugates) represent an emerging area of protein-based drugs. They consist of a recombinant antibody covalently bonded to a cytotoxic drug by a synthetic linker group. The goal is to combine the pharmacological potency of the small molecule cytotoxic drug and the high specificity of MAbs to target a particular set of cells. Antineoplastic drugs such as doxorubicin, daunomycin, vinca alkaloids, and taxoids are effective at killing cancer cells, but have low therapeutic indices because of their limited selectivity, and their high toxicity to normal cells. On the other hand, MAb drugs such as rituximab, trastuzumab, and panitumumab are therapeutically useful in malignancies, but require concurrent treatment with cytotoxic drugs to achieve significant clinical efficacy. MAb-drug conjugates may be able to overcome the deficiencies of the separate drugs. Several such conjugates are currently in the research stage or in clinical trials.

Formulation of Biopharmaceutical Drugs

Small molecule drugs can be easily converted and stored as solids, and formulated and dosed in solid or liquid dosage forms. By contrast, biopharmaceutical drugs (especially proteins) are almost always isolated from the biological host as an aqueous solution because protein tertiary and quaternary structures are best preserved in water.

Since proteins are usually expressed in fermentation media at concentrations significantly lower than those required for practical clinical use, they need to be concentrated. A variety of methods are used to concentrate proteins such as filtration, chromatography, lyophilization, dialysis or precipitation. All of these methods can potentially affect the stability of protein therapeutics.

For biological activity, protein drugs need to retain not only their primary structure but also their secondary, tertiary, and quaternary structures during manufacture, formulation, and storage. The active, folded structure of most proteins depends strongly on the environment (solvent, pH, temperature, and so forth) around the molecule. This restricts the types of solvents and excipients that can be used in protein formulation; many protein formulations are simple, buffered aqueous solutions. Good formulations can help the protein drug maintain its effective conformation, prevent aggregation, reduce oxidation, and help enhance stability.

However, the poor stability of these solutions often makes it impossible to give the product an adequate shelf life for clinical use. Even when refrigerated, many aqueous solutions of proteins do not have an adequate shelf life for practical use. Only a few biopharmaceuticals can be stored as aqueous solutions for 2 or more years at refrigerator temperatures.

Lyophilization technology allows solutions to be converted into solids, and is used for some biotech drugs, including vaccines, viruses, and blood products. Lyophilization (or freeze-drying) is the conversion of a liquid to a solid through the process of sublimation. A sterile solution of the protein is prepared, filled into primary containers, and frozen. The water is removed by directly converting it from frozen ice to water vapor. What remains in the container are the solids (drug, excipients) in the solid state; the 3D conformational structure of many proteins can be preserved in the lyophilized state. The process often requires inclusion of a *lyoprotectant*, an excipient added to prevent denaturation of the protein during lyophilization.

Water facilitates thermal instability of proteins, so that removing it to make dry protein powders dramatically improves protein stability. A dry powder is also safe from mechanical denaturation. When reconstituted with an appropriate solvent such as saline or a buffer, a successfully lyophilized protein will dissolve rapidly into its active, folded configuration; the resulting solution is then injected into the patient.

Examples of lyophilized biopharmaceuticals are etanercept (Enbrel®) and infliximab (Remicade®) for rheumatoid arthritis, interferon beta-1α (Avonex®) for multiple sclerosis and trastuzumab (Herceptin®) for breast cancer. Approximately 50% of all commercial biologic therapeutic protein products are lyophilized. Not all biotech drugs can be lyophilized; the 3D structure may not be preserved in the process, or the final solid may not be easily reconstituted.

Stability of Biopharmaceutical Products

Both physical and chemical instability can cause a biologic product to lose its activity or to develop a potential for toxicity. Instability can occur during production, purification, formulation or storage, and handling of the product. As mentioned earlier, the loss or change in the protein cannot always be detected by laboratory measurements, so strict control of process and handling is critical for biopharmaceutical products.

The primary structure of proteins, defined by peptide bonds between amino acids, is susceptible to degradation and cleavage by chemical reactions, causing *chemical instability*. Covalent bonds can be broken through hydrolysis reactions—either in the product or in vivo—and the protein can be cleaved into two or more chemically different molecules. Other chemical reactions often seen with proteins are oxidation, deamidation, and sometimes isomerization. This type of chemical stability problem is similar to that seen for small molecule drugs with

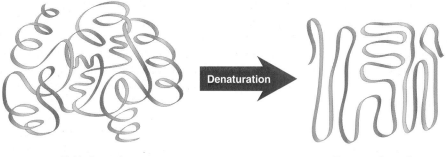

Folded protein   Denatured protein

Figure 18.9. Denaturation of a protein. The active, folded protein can be denatured to yield a partially or completely unfolded structure.

amide or ester bonds, and can often be minimized by appropriate choice of pH and buffer.

Physical instability issues are very important for proteins, so let us examine them more closely. Denaturation is defined as any modification of secondary, tertiary, or quaternary structure of the protein molecule. It is a process by which hydrogen bonds, hydrophobic interactions, and salt linkages are broken, and the protein goes from its native, folded state to an unfolded chain with no specific three-dimensional structure (Fig. 18.9). Because denaturation reactions are not strong enough to break peptide bonds, the primary structure remains unchanged.

Unfolding causes hydrophobic amino acid residues, previously buried inside the folded structure, to become exposed to water. This can have several other consequences. One is adsorption, in which the unfolded protein molecules stick to the sides of the product container, reducing their aqueous concentration. The composition of the product container (e.g., type of glass) is therefore very important in minimizing adsorption. Changes in the residues exposed on the surface can also cause aggregation of several protein molecules into a larger complex or aggregate. The aggregate may remain in solution, or may be insoluble enough to precipitate.

Aggregation increases as the concentration of protein in solution increases. Many MAbs require a high dose (1 to 2 mg/kg).

They need to be sufficiently concentrated to allow convenient dosing in a variety of settings such as in a hospital by intravenous injection or infusion or at home by subcutaneous injection. This poses formulation and stability challenges because of the propensity of antibodies to aggregate at higher concentrations. Many other peptide and protein therapeutics are also formulated at high concentration so that the volume of the injected solution can be kept small to reduce patient discomfort.

Physical instability can be minimized by using appropriate excipients (salts, sugars, amino acids, and glycerol) that protect the molecule. Many proteins denature and precipitate when solutions are agitated or shaken because of incorporation of air bubbles and adsorption of protein molecules to the air–liquid interface, where they can undergo conformational changes. Agitation of protein solutions is to be avoided during manufacture, shipping, and use. Aggregation is frequently increased at higher temperatures. Protein therapeutics thus needs to be shipped and stored under refrigeration, which adds a significant cost to the product.

Chemical and physical instability decreases the concentration of the native, active protein in the product as a function of time. For example, insulin rapidly aggregates and loses its activity when stored at temperatures greater than those encountered under refrigeration. In addition, the degradation products may cause serious adverse reactions owing to their immunogenic potential; we will discuss immunogenicity a little later. As a consequence of the greater instability of protein drugs as compared with small molecule drugs, protein drug solutions have a shorter shelf life and often need to be refrigerated. Freezing can further compromise protein physical stability, and is generally not appropriate for biotech drug solutions. Lyophilization, if possible for a particular protein, can greatly reduce all these stability problems because the product is kept dry until just before use.

ADME of Biopharmaceutical Drugs

Almost all conventional drugs are small molecules with MWs less than about 1,000; e.g., aspirin has a molecular weight of 180. They are usually relatively simple organic compounds containing a few functional groups. On the other hand, therapeutic proteins, the largest group of biopharmaceuticals, are made up of tens or hundreds of amino acids, each of which is as large as a conventional drug molecule. As an example, interferon beta-1a (Avonex®) has a molecular weight of approximately 22,500. These large polar drug molecules are handled differently than conventional drugs by our body.

Absorption

Being large polar molecules, most protein therapeutics cannot cross most epithelial tissues at the common sites of administration, and must be administered by injection. Most are typically administered by intravenous, subcutaneous, or intramuscular injection. Others, such as the drugs for macular degeneration, may be injected directly into the site of action (e.g., the eye) to achieve high enough concentrations in the intended organ. Although parenteral routes generally provide sufficient systemic exposure and are satisfactory for efficacy,

they are invasive and inconvenient, causing physiological stress, pain, and risk of infections as well as other implications. Recent research efforts suggest that inhalation, nasal, or delivery through the oral cavity (buccal or sublingual) will be viable administration routes in the near future.

Smaller polypeptide drugs may be given by these alternate routes. An example is calcitonin-salmon (Fortical®), a polypeptide hormone made by rDNA technology and administered as a nasal spray to treat osteoporosis. The bioavailability is about 3 to 5%, but is sufficient for therapeutic effect.

Distribution

Most biopharmaceutical drugs are large molecules. After entering the systemic circulation, they will tend to remain in the vascular space and exhibit low volumes of distribution. For example, the volume of distribution of adalimumab (Humira) is about 5 L and that of trastuzumab is 44 mL/kg (or about 3 L in a 70-kg individual). However, these low V_d values does not mean that these drugs do not enter tissues. Many protein drugs are recognized by transporters or carriers in capillary walls, particularly in the target tissues. Receptor-mediated or carrier-mediated transport or endocytosis into the target tissue allows relatively high tissue concentrations to be achieved, which are often necessary for efficacy. An example is the uptake of nartrograstim (a granulocyte-colony stimulating factor (G-CSF) derivative) into bone marrow, the target-tissue, by receptor-mediated endocytosis. This distribution mechanism is concentration dependent up to a point, after which the transporter becomes saturated. Because distribution is specific to the target tissue only, overall V_d values remain low.

Many biotech drugs are targeted to tumors. The structure of blood vessels in tumors is markedly different from that in normal tissues. For tumor cells to grow quickly, they must stimulate the formation of new blood vessels for nutritional and oxygen supply. These newly formed tumor blood vessels are usually abnormal in architecture, with poorly aligned, defective, endothelial cells and wide intercellular junctions. Because of these abnormalities macromolecules can distribute and accumulate in tumors more than in normal tissues.

Therapeutic proteins may bind nonspecifically to plasma proteins, just like conventional drugs. In addition, these drugs very commonly bind to specific endogenous "binding" proteins; in fact, such binding is often necessary for their transport and regulation. The binding may protect the drug from destruction or elimination, increasing its half-life, or may enhance elimination by making it more readily metabolized. For example, growth hormone is believed to have two specific binding proteins in plasma.

Elimination

Conventional, small molecule drugs are eliminated by excretion and metabolism, as discussed in earlier chapters. These pathways are available to biopharmaceutical drugs, too. In addition, the unique structures and properties of biotech drugs open up additional pathways such as receptor-mediated elimination and antibody-mediated elimination.

Metabolism. Peptides and proteins are eventually hydrolyzed to their amino acids by peptidases and other proteolytic enzymes; the process is also called proteolysis. These enzymes are present in all tissues of the body, which accounts for the relatively rapid metabolism of peptides. Blood, liver, and kidney, which contain a variety of peptidases, are probably the most important sites of peptide metabolism.

The lower the molecular weight of the peptide or protein, the more rapidly it is metabolized. Thus, a small peptide with a molecular weight of less than 4,000 has a plasma half-life of minutes, a protein with a molecular weight greater than 15,000 has a half-life of a few hours, while one with molecular weight of more than 50,000 would persist in the body for days.

Excretion. Most peptide and protein drugs are polar and water-soluble. Therefore, glomerular filtration can play an important role in the elimination of peptides and proteins, depending on their molecular size and charge. We know that a molecule with molecular weight of less than about 5,000 can be freely filtrated by glomerulus, whereas filtration of compounds with molecular weight of greater 60,000 is severely limited. For compounds with molecular weights between 5,000 and 60,000, charge and shape become progressively more important as determinants of filtration.

Although a molecular weight cut-off of serum albumin (~69,000) is commonly used to predict whether a drug is filtered by the glomerulus, molecular size after folding appears be a better predictor for the glomerular filtration of protein drugs. The "effective pore size" of the renal filter is presumed to be about 10 nm in diameter; so renal excretion plays an important role in the elimination of therapeutic proteins with molecular size below this.

Most small peptide drugs will be extensively filtered. In spite of this, rapid metabolism is the primary reason for their short half-life rather than extensive glomerular filtration. Even if the peptide were retained in plasma and completely filtered, its half-life would be about 20 minutes rather than the 4 to 5 minutes usually seen. Therefore, metabolism is much faster than excretion and the primary determinant of clearance of small peptides.

On the other hand, therapeutic proteins are metabolically more stable than peptides, so renal excretion may become more important in their clearance, depending on the molecular size. Filgrastim, a recombinant G-CSF with a molecular weight of 18,800 and a diameter of about

2.5 nm, is believed to be cleared in the urine, with renal clearance accounting for about 70% of elimination.

Receptor-Mediated Elimination. For conventional small molecule drugs, only a small, negligible fraction of the drug in the body is involved in receptor–drug binding, and binding is usually reversible. Thus, drug–receptor binding does not play a role in drug clearance. By contrast, biopharmaceutical drugs have an extremely high affinity to their target receptor, so that a significant fraction of the drug in the body may be involved in receptor binding. Further, receptor binding of therapeutic proteins and MAbs is irreversible, and often leads to internalization (by endocytosis) and subsequent degradation of the protein in the target cell. Thus, the process of receptor–drug binding contributes significantly not only to the efficacy, but also to the clearance of protein drugs; we call this pathway *target receptor-mediated elimination*. If the number of receptors or targets is small, target receptor-mediated clearance can be saturated at high doses of the protein drug.

Biopharmaceutical drugs also have the potential of binding to other, nontarget receptors on cells, which can then internalize the drug and eliminate it as described in the preceding text. In particular, glycoprotein receptors in the liver and spleen are presumed to be involved. The main function of these receptors is to regulate serum glycoproteins. In addition, they can contribute to the elimination of glycosylated protein drugs.

Antibody-Mediated Elimination. We shall see a little later in the chapter that biopharmaceutical drugs have the potential to cause an immune response. After taking a biotech drug, the patient's body produces neutralizing antibodies against the drug (antidrug antibodies, or ADAs). The ADAs bind to the drug and effectively prevent it from performing its function. Thus, production of ADAs against a protein drug may be considered to be an elimination process.

Pharmacological Considerations of Biopharmaceutical Drugs

Most, if not all, of the general concepts that describe the biological actions of small drug molecules are also applicable to biopharmaceuticals. Biopharmaceuticals, such as small drug molecules, produce their effect by interacting with another molecule in the body. In spite of their complex structures, the development of biopharmaceuticals as drugs and their subsequent actions in the body are still limited to influencing biochemical pathways and cellular events that already exist. Like small molecule drugs, biopharmaceuticals cannot create or confer a new biological function.

In our previous discussions on drug action, the focus was on the drug acting as a ligand and interacting with an endogenous target protein. In many instances, this principle holds true with biopharmaceuticals. However, for some biopharmaceuticals, this relationship is reversed; the drug may be a protein or an antibody that acts like a receptor in that it binds to the endogenous ligand and prevents it from interacting with its target. Even though this relationship is the opposite of our earlier discussions of drug action, the underlying concepts remain the same. That is, attractive forces, chemical bonding, the law of mass action and dose response relationships are important factors in determining ligand–receptor interactions and subsequent biological responses.

A potential advantage that therapeutic proteins and antibodies offer is another approach to treating illness with a specificity that sometimes cannot be achieved with small molecule drugs. Many conditions that cannot be adequately or safely treated with conventional drugs are now benefiting from the biopharmaceutical approach. It should be noted, however, that biopharmaceuticals are not magic bullets and do cause side effects and at times potentially dangerous adverse reactions.

Opportunities and Limitations of Biopharmaceuticals

Biopharmaceuticals are attractive as drugs because they represent naturally derived products for treatment of disease. However, the complexities of the manufacturing process, and the drugs themselves, represent some major challenges in their development and formidable limitations to their widespread use. Even if biotechnology can now successfully produce large quantities of the pure protein, controlling its 3D structure during manufacturing, handling, and storage is critical to safety and efficacy. Delivering the protein to the patient in a safe, accurate, convenient, and reproducible manner is difficult. Even if these problems are overcome, the body often treats proteins differently than it treats small molecules, limiting their use.

Immunogenicity of Biotech Drugs

The immune system is a defense against foreign organisms and proteins. It has evolved the capacity to recognize "self" and "nonself" structures. Although biopharmaceuticals are often designed to closely resemble "self" proteins, even slight differences can cause the immune system to view them as "nonself" (i.e., antigens) and mount an immune response.

The response is production of antibodies to the *epitope*, a specific part of the antigenic molecule. Most biologic drugs have the potential to be immunogenic; i.e., induce the formation of ADAs in the patient. ADAs not only reduce or eliminate the therapeutic activity of the drug but also can cause adverse reactions such as allergic shock and anaphylaxis. A potentially more serious problem is the cross-reactivity of ADAs; they may target and mount an immune response against other similar proteins. ADAs to a therapeutic protein may also neutralize the essential endogenous protein which it was intended to supplement or replace. An example is the ADA formation reported after the long-term administration of erythropoietin (epoetin, EPO); the patients' immune response produced ADAs that also neutralized endogenous erythropoietin. As EPO is essential for the erythropoiesis of bone marrow, its lack caused severe aplasia in these patients. Since many biopharmaceuticals are used in immunologically compromised patients, even a small amount of a potentially immunogenic substance may pose a serious risk.

Scientists initially believed that immunogenicity was a result of using nonhuman proteins, such as insulin derived from pigs and cows, or contaminants in the products. It was believed that the problem would disappear with the advent of recombinant technology that produces pure protein that is identical or nearly identical to human protein. However, although serious immune responses have been reduced, immunogenicity related to biopharmaceutical drugs still persists as a serious problem. Some of the common factors responsible for causing immunogenicity with the use of biopharmaceuticals are summarized here.

Sequence Differences

Therapeutic proteins derived from nonhuman sources may have a somewhat different amino acid sequence than the human protein. A greater degree of nonendogenous sequences generally correlates with increased immunogenicity. The immune response to a foreign protein is more likely to be of rapid onset and more likely to be irreversible than the response against a protein having significant homology to an endogenous counterpart. Sequence differences between the endogenous and human versions of the protein have been minimized by rDNA technology. A classic example is insulin which used to be obtained from porcine or bovine sources, but is now produced by rDNA technology.

However, even proteins with a sequence identical to the human version do sometimes show immunogenicity. Conversely, some proteins with a slightly different sequence from the human sequence may not lead to enhanced immunogenicity, which makes immunogenicity hard to predict.

The situation is similar with MAbs. Nonhuman MAbs elicit a rapid immune response and are appropriate only for single-use therapy or in immunosuppressed individuals, because subsequent exposures would lead to a rapid and progressing immune response. As increasing amounts of nonhuman sequences are replaced with the human counterpart (chimeric and humanized MAbs), there is progressively lower risk of sequence differences mediating an immune response. Fully human MAbs have the lowest, but not zero, immunogenic risk.

Epitopes for antibodies are often located at a small number of residues on the surface of a protein. If these can be identified and modified, it is possible to reduce immunogenic risk without affecting the efficacy of the protein.

Posttranslational Modifications

We have discussed the importance of posttranslational modifications in determining the biological activity of a protein. Glycosylation is a species-specific and cell-specific process; host cells used for recombinant protein manufacture have a significant bearing on immunogenicity. For example, natural interleukin 2 is less immunogenic than the one made by *E. coli*, in part because of the inability of bacteria to glycosylate proteins. The lack of glycosylation of glycoproteins, such as recombinant human granulocyte-macrophage colony-stimulating factor and

IFN-beta, induces antibodies because of the exposure of antigenic epitopes. Glycosylation often obstructs the epitope where an antibody would bind, and reduces immunogenicity. Glycosylation also may help the solubility, stability, and activity of the molecules.

Correct glycosylation is also important. If a protein therapeutic is not glycosylated in the same way as the endogenous human protein, it may not show biological activity and may be immunogenic. Thus, even recombinant human glycoproteins almost never have exactly the same glycosylation patterns as their endogenous counterparts, and will always carry immunogenic risk.

Stability Issues

Chemical instability of the protein can result in a product that could be perceived as foreign by the immune system, although not all changes result in immunogenicity. For example, oxidation or deamidation reactions could create a new conformation, or alter an epitope on the protein to increase or block recognition of that epitope. This could result in an increase or decrease in immunogenic potential.

Aggregation of a protein drug can make that protein more immunogenic, because the aggregate is more easily recognized by the immune system. Therefore, appropriate formulation and stabilization of the protein product is critical to not only its efficacy, but also its safety.

Drug Delivery Issues

If a protein is improperly formulated, it could undergo a change, such as oxidation or aggregation that would make the protein more immunogenic. Contaminants and impurities can either be immunogenic by themselves or could impart an adjuvant effect that results in the therapeutic protein becoming more immunogenic. When host cell proteins can be identified, it is then possible to develop methods to remove them from the drug product and eliminate their clinical impact.

In general, immunogenicity increases with the dose and total amount of drug given to the patient. Also, acute administration of biopharmaceuticals is less likely than chronic administration to be associated with immunogenicity. Route of administration can also influence immunogenicity. Studies have shown that intramuscular and subcutaneous administration of a protein tends to be slightly more immunogenic than intravenous administration. Presumably, this is due to lower exposure and contact time with phagocytic cells by the intravenous route. Intravenous injection is thus the favored route of administration, although the subcutaneous and intramuscular routes are used for some drugs for convenience.

Patient Susceptibility

Patient characteristics, including their general immune status, can play a major role in determining if a patient will develop an immune response. A patient, whose immune system is suppressed, either naturally or through the administration of some other drug, is less likely to mount an immune response against a therapeutic protein than one with a fully competent immune system. This is exemplified by the anti-B cell MAb rituximab (Rituxan®), which is strongly immunogenic in patients with rheumatoid arthritis, but not in cancer patients, in whom it is primarily used.

Furthermore, certain biotech drugs are designed to be immunomodulatory themselves, and the amount, frequency, and route of drug administration can affect their efficacy more than intrinsic antigenicity.

PEGylation of Biotech Drugs

Scientists have been examining ways to prolong the half-life of proteins in the body after administration. Therapeutic proteins have been modified chemically by the covalent addition of polymers, dextrans, or other sugars, or by cross-linking to other proteins. All of these modifications aim to extend circulation time or avoid immunogenicity or toxicity.

A solution to many problems in the disposition and toxicity of proteins is PEGylation, the attachment of one or more flexible strands of polyethylene glycol (PEG) to a protein, as shown in Figure 18.10. PEGs are neutral, water-soluble, nontoxic polymers available in a wide range of molecular weights. They are extensively hydrated in water and have a large exclusion volume, meaning that other molecules and cells cannot approach the hydrated structure too closely. PEGs used for PEGylation are approximately of the same molecular weight as the protein. PEGylation is achieved by forming covalent bonds between an amino or sulfhydryl group on the protein and a chemically reactive group (e.g., carbonate, ester, aldehyde) added to the PEG molecule. Random attachment can alter the biological activity of the protein, so careful consideration

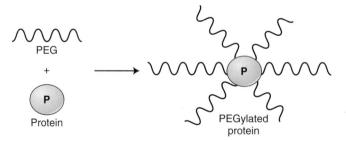

Figure 18.10. PEGylation, the covalent attachment of several polyethylene glycol molecules to a protein.

TABLE 18.4. Examples of Marketed PEGylated Protein Drugs

Brand Name	Drug	Indication
PEGasys®	PEG-interferon-alpha-2a	Hepatitis
PEGintron®	PEG-interferon-alpha-2a	Hepatitis
Neulasta®	PEG-filgrastim (granulocyte colony-stimulating factor)	Neutropenia
Adagen®	PEG-adenosine deaminase	Immunodeficiency
Oncaspar®	PEG-asparaginase	Cancer
Somavert®	PEG-visomant (growth hormone)	Acromegaly

must be given to the amino acid sites to which PEG is attached.

PEGylated proteins can be thought of as prodrugs because the protein–PEG linkage must be broken in the body to release the active protein drug. Examples of currently available PEGylated products include are shown in Table 18.4.

The advantages of protein PEGylation include enhanced solubility and physicochemical stability, improved distribution, reduced renal clearance, slower rate of metabolism, and longer plasma half-life. For example, attachment of one or two 10- to 20-kD PEG molecules can increase the circulating half-life of small proteins several fold. By increasing the biological half-life and improving the efficacy of therapeutic proteins in the body, PEGylation can reduce the frequency of injections a patient requires. Modifying proteins with multiple PEGs can also mask epitopes and prevent neutralizing antibody formation to the protein or MAb drug.

Nucleic Acid-Based Therapeutics

The increasing understanding of DNA and RNA structure and function, and the emergence of new biotechnological methods has opened opportunities to use functional nucleic acids as targets and tools to design innovative drugs. Nucleic acids are not only a valuable drug target; they can also be designed to act as drugs themselves. Antisense oligonucleotides and aptamers and ribozymes can be used to silence undesired gene expression. The common feature in all three strategies is that the synthesis of an undesirable protein is inhibited at the level of the mRNA.

Antisense Oligonucleotides

An oligonucleotide is a short sequence of nucleotides (DNA or RNA), typically with 25 or fewer base pairs and molecular weights in the range of 6,000 to 8,000. Our genes consist of long strings of nucleotides along the DNA in our chromosomes. When we need a particular gene to be expressed, transcription leads to the production of an mRNA message from that gene, which then translates it into a protein. Unlike double-stranded DNA, mRNA molecules are single-stranded and will bind to complementary nucleic acid strands. Therefore, if a single-stranded oligonucleotide drug with a sequence complementary to targeted mRNA (the antisense sequence) enters the cell, it will bind to that mRNA, creating a duplex that is not suitable for translation, as illustrated in Figure 18.11.

In principle, antisense technology will be able to target almost any cellular process with complete specificity. If a protein is helping a cancer cell to grow, then the appropriate antisense oligonucleotide could be used to prevent that protein from being made. Antisense oligonucleotides are extremely specific, so it is unlikely that they would affect the production of

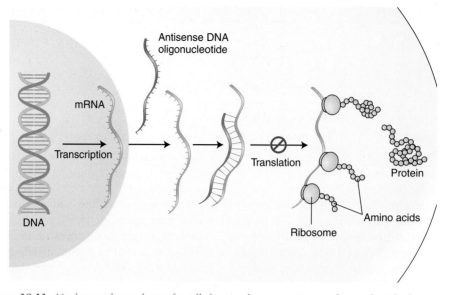

Figure 18.11. Nucleus and cytoplasm of a cell showing how an antisense oligonucleotide drug can target mRNA and prevent translation and, therefore, protein synthesis.

any other protein in the body. This specificity is expected to reduce the side effects often seen with conventional cancer treatments. Because the target is protein synthesis, antisense drugs are expected to have a slow onset of action (24 to 48 hours), which will limit their utility in acute, life-threatening diseases such as sepsis and cardiovascular events.

One antisense-based drug has been approved to date, fomivirsen sodium (Vitravene®) for the treatment of cytomegalovirus retinitis in AIDS patients. Vitravene is delivered by local injection into the vitreous of the eye.

Aptamers

An aptamer is a single-stranded oligonucleotide that binds to and inactivates a specific target, usually a protein. Several properties of aptamers make them attractive therapeutic agents similar to, but potentially better than, antibodies. They act in the same way as MAbs by folding into a three-dimensional structure based on their nucleic acid sequence to bind to their target. The smaller size of aptamers compared with MAbs might enable them to easily reach targets that are not readily exposed on the cell surface.

Because their small size results in rapid renal clearance (half-life of a few minutes) minutes, aptamers must be modified, e.g., by PEGylation. An aptamer drug on the market is pegaptanib sodium (Macugen®), a pegylated aptamer that adopts a three-dimensional conformation that enables it to bind to extracellular VEGF. In age-related macular degeneration (AMD), an isoform of VEGF is overexpressed, promoting growth of new blood vessels. Macugen specifically binds and inhibits the isoform of VEGF, leading to reduced pathologic vessel growth. It is delivered locally to the eye by intraocular injection for the treatment of wet AMD.

Gene Therapy

Gene therapy is still an experimental technique that uses genes to treat or prevent disease. In the future, this technique may allow the treatment of a disorder by inserting an appropriate gene into a patient's cells. Researchers are testing several approaches to gene therapy, including.

- Replacing a mutated gene that causes disease with a healthy copy of the gene
- Inactivating, or "knocking out," a mutated gene that is functioning improperly
- Introducing a new gene into the body to help fight a disease
- Repairing a gene with antisense drugs

Although gene therapy is a promising treatment option for a number of diseases (including inherited disorders, some types of cancer, and certain viral infections), the technique remains risky and is still under study to ensure that it will be safe and effective. Gene therapy is currently only being tested for the treatment of diseases that have no other cures. The ultimate goal of gene therapy is the permanent treatment or cure of disease, hopefully with few or no side effects.

Successful gene therapy requires two main components: the therapeutic gene and a suitable gene delivery system—a way to get the correct genes into the correct cells. Although several therapeutic genes have been identified, all gene therapy strategies share a common problem— the need for a selective gene delivery system, containing a "vector" to introduce genes into the desired cells. If the target cells are accessible and can be extracted from the patient (e.g., bone marrow or liver), an ex vivo approach can be used, as illustrated in Figure 18.12A. However, target cells are usually inaccessible, so the gene delivery system is given directly to the patient, an in vivo approach, with the hope that it will reach the target cells (Fig. 18.12B).

The most successful delivery vectors so far have been viruses; particularly adenovirus, a group of DNA-containing viruses that can readily infect most cell types. Viruses, although the vector of choice in most gene therapy studies, present several potential problems for the patient: toxicity, immune and inflammatory responses, and gene control and targeting issues. In addition, there is the concern that the viral vector may recover its ability to cause disease once inside the patient. This has reduced

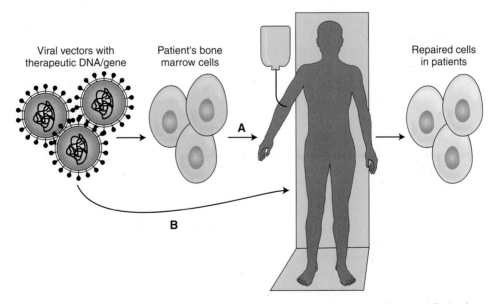

Figure 18.12. Examples of ex vivo (**A**) and in vivo (**B**) gene therapy. In ex vivo therapy, cells (such as bone marrow cells) are removed from the patient, and the desired gene or DNA is inserted into them using recombinant techniques. The modified cells are then injected into the patient. In vivo gene therapy involves injecting a vector containing the therapeutic DNA directly into the patient.

their initial popularity as gene delivery vectors. Nonviral or synthetic vectors (e.g., liposomes and polycationic carriers) are getting increasing attention for gene delivery. Their major challenge is overcoming the many biological barriers before and after reaching the target cells.

Even when the gene is successfully introduced into target cells, it must be integrated into the genome and remain functional. The altered cells must be long-lived and stable. These limitations prevent gene therapy from achieving guaranteed long-lasting benefits, and patients will need multiple rounds of gene therapy before it cures a disease.

Monogenic disorders (arising from defects in a single gene) are the best candidates for gene therapy. Unfortunately, most commonly occurring disorders, such as heart disease, high blood pressure, Alzheimer's disease, arthritis, and diabetes, are polygenic (caused by variations in many genes) and will be especially difficult to treat effectively with gene therapy.

Stimulating the immune system in a way that reduces the effectiveness of gene therapy is a potential risk. Furthermore, the immune system's enhanced response to foreign materials makes it difficult for gene therapy to be repeated in patients.

Key Concepts

- Biopharmaceuticals are therapeutic agents manufactured by biotechnology methods (using living organisms or parts of living organisms) rather than by chemical synthesis.
- Most biopharmaceuticals are made using rDNA techniques using bacterial, yeast, or mammalian cells as hosts. Transgenic plants and animals are also being used to make biopharmaceuticals.
- Glycosylation differences among various hosts need to be taken into account when making a human biopharmaceutical.
- Therapeutic proteins are naturally occurring or slightly modified proteins that are administered to patients as biopharmaceutical drugs for replacement or facilitative therapy.
- Therapeutic antibodies are proteins made in response to an antigen, and are used as biopharmaceuticals or as drug-targeting systems.
- Monoclonal antibodies (MAbs) are made using hybridoma technology.

- MAbs may be animal in origin, or may be partially human as in chimeric, humanized, or human antibodies.
- Biopharmaceuticals are large molecules with chemical and physical stability problems.
- Biopharmaceuticals are difficult and expensive to make; and their identity and purity is difficult to test.
- Most biopharmaceuticals are available as aqueous solutions or as lyophilized solids designed to be reconstituted before use.
- Most biopharmaceutical solutions must be given by injection because of poor stability and permeability.
- Immunogenicity is one of the major safety issues with biopharmaceuticals.
- Nucleic acid-based therapeutics are a new area of biotech drugs.
- Gene therapy is the transfer of genetic material into the cells of an individual with the objective of fixing a defective gene.

Review Questions

1. How are proteins used as drugs in therapy?
2. Explain the terms biotechnology, biologics, and biopharmaceuticals.
3. Describe the steps in making a therapeutic protein by recombinant DNA technology.
4. Compare different host cell types for the manufacture of recombinant proteins. What advantages do transgenic animals provide in the manufacture of recombinant proteins?
5. Describe the structure of a monoclonal antibody. What is the difference between monoclonal and polyclonal antibodies?
6. Outline the manufacture of monoclonal antibodies using hybridoma technology.
7. What are the differences between murine, chimeric, humanized, and human MAbs? Their relative advantages and disadvantages.
8. Why are most biopharmaceuticals administered by injection?
9. Explain the sources of protein instability and how formulation techniques can minimize instability.
10. Briefly describe the denaturation process and its consequences.
11. What factors are responsible for the short duration of action and immunogenicity of biopharmaceuticals?
12. What are the differences between in vivo and ex vivo gene therapy?
13. Why are vectors needed to transport DNA during gene therapy?

Additional Readings

Crommelin D, Sindelar RD, Meibohm B (eds). Pharmaceutical Biotechnology: Fundamentals and Applications, 3rd ed. Informa Healthcare, 2007.

Grewal IS. Emerging Protein Biotherapeutics. 1st ed. CRC Press, 2009.

Meibohm B (ed). Pharmacokinetics and Pharmacodynamics of Biotech Drugs: Principles and Case Studies in Drug Development. 1st ed. Wiley-VCH, 2007.

Van de Weert M, Moeller EH (eds). Immunogenicity of Biopharmaceuticals (Biotechnology: Pharmaceutical Aspects). 1st ed. Springer, 2008.

CHAPTER 19

Drug Discovery and Approval

Every pharmaceutical and biopharmaceutical product undergoes rigorous scientific testing and scrutiny, to ensure safety and efficacy for its intended use, before receiving approval for marketing in the United States. For every 10,000 compounds synthesized or isolated as potential drugs, only one, on average, will successfully complete all the requirements to make it to the market. Compounds are eliminated for several reasons, the most common ones being:

- Lack of the desired level of efficacy
- Unacceptable toxicity
- Poor pharmaceutical properties, such as instability, low aqueous solubility, poor cell permeability, and unacceptably high clearance
- Poor market potential or extensive competition

Pharmaceutical companies try to identify and eliminate potentially problematic compounds from the development process as early as possible. The estimated average cost of bringing a new drug to market is $800 million, and the average length of time from discovery to use in patients is 10 to 15 years. As lengthy and complicated as the process is, however, it has been remarkably successful in bringing safe and effective drugs to market.

The FDA

In the United States, the Food and Drug Administration (FDA) regulates the development of new drug products and their subsequent marketing. One of the FDA's functions is to promote and protect public health by helping safe and effective drug products reach the market in a timely manner, and to monitor these products for continued safety after they are in use. In addition to conventional and biologic drugs, the FDA regulates related products such as tissues for transplantation, medical devices, veterinary drug products, as well as most food products (except meat and poultry), animal feed, and tobacco products. In addition, the FDA monitors the safety of cosmetics, medical and consumer products, and devices that emit radiation (such as cell phones, microwave ovens, and lasers). The FDA also has responsibilities in response to bioterrorism by ensuring adequate and timely supplies of therapeutic agents to treat the injured.

FDA Centers

The FDA is divided into several centers each with its own responsibility; the major centers are shown in Figure 19.1. Of these, the Center for Drug Evaluation and Research (CDER) and the Center for Biologics Evaluation and Research (CBER) are most relevant for us because

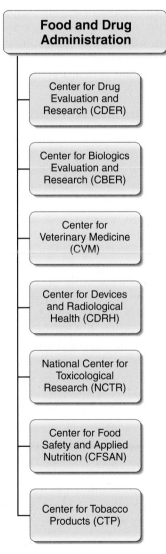

Figure 19.1. Major centers of the US Food and Drug Administration. CDER is responsible for human drugs, including most biopharmaceuticals, whether prescription, generic, or over-the-counter (OTC). The CBER regulates some biopharmaceuticals and other biologics such as vaccines, blood products, and gene therapy.

they are involved in the review, approval, and monitoring of human drug products.

Evolution of FDA Drug Regulations

The drug regulatory system in the United States is continuously evolving. Drug product regulations introduced in the early years came about as a result of public demand that caused Congress to pass a series of bills. The current FDA authority to regulate pharmaceutical products comes from the 1938 *Federal Food, Drug, and Cosmetic Act*, a law that has undergone many changes over the years. The Code of Federal Regulations, or CFR, is the book in which all final regulations are codified.

Some of the major milestones that came before and after the 1938 Act are summarized here.

- *Food and Drugs Act (1906):* This first drug law mandated that marketed drug products meet standards of strength and purity, but did not require evidence of safety or effectiveness. The FDA had to prove a product's labeling was false and fraudulent before it could be removed from the market.
- *Federal Food, Drug, and Cosmetic (FD&C) Act (1938):* The 1906 Act was revised by Congress in 1938. The revision was prompted by the death of 107 people from a poisonous ingredient in the product "Elixir Sulfanilamide." Pharmaceutical manufacturers now had to prove that a drug product was safe before it could be marketed.
- *Durham-Humphrey Amendment (1951):* This amendment to the Act separated prescription and nonprescription drugs, requiring that certain pharmaceutical products be labeled "for sale by prescription only." It defined prescription drugs as those unsafe for self-medication and which should be used only under a doctor's supervision.
- *Kefauver-Harris Drug Amendments (1962):* Congress passed these amendments to

tighten control over marketed drugs. A pharmaceutical company now had to prove not only the safety but also the effectiveness of the drug product for its intended use. In addition, the company was required to send to the FDA all adverse reaction reports about the drug product. Pharmaceutical advertisements in medical journals were required to provide complete information about the drug, including its risks. The amendments also required informed consent from subjects who participate in clinical trials.

- *Orphan Drug Act (1983):* An "orphan" disease is a condition affecting fewer than 200,000 people in the United States; examples are Huntington's disease, Tourette's syndrome, and muscular dystrophy. This act was passed to encourage development of drugs for orphan diseases, by providing financial incentives to pharmaceutical companies, and exclusive rights to market these medicines for a period of time.
- *Drug Price Competition and Patent Term Restoration Act (1984):* This legislation ensured that less expensive generic versions of approved drugs could be brought to market quickly. A less stringent, abbreviated application process was introduced for approval of generic drug products. In return, patents of new drugs were extended by some of the time lost during their FDA approval process.
- *Prescription Drug User Fee Act (PDUFA, 1992):* This legislation established a system whereby prescription drug manufacturers pay fees to have their new drug applications reviewed by the FDA. The system provided additional funds to help FDA accelerate its review of applications.
- *Food and Drug Administration Amendments Act (FDAAA, 2007):* This act reauthorized the PDUFA, and two other important laws: Best Pharmaceuticals for Children Act (BPCA) and Pediatric Research Equity Act (PREA). Both are designed to encourage more research and development into pediatric treatments.

New Drug Development

Drug discovery and development efforts typically emerge from basic research and then gradually move on to specific sequential tasks, which—if successful—culminate in a new drug product for the treatment of a human disease. The overall pathway has well-delineated milestones, which include selection of the drug target, identification of a lead compound, its modification to a compound suitable for toxicity testing in animals, and selection as drug candidate for clinical testing.

Lead Compound Selection

The process starts with a *sponsor*, usually a pharmaceutical company, seeking to develop a new drug it hopes will be useful to patients and profitable in the market. Extensive initial research goes into studying the disease process and identifying potential targets (receptors, enzymes), as discussed in Chapter 2, Drugs and Their Targets. A series of promising compounds is identified on the basis of a favorable affinity for and interaction with the desired drug target. These compounds are then screened for efficacy and potential toxicity in several suitable cellular models; the best one, called the *lead compound*, is selected for further preclinical studies. The lead compound then goes through an extensive process of research and modification (*lead optimization*) to make it more "drug-like." In this process, the chemical structure of the compound is progressively modified to optimize efficacy, toxicity, and ADME (absorption, distribution, metabolism, and excretion) properties. The final compound is now called a preclinical drug candidate.

Preclinical Testing

The goal of early preclinical development is to determine whether a preclinical candidate is reasonably safe for initial, small-scale clinical studies in humans, and whether it has sufficient pharmacological activity in animals to justify further development.

Primary activities during preclinical testing are in vitro and in vivo laboratory animal experiments to evaluate the compound's toxicological, pharmacological, and ADME characteristics. Additional laboratory studies include characterization of the chemical structure, purity, and physicochemical properties. A formulation for use in early human trials is designed and manufacturing processes for the drug compound and dosage forms are developed. Thus, preclinical development encompasses almost all of the concepts we have discussed in earlier chapters.

The major question that arises during preclinical testing is whether the results in animals will correlate with those in humans; disease processes and ADME are often different between commonly used laboratory animals and humans. Design of the appropriate animal model is a very important consideration in preclinical development. An animal model that is best to study the pharmacological action of the compound in a particular disease state is often not suitable for studying its ADME behavior, and vice versa. Decisions about extrapolating animal data to justify the first use of a drug candidate in humans are difficult, and testing at this stage can take from 1 to 5 years. Of every 1,000 new candidates tested preclinically, on average only one enters clinical trials—a success rate of only 0.1%.

The activities during lead optimization and preclinical testing are shown in Figure 19.2.

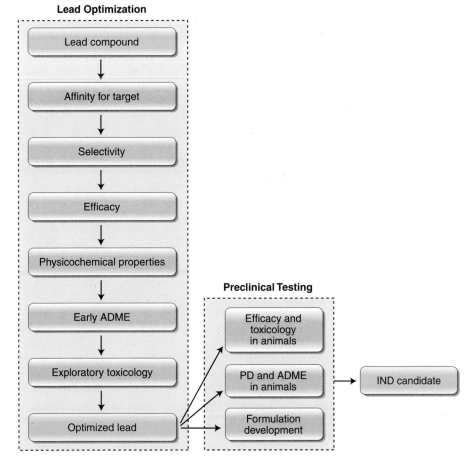

Figure 19.2. The process for lead optimization, preclinical testing, and selection of a drug candidate for clinical development. This process can take anywhere from 2 to 10 years.

Investigational New Drug

If results from laboratory and animal studies show promise, the sponsor can apply to the FDA to proceed to the next stage of development—testing the drug in humans. At this point, the compound changes legal status and becomes an investigational drug. The Investigational New Drug (IND) application is a proposal from a sponsor to the FDA requesting permission for clinical testing of a drug in humans. The IND application must contain information in five broad areas as shown in Table 19.1. By law, the FDA has 30 days to review the submitted IND documentation; the IND application is considered approved if the FDA does not disapprove it within 30 days.

However, before human clinical trials can begin, the IND must also be reviewed and approved by an Institutional Review Board (IRB) at the site (e.g., a hospital or medical center) where the proposed clinical studies will be conducted. An IRB is a group that has been formally designated to review and monitor biomedical research involving human subjects. Its primary aim is to ensure the rights and welfare of people participating in clinical trials both before and during their trial participation. The IRB reviews the sponsor's clinical trial protocol, informed consent documents, investigator brochures, and other documents related to the trial. The IRB has the right to approve, disapprove, or require changes to the study.

Clinical Trials

To demonstrate safety and efficacy, a new drug must pass through three distinct phases of controlled testing in humans. The phases progressively involve more human subjects tested for longer times. All trial subjects must be provided with sufficient information about the trial and the drug to give informed consent, freely and without coercion, before trial participation. The FDA has issued many guidelines related to the conduct of clinical trials and may meet with sponsors during the clinical trial process.

In a *controlled* clinical trial, subjects are divided into the treatment group (those given the investigational drug) and a

TABLE 19.1. Information Needed to Support IND Filing	
Information	*Details*
Chemistry, manufacturing, and control (CMC)	Compound with acceptable stability and formulation
	Controlled production under cGMP (current good manufacturing processes)
Absorption, distribution, metabolism, and excretion (ADME)	Route of administration, half-life
	Metabolic pathways
	Potential drug–drug interactions (including effects on cytochrome P450 enzymes)
Toxicology	Systemic and organ toxicity: gross and microscopic changes; two animal species, covering time periods of intended human exposure
	Estimated safety window between efficacious dose and "no observed adverse effect level" (NOAEL)
	Initial data on potential genotoxicity and cardiotoxicity
Mechanism of action and pharmacology	Effects on receptor in vitro
	Efficacy in animal models in vivo
Clinical development plans	Detailed protocol of initial studies

control group. Depending on the purpose of the trial, patients in the control group get no treatment, a placebo (an inactive product resembling the investigational drug), another drug known to be effective, or a different dose of the drug under study. Treatment and control groups must be as similar as possible in characteristics that can affect treatment outcome. For example, all patients in both treatment and control groups must have the disease the drug is meant to treat. Treatment and control groups should also be similar in age, weight, general health, and in other characteristics that could affect the outcome of the trial. In a process called *randomization*, subjects are randomly assigned to treatment or control groups rather than deliberately selected for either group. If the sample population is large enough, randomization creates treatment and control groups that are similar in important characteristics.

Along with randomization, another feature known as *blinding* limits bias in the conduct of a clinical study or interpretation of its results. In a *single-blind* study, patients do not know whether they are receiving the investigational drug or a placebo. In a *double-blind* study, patients, investigators, and data analysts do not know which patients received the investigational drug. Only when the assignment code is broken, usually at the end of the trial, is it possible to identify treatment and control patients in a double-blind trial.

Phase I Trials

Phase I testing refers to the first series of human trials of an IND. Single doses of the drug are administered to between 20 and 100 healthy human volunteers, starting at low doses and progressively increasing to higher doses. The emphasis in this phase is the acute safety profile and ADME behavior of the drug in humans. No determination of efficacy is usually possible at this stage. Phase I trials are generally not blinded and take about 1 year to complete.

Phase I studies identify a drug's primary adverse effects and establish a safe dosage range. Volunteers are closely monitored for adverse reactions. If the drug is well tolerated at the end of Phase I clinical trials and no major problems such as unacceptable toxicity are seen, the sponsor can move to Phase II clinical testing.

Phase I trials also provide important information about the ADME of a drug. Blood, urine, and other biological samples are monitored to determine how the drug is absorbed, distributed, metabolized, and excreted in humans. In particular, data on absorption and bioavailability of the drug product are used to modify the dosage form to improve any deficiencies. Information about the elimination pathways and pharmacokinetics of the drug in humans is used to design appropriate dosing regimens for Phase II clinical trials.

Approximately 70% of drug candidates entering Phase I are found safe enough to progress to the next phase. The 30% that do not proceed usually fail because they are not well tolerated, or because blood levels are lower than those thought to be necessary for efficacy.

Phase II Trials

Phase II trials follow after successful completion of Phase I. Some trials are exploratory studies to determine if the drug has clinical efficacy. They are carried out in a small group of patients with the target disease or condition. During these clinical trials, a "clinical endpoint"—defined by the FDA as a characteristic that reflects how a patient feels, functions, or survives—is recommended to determine a drug's efficacy. Dose-ranging studies are done to determine the optimum dose for efficacy, and the most appropriate method of administration. Phase II trials also study the pharmacodynamics and mechanism of action of the drug in more detail.

Most Phase II trials are double-blinded and randomized; many also have a *crossover* design, in which a second part of the trial has the group initially receiving placebos now receiving the investigational drug, and vice versa. On average, Phase II studies involve 100 to 300 patient volunteers and take about 2 years to complete.

Approximately 40% of drugs entering Phase II will proceed to the next phase. This occurs if the drug shows efficacy, a safe dose that is therapeutically effective is found, and the drug has acceptable pharmacokinetics for further development. Information collected at this stage of development is often used to further fine-tune the dosage form for better absorption and bioavailability, and to select an appropriate dosage regimen for Phase III trials. Investigational drugs that drop out during Phase II are either not sufficiently effective or reveal unacceptable side effects not seen in Phase I trials.

Phase III Trials

In Phase III, the sponsor conducts "pivotal" trials to get statistically significant evidence of efficacy and safety required for approval by the FDA. The drug is studied in a larger (1,000 to 3,000) and more diverse (in age, sex, health, and so forth) group of patients to confirm efficacy and safety. Furthermore, the trials are conducted at multiple centers and often in worldwide. This larger group of diverse patients enables clinicians to identify adverse events that may occur in only one or two patients per thousand, or in one type of patient subgroup. Phase III studies are also longer in duration to provide reassurance regarding long-term safety. Additional data regarding the risk versus benefit of the drug, dosing regimens, and other information contained in the package insert are also obtained at this stage.

About 70% of the drugs entering Phase III are successful in clearing this hurdle. The failure of an IND at this stage often opens up new avenues for drug discovery studies. Scientists try to understand why the compound failed in humans, and go back to study other closely related compounds to see whether another analog might be a more viable drug candidate.

Biomarkers and Surrogate Endpoints

The most difficult, time-consuming and, therefore, expensive aspect of clinical trials is demonstrating efficacy with a clinical end point; a statistically significant improvement in how a patient feels, functions, or survives. The use of biomarkers is increasingly being considered to predict efficacy more quickly than by these conventional clinical criteria. A biomarker is a quantitative measure that allows us to diagnose and assess the disease process and monitor response to treatment. A biomarker accepted by the FDA for use in clinical trials is called a surrogate end point; a laboratory measurement or a physical sign used as a substitute for a clinical end point. A surrogate end point is expected to predict clinical benefit (or harm, or lack of benefit) based on epidemiologic, therapeutic, pathophysiologic or other scientific evidence.

An example is osteoporosis, a disease of bones in that leads to an increased risk of fracture. Low bone mineral density is a biomarker for osteoporosis. The clinical end point for a drug to treat osteoporosis is fewer fractures, requiring clinical trials that are either very large or very long to demonstrate this antifracture efficacy. Improvement in bone mineral density is a surrogate end point that is more easily monitored in patients to determine if the drug has efficacy against osteoporosis. Another example is elevated cholesterol and its link to heart disease. The clinical end point is reduced deaths from heart disease, the surrogate end point is serum cholesterol levels. Many statin drugs (e.g., simvastatin) were approved based on their effectiveness at reducing serum cholesterol, without showing directly that they prevent death from heart disease. The FDA often requires the sponsor to carry out additional studies after approval to confirm that the drug product does produce the intended clinical end points.

Biomarkers have shown great potential in the developing field of individualized medicine. Biomarkers can predict how an individual will react to a drug before it is administered. Biomarkers also offer hope for speeding up new drug development by early identification of the efficacy and safety potential of a compound.

NDA Review and Approval

After successful completion of all three phases of clinical trials, the sponsor may file a New Drug Application (NDA) with the FDA. An NDA requests permission from the FDA to market the drug commercially. It details the entire history and experience with the drug product, including preclinical studies, animal studies, human clinical trials, and information about manufacturing and labeling of the drug product. NDAs typically run 100,000 pages or more. All NDAs are reviewed by a CDER review team comprising chemists, pharmacologists, physicians, field inspectors, statisticians, and other experts necessary for a particular drug. This team is responsible for reaching a decision regarding approval of the product.

Type of Review

First, the review team determines whether the application should get a standard or priority review, using letters: P is for priority; S is for standard. A priority (P) rating is given to products that

- Represent a therapeutic advance because no other effective drugs are available
- Is more effective and/or safer than current products
- Has significant other advantages over current products (convenience, reduced side effects, improved tolerance)

A standard (S) rating means that the product may have only minor advantages over existing marketed therapies. To further determine priority, each new NDA is also assigned a number, indicating the type of drug product as follows:

1. New molecular entity (NME)
2. New salt, ester or other noncovalent derivative of approved drug
3. New dosage form or formulation
4. New combination of existing drugs
5. New manufacturer of approved drug product
6. New indication of approved drug product
7. Drug already marketed without approved NDA
8. Over-the-counter (OTC) switch of approved drug product

These classifications are not mutually exclusive; e.g., a new formulation may also contain a new salt. The sponsor will suggest a classification, but the FDA finally determines it. The final letter-number classification will determine the priority the FDA gives to reviewing the NDA.

The review team examines the NDA carefully to determine whether the results of the well-controlled clinical studies provide substantial evidence of the drug's effectiveness, and whether the results show that the product is safe under the conditions of use proposed in the labeling. Typical information that must be on a drug product label, usually supplied as a package insert for prescription drugs, is shown in Table 19.2.

FDA Advisory Committees

The FDA or sponsor may request that a non-FDA advisory committee review the information about a drug product to have the benefit of wider national expert input. Advisory committee members are scientific experts such as physicians, statisticians, pharmacologists, and epidemiologists, as well as consumer representatives who represent the patients and the

TABLE 19.2. Typical Information Contained in Drug Product Labeling, Usually Included as a Package Insert with Prescription Drug Products

Boxed warnings
Very serious and potentially life-threatening adverse effects of drug; highlighted in a black box at top of package insert

Description
Chemical structure, molecular weight, physicochemical properties of drug; dosage form, formulation including inactive ingredients; route of administration

Clinical pharmacology
Mechanism of action(s), pharmacokinetics (including bioavailability and ADME); brief summary of clinical trial results; age, sex, or population differences, if any

Indications
Clinical uses, i.e., indications for which drug is approved; use in special populations; use in pediatric and geriatric patients; genetically linked differences in drug behavior; use in patients with impaired organ function (e.g., hepatic or renal disease)

Contraindications
Situations or patient characteristics in which drug should not be used, e.g., prior allergic reaction to a similar class of drugs

Warnings
Serious risks of using drug; situations in which drug should be discontinued; most serious are in bold black type

Precautions
Actions to be taken during therapy to ensure safety and efficacy; includes drug interactions, food interactions, hypersensitivity; precautions for pregnant women or nursing mothers

Adverse reactions
All significant side effects seen with recommended doses of drug during clinical trials

Overdosage
LD_{50} of drug; symptoms of an overdose, recommended actions

Drug abuse and dependence
Potential for abuse, or for psychological or physical dependence

Dosage and administration
Specific age categories for dosing; recommended doses (initial and maximum) and frequency for approved conditions; directions on administration of drug; storage conditions (temperature, protection from light, heat, and air)

How supplied
Route of administration, dosage forms (including descriptions of color, shape, and markings), strengths, and units per package

---

public. This group weighs the available evidence, assesses risk versus benefit, and provides advice on the approval of a drug product. The FDA usually agrees with the advisory committee recommendations, although they are not binding. Advisory committees play a prominent role at the product approval stage, but may be used earlier in the product development cycle or during postmarketing monitoring.

Drug Approval

The FDA's goal is to complete the NDA review of a priority drug within 6 months after it has been filed; for drugs with a standard designation the goal is 10 months. However, actual approval times may vary.

The NDA review team takes one of three actions on the NDA after their review is complete.

- *Approved*: The sponsor may now market the drug product in the United States.
- *Not approved*: The product may not be marketed in the United States and provides a detailed explanation of the reasons for the decision.
- *Approvable*: FDA is prepared to approve the NDA after the sponsor rectifies identified deficiencies and satisfies conditions specified in the complete response letter.

Once the FDA approves an NDA, the sponsor can introduce the drug product to the market and make it available for physicians to prescribe. Note that the approval is restricted to the specific drug product (active ingredient, route of administration, dosage form, formulation, strength, manufacturer, and so forth), and the indication (disease, illness) specified in the NDA. Any changes in these parameters require another FDA review.

Early Access

The FDA has designed *early access* programs to allow patients with life-threatening conditions to begin using promising new therapies before formal FDA approval. Under early access, patients may receive investigational drugs that have shown promise in Phase II clinical trials. Patients are informed that they accept some risk in using drug products not yet FDA-approved, but seriously ill patients are typically willing to accept more risk. Examples of early access are the *treatment IND* and the *parallel track* programs that were designed for individuals with AIDS whose condition prevented them from participating in clinical trials.

Postmarketing Surveillance

After FDA approval, the drug product enters the postmarketing surveillance phase that encompasses the entire duration of the product's life on the market. The FDA continues to monitor all drugs that are on the market throughout their lifetime; the Office of Drug Safety (ODS) in the CDER performs this function. The MedWatch Reporting Program of the ODS is a spontaneous method for reporting adverse events and problems with a drug product so that significant health hazards can be rapidly identified. It is a voluntary program for health care practitioners (pharmacists, physicians, nurses) and patients; reporting is mandatory for pharmaceutical companies.

If an adverse event or problem is identified with a marketed drug, the ODS can take any one or more of the following actions:

- *Labeling changes:* requires manufacturer to add new information to the product's package insert.
- *Boxed warnings:* addition of a boxed warning to the product package insert.
- *Product recalls or withdrawals:* these are the most serious FDA actions. Recalls involve the removal of one or more batches of product from the market; withdrawals require taking the product off the market permanently.
- *Medical and safety alerts:* the ODS provides important new safety information about the drug product to health professionals, trade, and media organizations.

Figure 19.3 and Table 19.3 summarize the phases of the new drug development process. It is estimated that the average cost of developing a new drug today is about $800 million.

Phase IV Trials

For some drug products, the FDA requires the sponsor to perform additional studies after the drug is in general use (Phase IV) to evaluate long-term effects. This is because all possible effects of a drug cannot always be evaluated during Phase I, II, and III clinical

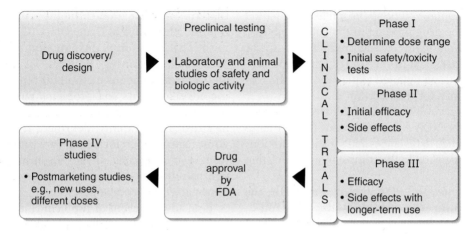

Figure 19.3. The stages of new drug development, starting with preclinical testing and ending with activities monitoring a marketed drug product.

trials. An NDA typically includes safety data on several hundred to several thousand patients. If an adverse event occurs in 1 in 5,000 or even 1 in 1,000 users, it could be missed in clinical trials, but could pose a serious safety problem when the drug is used by hundreds of thousands of patients after marketing. Phase IV studies may address a variety of other issues such as drug interactions, alternate dosing schedules, or response in specific patient subpopulations.

Pharmaceutical companies may also conduct postapproval clinical trials studies to expand the list of approved indications, optimize dosing schedules, or add other new information to product labeling. These studies can provide important marketing information for the product, e.g., fewer adverse effects or better clinical efficacy compared with a competitor drug. Outcomes research is also begun after marketing to measure a drug's cost-effectiveness and therapeutic

TABLE 19.3. Activities, Duration, and Success Rates of Various Stages in New Drug Development				
Activity	*Test Population*	*Duration*	*Purpose*	*Success Rate*
Preclinical	Laboratory studies Animal studies	3 to 5 years	Effectiveness, safety, ADME in animals	5,000 compounds tested
IND Submission				
Phase I	20 to 100 healthy volunteers	1 to 1.5 years	Acute safety, ADME dose	Five drug candidates enter Phase I
Phase II	100 to 300 patient volunteers	1.5 to 2 years	Effectiveness, short-term safety	
Phase III	1,000 to 3,000 patient volunteers	2 to 4 years	Long-term safety, confirm effectiveness	
NDA Submission				
FDA review		1 to 4 years		One drug approved
NDA Approval				
Phase IV	All patients taking drug	Long term	Postmarketing surveillance	

value compared with other drugs, and with other interventions such as surgery or hospitalization.

Supplemental NDA

After approval of an NDA, a sponsor may not usually make any changes in the drug (chemical form, crystallinity, particle size, etc.) or the formulation (excipients, amounts of excipients, etc.), or the manufacturing process. If a change is desired, the manufacturer must submit a supplemental NDA demonstrating that the modified product is therapeutically identical to the approved product. Supplemental NDAs also get assigned a classification and priority, as discussed earlier in this chapter.

International Harmonization of Drug Development

In the past, the requirements for new drug approval were significantly different from country to country, so that clinical trials and even preclinical studies often had to be repeated in each country before a new drug could be approved and made available to patients. The International Conference on Harmonization (ICH) brought together government regulators and drug industry representatives from the United States, the European Union, and Japan to make the international drug regulatory process more efficient and uniform. The regulatory systems in these regions share the same fundamental concerns for the safety, efficacy, and quality of drug products. The goals of this effort are to

- Make new drugs available with minimum delay to American consumers and those in other countries.
- Minimize unnecessary duplicate testing during the research and development of new drugs.
- Develop guidance documents that create consistency in the requirements for new drug approval.

Generic Drug Development and Approval

An FDA-approved generic drug product is identical to a brand name drug in dosage form, strength, route of administration, quality, performance characteristics, and intended use.

Drug sponsors are required to submit an abbreviated new drug application (ANDA) for approval to market a generic product. The ANDA process allows generic sponsors to skip time-consuming and expensive animal testing and Phase I through III clinical trials for drugs approved by the FDA, since this testing has already been done by the original innovator drug company.

The ANDA requirements for approval of a generic drug product are that it must

- Contain the same active ingredients as the innovator drug; inactive ingredients may vary.
- Be identical in strength, dosage form, and route of administration to the innovator drug.
- Be bioequivalent (see definition in the following text) to the innovator drug.
- Meet the same standards for identity, strength, purity, and quality as the innovator drug product.
- Be manufactured under the FDA's good manufacturing practice regulations required for innovator products.

If all these conditions are met, it is assumed that the generic product will have the same therapeutic profile as the innovator product, and can be used interchangeably in most patients.

Two products are considered bioequivalent if the rate of absorption, maximum plasma concentration (C_{max}), extent of absorption, and area under the time–plasma concentration curve (AUC) of the drug from the two products are not statistically different. In other words, bioequivalency means the plasma level curves of the generic and innovator companies are *superimposable*. Bioequivalency is usually demonstrated in single-dose bioequivalency clinical trials in a small (24 to 36) group of healthy volunteers that compares the plasma level curves of generic product against the innovator product. Bioequivalency testing is the only clinical trial requirement for an ANDA.

Certain drug products such as solutions and others without a known or potential bioequivalence problem may be eligible for a waiver of in vivo bioequivalency study requirements. No clinical studies are necessary for approval of the generic version of such drugs; in vitro laboratory studies such as dissolution testing may suffice for demonstration of therapeutic equivalency. A detailed discussion of bioequivalency requirements is outside the scope of this book.

Pharmacogenomics in Drug Development

Chapter 17, Pharmacogenomics, discussed the impact of a patient's genetic information on appropriate therapy choice. The knowledge that genetic diversity makes drugs ineffective or toxic in certain individuals is being exploited in the preclinical and clinical testing of investigational drugs. Biomarkers or gene markers can be used to identify patients more receptive or more susceptible to a particular drug. Suitable clinical trial participants can be tested to provide information on metabolic status, drug target polymorphism, and disease susceptibility. Patient testing in early clinical trials can permit selection of patients who are biochemically predisposed to respond favorably to the drug. Other patients, such as slow metabolizers who are expected to show predictable adverse effects, can be excluded from trials.

The benefits of a pharmacogenomic approach to clinical trial design are as follows:

- Pharmaceutical companies will be able to discover potential therapies more easily using genomic targets. Previously failed drug candidates may be revived as they are matched with the niche population in which they work.
- Even small groups of subjects selected in this way can yield statistically significant results. This could reduce the number of patients required for clinical trials of an investigational drug.
- The risk to clinical trial participants will be reduced because individuals with predictable adverse effects will be excluded, and only those persons capable of responding to a drug will be selected.
- The failure rate of drugs in clinical trials will decrease as trials are targeted for specific genetic population groups, providing greater degrees of success.
- The drug review and approval process will be shorter because data from clinical trials will be more uniform and cohesive.
- Therapies for diseases with a small patient population will be more likely to be developed.
- There will be decrease in the number of drugs a patient must try to find an effective therapy; a trial and error approach to therapy will not be the norm.
- An increase in the range of possible drug targets will decrease the overall cost of health care.

Today, a drug that helps only 20% of the subjects in clinical trials would probably not be approved, but a drug that *always* helps 20% of the population with the same genetic marker or biomarker might be approved for that limited population.

Over-the-Counter Drugs

OTC or non-prescription drugs are medications that do not require a physician's prescription. The first method of developing and marketing an OTC drug product is the process we have already discussed earlier, in which a sponsor company performs preclinical research, conducts clinical trials, and so forth, and submits an NDA for an OTC drug.

The second and more frequently used mechanism is the *prescription to OTC switch*. In this process, the sponsor of an approved prescription drug submits a supplemental application to the FDA, requesting a switch of the drug's status from prescription to OTC. The OTC product suggested is usually lower strength than the prescription version. The FDA reviews the drug's performance as a prescription drug, including information obtained during postmarketing surveillance. There are three man considerations in making this switch:

- The potential toxicity and side effect risk
- Adequate self-diagnosis of the condition without a health care professional
- Ease of use in a safe and effective manner

The prescription to OTC switch provides consumers with easy access to safe and effective products without the assistance of a health care professional.

The third mechanism for marketing OTC drugs is the *OTC drug review process* in which products are marketed without an application as required in the first two mechanisms. Here, the FDA and an advisory panel of experts establish that the active ingredients in a product, rather than the product itself, are safe and effective for OTC use.

Key Concepts

- In the United States, the FDA regulates marketed drugs. In particular, the CDER and the CBER regulate human drugs and biologics.
- Several congressional acts have established and improved drug regulations over the years.
- Preclinical studies (laboratory and animal) on a group of drug candidates select the best compound to move forward into initial testing in humans.
- The IND application is a proposal from a sponsor to the FDA requesting permission for clinical testing of a drug in humans.
- Phase I trials characterize the acute safety profile and ADME behavior of the drug in healthy human volunteers.
- Phase II trials in patients are designed to investigate efficacy

- and to determine an appropriate dosing regimen.
- Phase III trials involve a larger and more diverse patient population and are carried out to confirm efficacy and long-term safety.
- The sponsor may file an NDA with the FDA after completion of clinical trials. The FDA may deem the drug product approved, not approved, or approvable.
- The FDA's postmarketing surveillance monitors all marketed drugs throughout their lifetime; sponsors may be required to conduct Phase IV clinical trials after marketing.
- Generic products may be approved under an ANDA.
- Clinical trials are now being designed using a pharmacogenomic approach to select the appropriate trial subjects and analyzing data.

Review Questions

1. What are the specific responsibilities of the CDER and the CBER?
2. What information does the FDA require in an IND application?
3. Why is an IRB review necessary before a clinical trial is begun?
4. Why are clinical studies randomized and blinded? What does single and double blinding mean?
5. What are the goals of Phase I, II, and III trials? How many subjects are involved in each, and how long does the process take?
6. How are surrogate end points used to make clinical trials shorter and less expensive?
7. What is the purpose of an NDA? What is involved in the review and approval of an NDA?
8. How are NDA submissions prioritized for review by the FDA?
9. Why is postmarketing surveillance necessary? When and why are Phase IV trials conducted?
10. How does an ANDA differ from an NDA? What studies are required for approval of generic drug products?
11. How will a pharmacogenomic approach improve the development of new drugs?
12. What is the difference between a prescription and an OTC drug product? What is the process for switching a drug from prescription-only to OTC status?

Additional Readings

Cayen MN. Early Drug Development: Strategies and Routes to First-in-Human Trials, 1st ed. Wiley, 2010.

Friedhoff LT. New Drugs: An Insider's Guide to the FDA's New Drug Approval Process for Scientists, Investors and Patients. PSPG Publishing, 2009.

Mathieu M. New Drug Development: A Regulatory Overview. Parexel Intl Corp, 2008.

Ng R. Drugs—From Discovery to Approval, 2nd ed. Wiley-Liss, 2008.

NOTE: Page numbers in italics designate figures; page numbers followed by letter "t" designate tables.

A

ABCB1 gene, 305
Absolute bioavailability, 193
Absorption, 3, 281–282
    rate and extent, 186–189
    rate constant, 187
Absorption, distribution, metabolism, and excretion
        (ADME), 263
    behavior, 252
    processes, 9, 267
ACE (*see* Angiotensin-converting enzyme (ACE))
Acetylation, 168, *168*
Acetylcholine (ACh) receptors, 215
N-Acetyl-transferase-2, 303
Acid dissociation constant, 30
Acquired mutation, 308
Acquired resistance, 270–271
Active ingredient, 5, 106
Active sites, 10
Active transport, 75
Additive, 286
ADH (*see* Antidiuretic hormone (ADH))
Administration with meals, 287
ADR (*see* Adverse drug reactions (ADR))
Adsorption, 280–281
Adult-onset diabetes, 299
Adverse drug reactions (ADR), 256, 278
Affinity, 231–232
Agonists, 227–229
    drugs, receptor targets, and conditions, 229t
    of epinephrine, *229*
    of histamine, *229*
    potency of, 254
Alcohol, 287
Aldosterone, 268
Alleles, 295
Allergic effects (*see* Idiosyncratic reactions)
Allergy, 272–273
    antibiotics, 272
    penicillin allergy, 272–273
    sensitization, 272
Allosteric agonists, 230
Allosteric antagonism, 236
Allosteric drugs, 229–230
Allosteric modulation, 222
Allosteric modulators, 230
Alpha- and beta-adrenergic receptors, *13*
Alzheimer's disease, 299–300
Amino acid conjugation, 167–168
    glycine and glutamine, *167*
    process of, *168*

Amiodarone, 53
Amoxicillin, 272
Amphetamine, 151, 237
Amphiphiles, 53
Amphiphilicity, 53
    micelle formation, 54
    surface tension effect, 54
Ampholytes, 27, 38
Amphoteric compounds, 38–39
    amino acid glycine, *39*
    ionization schemes for, *38*
Ampicillin, 150, 272
Amplification, 213
Analogs, 12
Anaphylactic shock, 272
Anaphylaxis, 272
Antibody-drug conjugates, 326
Anatomical barriers, 8
Anchoring junctions, 80
Angiotensin, 268
Angiotensin-converting enzyme (ACE), 238–239, 305
Anonymous SNP, 298
Antacids, 283
Antagonism, 286
    allosteric and noncompetitive, mechanisms of,
        231
    chemical antagonist, 237
    competitive antagonists, 235–236
    functional antagonists, 236–237
    noncompetitive antagonist, 236
Antagonists, 227–229, 249
    drugs, receptor targets, and conditions, 230t
    of epinephrine, *229*
    of histamine, *229*
    and inhibitors, 248–252
    mechanisms of action, 235
Antibody, 316
    fragments, 325–326
    monoclonal, 323–324
    structure, 322–323
Antisense oligonucleotide drug, 336
Anthracyclines, 271
Antibiotics, 272
Antidiuretic hormone (ADH), 205
Anti-Parkinsonian activity, 17
APOE gene, 300
Aptamers, 336
Area under curve (AUC), *192*, 192–193
Aspirin, 241
Asthma, 299
Astrocytes, 125

ATryn®, 321
Autacoids, 208
    structures of, 209
Autocrine signaling, 208
Autosomes, 295
Aztreonam, 273

B
BBB (see Blood-brain barrier (BBB))
Benzodiazepine receptor, 230
Benzylpenicillin, 272
Biliary excretion, 149–150
    processes of, 150
Biliary secretion, 172
Binding and response curves, 246–248
Bioavailability, 188–189
Biochemical barriers and targets, 8
Bioisosterism, 17
Biological buffers, 34–35
Biological markers, 301
Biological targeting systems, 114
Biopharmaceuticals drugs, 314
    ADME of, 329–331
    advantages of, 315–316
    formulation of, 326–327
    nucleic acid-based, 335
    opportunities and limitations of
    pharmacological considerations of, 331–332
    stability of, 327–329
    types of, 316–322
Biotechnology and Genetic Engineering, 314–315
    drug delivery issues, 333
    immunogenicity of, 332–333
    posttranslational modifications, 333
    stability issues, 333
Biotransformation, 4, 283–285
Blood, 121
    composition of, 121
    flow, 127–128
    vessels, 122
Blood-brain barrier (BBB), 84–85, 125
    features of, 126
Breast milk, excretion by, 151
Breathalyzer test, 151
Buffer capacity, 34
Buffered solution, 34

C
Capillary exchange, 122–123
Carbacephems, 273
Carbapenems, 273
Cardiac glycosides, 150
Cardiac output, 121
Carrier, 73
    groups, 12
    proteins, 63–64
Carrier-mediated absorption, 282
Carrier-mediated transport, 72–77, 82
    rate of, 74
    representation of, 73

transporters, 73–74, 75
    types of, 74–77
Catecholamines, 206–208, 268
Catechol-O-methyltransferase (COMT), 238
Cefprozil, 273
Ceftriaxone, 150
Cefuroxime, 273
Celecoxib, 241
Cells
    junctions, 79–80
    signaling, 201–202
Cell membrane, 60–78, 64
    components of, 60
        cellular proteins, 62–64
        lipid bilayer, 61–62
    mechanisms of transport, 64
        carrier-mediated transport, 72–77
        endocytosis and exocytosis, 77–78
        passive diffusion, 65–72
Cell-surface receptors, 215–219
    enzymatic receptors, 218–219
    G protein-coupled receptors (GPCR), 217–218
    ion-channel receptors, 216, 216–217
Cephalexin, 273
Cephalosporins, 238, 273
Certain safety factor (CSF), 258–259
Cetirizine, antiallergy drug, 10
Channel proteins, 63
Chelation, 279–280
Chemical antagonist, 237
Chemical barriers, 8
Chemical shelf life, 115
Chemical stability, 114
Chinese hamster ovary (CHO) cells, 320
Chiral center, 15, 15–16
Chiral recognition, 15
Chloramphenicol-3-palmitate, 43
Chromosomes, 294–295
Chyme, 93
Circadian rhythms, 268–269
Circulatory system, 120–124
    branching arrangement, 122
    cardiovascular system
        blood, 121
        blood vessels, 122
        capillary exchange, 122–123
        fluids exchange, 123
        heart and cardiac output, 121
    lymphatic system
        functions of, 124
        lymph, 123–124
        lymphatic vessels, 123
Clindamycin, 150
Clinical therapeutic index, 257
Cocaine, 151
Codons, 295
Compartmental modeling, 185
Competitive antagonists, 235–236, 249–250
    mechanisms of action, 235
Competitive enzyme inhibitors, 239–240

Competitive inhibition, 175
Complementarity
    electrostatic, 13
    physicochemical, 12–14
        alpha- and beta-adrenergic receptors, *13*
        ionic and hydrophobic interactions, 13
        pharmacophore, *13*
        protein–ligand binding, 13
        regions role in binding, 13–14
    steric, 14–17
        chiral center, *15, 15*–16
        enantiomers and chirality, 14–15
        geometric isomers, 16, *16*
        hypothetical enantiomers, binding, *15*
        racemic mixtures, 16–17
        stereoisomers, 14
COMT (*see* Catechol-O-methyltransferase (COMT))
Concentration gradient, 65, 110
    plot of, *109*
Concentration ratio, 250
Concentration–response curve, 247, *247*, 248, 250
    for agonist, *249*–252
        substrate concentration and fractional response,
            248
Conjugate acid-base pair, 30
Conjugation reactions, 160–161, 164–165
Contact-dependent signaling, 208
Continuous capillaries, 125–126
Controlled-release products, 111–113
Cordarone®, 53
Cortisol, 268
Cosolvents, 46
COX (*see* Cyclooxygenase (COX))
Creatinine clearance, 147–148
Cross-resistance, 270
Crosstalk, 213
Crystal lattice, 43
CSF (*see* Certain safety factor (CSF))
Cyclooxygenase (COX), 241
CYP3A4, 287
CYP3A Inducers, 285t
CYP3A Inhibitors, 285t
CYP2D6 activity, 303
CYP2D6 polymorphism, 304
CYP enzymes, 303
CYP450 enzymes, 287
CYP450 isozymes, 283
Cystic fibrosis (CF), 297, 299
Cytochrome P450 (CYP), 161–163
    enzymes, 162–163
        drug substrates, 163t
        strong enzyme inhibitors and inducers, 177t
    nomenclature of, 161, *162*
    phase I oxidative metabolism reactions, *162*

D
Dactinomycin, 271
DAG (*see* Diacyl glycerol (DAG))
Degradation reactions, 115
Degree of ionization, 36t

Delayed hypersensitivity (*see* Drug allergy)
Depression, 299
Diacyl glycerol (DAG), 236
Diazepam, 286
Dicloxacillin, 272
Diffusion coefficient, 65, 111
Diffusion layer, 107
Diffusion layer thickness, 111
Digoxin, 151
Dipole–dipole interaction, 45
Dipole-induced dipole interaction, 45
Discontinuous capillaries, 126–127
Dispersions, 106
Dissolution rate, 107–108
Distomer, 16
Distribution, 282–283
Distribution rate, 189–190
DNA configuration, 295
Dosage forms, 105–107
    need for, 106
    types of, 106–107
Dose-response curve (DRC), 252–253, 258–259
Dose-response relationships, 252
    concentration–response
        antagonists and inhibitors, 248–252
        binding and response curves, 246–248
        logarithm scales, 248
    graded dose-response curves, 253–254
    quantal dose-response curves, 254–255
    selectivity and toxicity, 255
        certain safety factor, 258–259
        risk *versus* benefit, 259
        therapeutic index, 256–258
Doxycycline, 150
DRC (*see* Dose-response curve (DRC))
Drug
    administration, 3–4
    amphiphilicity, 53
        micelle formation, 54
        surface tension effect, 54
    definition, 1–2
    design, 3
    development and approval process, 5
    distribution, 4
        circulatory system, 120–124
        processes, 124–130
        volume of, 130–133
    ionization of
        electrolytes and nonelectrolytes, 26, 27
        multiple ionizable groups, 38–39
        pH and, 33–37
        salts of weak acids and bases, 32–33
        strong acids and bases, 28–29
        unbuffered solutions, 37–38
        water as solvent, 27–28
        weak acids and bases, 29–32
        weak electrolytes, 27
    lipophilicity
        apparent partition coefficient, 51–53
        partition coefficient, *50, 50*–51

Drug (*Continued*)
    pharmacogenomics, 5
    pharmacotherapeutics, 4
    physicochemical properties, 17–21
        bioisosteric applications, 18–19, *19*
        bioisosteric equivalents, 17–18, *18*
        bioisosterism, 17
        ionization, 20–21, *20*, *21*
        lipophilic–hydrophilic balance, 19–20, 20t
    site of action, 2–3
    solubility
        principles, 42–43
        solid-state structure, 43–44
        solvent, 44–46
        water solubility, 46–50
    targets and biological activity, 8–9
        anatomical barriers, 8
        binding to, 12–17
        biochemical barriers and targets, 8
        chemical barriers, 8
        physicochemical properties, 17–21
        protein–ligand interactions, 11, *11*
        proteins, 9–11
        structure–activity relationships, 21–22
Drug absorption, 89
    routes of administration, classification, 90t
    systemic administration
        local administration, 101–102
        macromolecular drugs, 100–101
        nonoral routes for, 98–100
        oral administration, 92–98
        rate of absorption, 90–92
Drug action
    antagonism, mechanisms of
        allosteric and noncompetitive, mechanisms
            of, *231*
        chemical antagonist, 237
        competitive antagonists, 235–236
        functional antagonists, 236–237
        noncompetitive antagonist, 236
    interaction with enzymes
        enzymatic and receptor processes, terms and
            events, 242t
        enzyme inhibitors, 238–241
        receptors and, 242
        selectivity in enzyme inhibition, 241–242
    nonreceptor-based, 242
    receptor interactions, 230
        affinity, 231–232
        efficacy, 234
        intrinsic activity, 233–234
        occupation theory, 232–233
        spare receptors, 234–235
    stereoselectivity in, 237–238
    theory of, 226
        agonists and antagonists, 227–229
        allosteric drugs, 229–230
        two-state receptor model, 226, *227*–228
Drug allergy, 272–273 (*see also* Allergy)
Drug binding to plasma proteins, 128–129

Drug candidate, *12*
Drug compliance, 273
Drug concentrations
    in body fluids, 183–184
        pharmacokinetic compartments, 185, *185*
        plasma, 184
        tissues, 184–185
Drug delivery
    approaches to, 111–114
        controlled-release products, 111–113
        immediate-release products, 111
        targeted drug delivery, 113–114
    characteristics of, 106
    dosage forms, 105–107
    macromolecular drugs, 116
    release and dissolution, 107–111
    stability, 114–116
    transport across biological barriers, 59
        cell membrane, 60–78
        multiple transport pathways, 85
        tissue, 78–85
Drug development, 342–347, 351
    activities, duration, and success rates in, 350t
    approval, 351–352
    biomarkers and surrogate endpoints, 346–347
    clinical trials, 344–346
    investigational new drug, 344
    lead compound selection, 342
    new drug application (NDA), 347
    over-the-counter drugs, 352–353
    pharmacogenomics in, 352
    preclinical testing, 342–343
Drug discovery, 307, 340
Drug distribution processes
    dynamics of, *124*
    intracellular fluid, 129
        body fluids, relative volumes of, *130*
        protein-bound drug, *130*
    out of capillaries, 124
        binding to plasma proteins, 128–129, 129t
        blood flow, 127–128
        continuous capillaries, 125–126
        discontinuous capillaries, 126–127
        fenestrated capillaries, 126
        physicochemical properties, 127
        protein-bound drug, *128*
        type of, 125
    tissues to plasma, 129–130
Drug–drug interactions, 279
    pharmaceutical drug interactions, 279
        adsorption, 280–281
        chelation, 279–280
        gastric pH, alteration of, 281
        incompatibilities, 281
    pharmacodynamic drug interactions, 286
        additive, 286
        antagonism, 286
        synergistic, 286
    pharmacokinetic drug interactions, 281
        absorption, 281–282

biotransformation, 283–285
distribution, 282–283
excretion, 283
Drug efflux, 75–76
Drug excretion, 139t
breast milk, 151
expired air, 151
kidneys, 138
nephron and its blood supply, 141
renal clearance, 146–149
renal excretion, 144–146
schematic view of, 139
structure of, 139–140, 140
urine formation, 140–144
liver
biliary excretion, 149–150
enterohepatic recirculation, 150
saliva, 151
sweat, 151
Drug-food interaction, 288t
Drug–herbal interactions, 288–289, 289t
Drug interactions in elderly, 290t
Drug ionization, 33–37
Drug metabolism
enzymes, 157–158
factors altering, 174–177
competitive inhibition, 175
enzyme induction, 176–177
enzyme inhibition, 174–175
genetic variability, 177
noncompetitive inhibition, 175–176
kinetics of, 159
lipophilic drugs elimination, 155, 156
metabolites, 158–159
phases of, 160
sites of
first-pass metabolism, 173
in intestines, 173
in liver, 169–172
presystemic metabolism, 172–173
total body clearance, 174
types of reactions, 160
phase I reactions, 161–164
phase II reactions, 164–169
xenobiotics, 156
Drug-metabolizing enzymes, 302–304
Drug–protein interactions, 9
Drug release and dissolution, 107–111
dissolution rate, 107–108
dosage forms
concentration gradient, 110
diffusion coefficient, 111
diffusion layer thickness, 111
particle size, 110–111
pH of medium, 110
solid state structure, 109–110
solubility, 109
solubility in absorption rate, role of, 110
schematic diagram of, 107
Drug resistance, 270–271

Drug salts, 48–50
product of, 48–50
unbuffered solutions, solubility, 48, 49
Drug selectivity, 256
antibiotic drugs development, 257
Drug stability, 114–116
chemical stability, 114
degradation reactions, 115
shelf life, 115
microbiological stability, 115
physical stability, 116
Drug tolerance, 269–270
Durham-Humphrey Amendment, 341

E
Efficacy, 234
Efflux proteins, 76
EIS complex (*see* Enzyme–inhibitor–substrate (EIS) complex)
Electrolytes and nonelectrolytes, 26
nonelectrolyte functional groups, 27
strong electrolyte, 26
weak electrolyte, 26
Electrostatic complementarity, 13
Elimination rate constant, 190–191
Enalapril, structures of, 159
Enalaprilat, 158–159
structures of, 159
Enantiomers and chirality, 14–15
Endocrine signaling, 205, 205
Endocytosis, 77–78
mechanisms of, 77
Endogenous ligands
hydrophilic ligands, interaction of, 203
ligands classification, 202–203, 203t
modes of intercellular signaling, 203–209, 204t
autocrine signaling, 208
endocrine signaling, 205
hormones, 205–208
juxtacrine signaling, 208
local signaling, 208–209
paracrine signaling, 208
Endothelium tissue
drug transport across, 83–85
Enterocytes, 93
Enterohepatic recirculation, 150
Enzymatic receptors, 218–219
Enzymes, 11
in drug metabolism, 157–158
classification of, 157t
specificity, 157–158
inducers, 176
induction, 176–177
inhibition, 18, 174–175
selectivity in, 241–242
inhibitors, 238–241
Enzyme induction, 284
Enzyme inhibition, 284
Enzyme–inhibitor–substrate (EIS) complex, 240

Epipodophyllotoxins, 271
Epithelial tissue
    cell junctions, 79–80
    drug transport across, 81–83
    structure of, *79*
    tight junctions role, 80–81
Erythromycin, 150–151
Escherichia coli, 319
Etanercept (Enbrel), 327
Ethanol, 151
Eutomer, 16
Excipients, 105
Excretion, 138–151, 283 (*see also* Drug excretion)
Exocytosis, 77–78
    illustration of, *78*
Expiration date, 114
Expired air, excretion by, 151
Extracellular fluid, 123

F

Facilitated diffusion, 74–75
Federal Food, Drug, and Cosmetic (FD&C)
        Act, 341
Fenestrated capillaries, 126
Fick's law of diffusion, 65, 90
5-fluorouracil (5FU), 238
Fluoxetine, 11
Flurbiprofen, 237
Flux, 65
Food and Drugs Act, 341
Food and Drug Administration (FDA), 321, 340–341
    centers, 341
    evolution of, 341–342
Food–drug interactions, 286
    administration with meals, 287
    alcohol, 287
    food ingredients, 287–288
    grapefruit juice, 287
Food ingredients, 287–288
Free fraction, 129
Free (unbound) drug, 184
Functional antagonists, 236–237
Functional membranes, 59
Functional proteome, 308
Fusion proteins, 328

G

Gap junctions, 80, 208
Gastric pH, alteration of, 281
Gene amplification, 302
Gene deletion, 302
Gene expression, 296
Genes, 295
Gene therapy, 316, 336–338, *337*
Genetic code, 295
Genetic engineering, 315
Genetic polymorphisms, 297–298, 302
Genetic variability, 177
Genetic variation and disease, 296
    linkage, 300–301

monogenic diseases, 299
polygenic diseases, 299–300
types
    genetic polymorphism, 297–298
    mutation, 296–297
Genetic variation and response to drugs, 301
    consequences of, 302
    drug-metabolizing enzymes, 302–304
    drug targets, 304–305
    transporters, 305
    pharmacogenetics, 301–302
    pharmacogenomics, 302
Genome sequencing, 308
Genotyping of infectious agents, 304
Germline mutation, 308
GFR (*see* Glomerular filtration rate (GFR))
GI motility, 281–282
GIP (*see* GPCR-interacting proteins (GIP))
Glomerular filtration, 140, 142
    barrier, 141–142
    of drugs, 144
    schematic diagram, *143*
Glomerular filtration rate (GFR), 142
Glucose-6-phosphate dehydrogenase (G6PD), 297
Glucuronidation, 165
    glucuronic acid, structure of, *165*
    phase II reactions, *166*
Glucuronides, 165
Glutathione conjugation, 167
Glutathione S-transferases (GST), 167
GLUT transporters, 73
Glycine, amino acid, *39*
Glycolipids, 64
Glycoproteins, 64
    illustration, *318*
    GPCR (*see* G protein-coupled receptors
        (GPCR))
    GPCR-interacting proteins (GIP), 222
    G protein-coupled receptors (GPCR), *217*,
        217–218
    Graded dose-response curves, 253–254
    potency, affinity, and efficacy, 253–254
Granulocytopenia, 17
Grapefruit juice, 287
Guanine nucleotide-binding protein, 218

H

Half-life, 191–192
    plasma concentration, 191t
Heart and cardiac output, 121
Heart disease, 299
Hemophilia, 299
Henderson–Hasselbalch equation, 33–34
Hepatic clearance, 171
Hepatic extraction ratio, 171
Hepatic first-pass metabolism, 173
Hereditary mutation, 308
Histamine receptors, 18, *19*
Hormones, 205–208
Human genome, 295–296

Human Genome Project, 308
Huntington's disease, 299
Hydrogen bonding, 45, 295
Hydrolysis, 164 (*see also* Drug metabolism)
  phase I, *164*
Hydronium ion, 27
Hydrophilic pores, 66
Hydrophobic effect, 46
Hydrophobic hormones, 206
Hydrophobic interaction, 54
3-hydroxy-3-methylglutaryl coenzyme, 305
Hyperresponsive receptor, 304
Hypothetical enantiomers, binding, *15*

I
Ibuprofen, 9, 237, 241
ICF (*see* Intracellular fluid (ICF))
Idiosyncrasy, 268
Idiosyncratic reactions, 256
  response, 268
Imipenem, 273
Imipramine, 53
Immediate hypersensitivity, 272 (*see also* Drug
  allergy)
Immediate-release products, 111
Immediaterelease systems, 111
Immunoglobins (Igs)
  constant, 323
  variable, 323
Immunological variability, 271
Incompatibilities, 281
Individualization of therapy, 273
  factors causing variability, *274*
Indomethacin, 27, 150
Insulin, 43–44
  overview of, *315*
Integral proteins, 63
Interindividual variability, 306
Interstitial fluid (ISF), 122, 184
Intestinal drug efflux, 97
Intestinal flora, 282
Intracellular fluid (ICF), 59, 184
Intracellular receptors, 219–221
  intracellular enzymes, 220–221
  transcriptional regulation receptors, 219–220
Intrinsic activity, 233–234
Intrinsic aqueous solubility, 46–47
Intrinsic dissolution rate constant, 108
Intrinsic resistance, 270
Intrinsic solubility, 47
Inulin clearance, 147
Inverse agonist, 227
Ion channel proteins, 10–11
Ion–dipole interaction, 45
Ionic and hydrophobic interactions, 13
Ionization, *20,* 20–21, *21*
Ion trapping, 71–72
Irreversible enzyme inhibitors, 240–241, *241*
ISF (*see* Interstitial fluid (ISF))
Isoelectric point, 38

J
Juxtacrine signaling, 208

K
Kefauver-Harris Drug Amendments, 341–342
Ketoprofen, 237
Kidneys
  excretion by, 138
    renal clearance, 146–149
    renal excretion, 144–146
    structure of, 139–140
    urine formation, 140–144
Kinetics of elimination, 190

L
β-Lactams, 272
Lacteal, 94
Lactobacillus acidophilus, 287
L-DOPA, structures of, *158*
Lead optimization process, 343
Ligands, 11
  concentration, 222
Ligand-receptor interactions, 210
Lipid bilayer, 61–62
  solutes and ions transportation, *66*
    cellular proteins, 62–64
    characteristics, 62
    phosphatidylcholine structure, *61*
    phospholipid structure of, *61–63*
Lipid solubility, 18
Lipophilic drugs elimination, 155, *156*
Lipophilicity and hydrophilicity, 19–20, 20t,
  67–68
Liposomes (*see* Vesicles)
Lithium, 151
Liver
  drug excretion by
    biliary excretion, 149–150
    enterohepatic recirculation, 150
  drug metabolism in, 169–172
    biliary secretion, 172
    blood circulation, *170*
    blood flow, 172
    hepatic clearance, 171
    hepatic extraction ratio, 171
    lobule diagram of, *170*
    metabolic efficiency, 171–172
    plasma protein binding, 172
    structure and function, 169–171
Local signaling, 208–209
Logarithm scales, 248
Lymph, 123–124
Lymphatic vessels, 123
Lyophilization technology, 327–328

M
Macromolecular drugs, 116
Marker proteins, 63
Maximum safe concentration (MSC), 195
MDR1 (*see ABCB1* gene)

MDR transporter (*see* Multidrug resistance transporter (MDR transporter))
MEC (*see* Minimum effective concentration (MEC))
Median effective concentration, 248
Median toxic dose, 257
Membrane proteins, 63
6-mercaptopurine (6MP), 238
Metabolic poison, 75
Metabolic rate constant, 159
Metabolites
    in drug metabolism, 158–159
Methylation, 168, *169*
Metronidazole, 150
Micelle formation, 54
    organization of, *54*
Michaelis constant, 302
Michaelis-Menten constant, 74
Michaelis-Menten kinetics, 159
Microbiological stability, 115
Micronization, 111
Microsomal enzymes, 161
Microsomal oxidation, 161
Microsomes, 161
Migraine, 299
Minimum effective concentration (MEC), 195
Minimum toxic concentration (MTC), 195
Mitomycin C, 271
Molecular farming, 320
Monoamine oxidase (MAO), 287–288
Monobactams, 273
Monoclonal antibodies, 323–325
Monogenic disorders, 299–299t, 338
    and polygenic disorders, *301*
Morphine, 150–151
Motrin®, 9
MRP (*see* Multidrug resistance protein (MRP))
MTC (*see* Minimum toxic concentration (MTC))
Multidrug efflux, 76–77
    illustration of, *76*
Multidrug resistance (MDR), 270–271
Multidrug resistance protein (MRP), 76
Multidrug resistance transporter (MDR transporter), 76
Multiple dosing, 196
Multiple transport pathways, 85
Mutant allele, 299
Mutation causing cystic fibrosis (CF), *297*

N

N-Acetyltransferases (NAT), 168
Nafcillin, 272
Naproxen, 241
Nephron, *141*
Neuropeptides, 206
Neurotransmitters (*see* Local signaling)
New drug application (NDA)
    drug approval, 348–349
    FDA advisory Committees, 347–348
    postmarketing surveillance, 349–350
    review and approval, 347
    supplemental, 351

Noncatalytic and catalytic receptors, 210–211
Noncompetitive antagonist, 236, *236,* 249, 251
Noncompetitive enzyme inhibitors, 240
    rate of enzymatic reaction, effect, *240*
Noncompetitive inhibition, 175–176
Non-CYP oxidation, 163
Nonelectrolytes, 68
Nonpolar solvents, 46
Nonsteroidal anti-inflammatory drugs (NSAID), 237, 241
Nonsynonymous SNP, 298
Nonviral/synthetic vectors, 338
Norvir®, 44

O

Oligonucleotides, antisense, 335–336
Oral administration, 92–98
    drug absorption, 95–98
    gastrointestinal tract, 92–93
    large intestine, 94–95
    small intestine, 93–94
    stomach, 93
Oral drug absorption, 95–98
    intestinal drug efflux, 97
    passive transcellular diffusion, 95–96
    transcytosis, 97
Oral formulations, *194*
Orphan Drug Act, 342

P

PABA (*see* Para-aminobenzoic acid (PABA))
p-Aminohippuric acid clearance, 148
Panitumumab, 326
Para-aminobenzoic acid (PABA), 18
Paracrine signaling, 208
Parkinson's disease, 238
Partial agonist, 227
Partition coefficient, *50,* 50–53
    importance of, 53
    weak acid and weak base, *52–53*
Passive diffusion, 65–72
    equilibrium conditions for, *71*
    hydrophilic pores, 66
    initial and equilibrium conditions, *69–70*
    ion trapping, 71–72
    lipid bilayer, 66
    lipophilicity and hydrophilicity, 67–68
    nonelectrolytes, 68
    pH and pK_a influence, 68–71
    rate of, 66–67
    schematic representation of, *67*
    weak acid and weak base, *69*
Passive transcellular diffusion, 81–82, 95–96
PEGylation process, *334*
Penetration enhancer, 101
Penicillamine, 17
Penicillin allergy, 272–273
Penicillin G, 272
Penicillin V, 272
Perfusioncontrolled distribution, 127

Peritubular capillaries, 140
Permeability coefficient, 82
Permeation rate constant, 91
P-glycoprotein (P-gp), 64
    expression of, 271
pH
    buffered solution, 34
        biological buffers, 34–35
        buffer capacity, 34
    concept, 28
    drug ionization, 33–37
    Henderson–Hasselbalch equation, 33–34
    ionization profiles, 35–37
        degree of ionization, 36t
    medium, 110
    pharmaceutical systems, 28
    and pK_a influence, 68–71
    solubility profiles, 48
Pharmaceutical drug interactions, 279
    adsorption, 280–281
    chelation, 279–280
    gastric pH, alteration of, 281
    incompatibilities, 281
Pharmaceutical interactions, 279
Pharmaceutical toxicology, 1
Pharmaceutics, 1
Pharmacodynamic drug interactions, 286
    additive, 286
    antagonism, 286
    synergistic, 286
Pharmacodynamic interactions, 279
Pharmacodynamics, 1
Pharmacodynamic variability, 267–271
    circadian rhythms, 268–269
    drug resistance, 270–271
    drug tolerance, 269–270
    idiosyncrasy, 268
    sex-related differences, 267–268
Pharmacogenetics, 265
    genetic variation and response to drugs, 301–302
Pharmacogenomics, 1, 294
    benefits of, 306
    clinical applications, 305–307
    drug, 5
    genetic review
        chromosomes, 294–295
        gene expression, 296
        genes, 295
        human genome, 295–296
    genetic variation and response to drugs, 302
    promise of, 309
    proteomics, 308–309
Pharmacokinetic compartments, 185, *185*
Pharmacokinetic drug interactions, 281
    absorption, 281–282
    biotransformation, 283–285
    distribution, 282–283
    excretion, 283
Pharmacokinetics, 1
    interactions, 279
    and pharmacodynamics, 183, *184*

PK–PD correlation, *194*
    relationship, 193–195
Pharmacokinetic variability, 264–267
    age, 265–266
    body weight and composition, 265
    elderly, 266
    health and disease, 267
    infants and children, 266
    interindividual effect, *264*
    pregnancy and lactation, 267
    sex-related differences, 266–267
Pharmacological therapeutic index, 257
Pharmacology, 1
Pharmacophore, *13*
    analog, 12
    for drugs, *13*
Pharmacotherapeutics, 4
    drug, 4
Phase II reactions (*see* Conjugation reactions)
Phase I oxidation, 161
Phase I/phase II reactions, 161–169
Phenergan® (*see* Promethazine)
Phenytoin, 151
Phosphate buffer system, 35
Phospholipid bilayer
    with membrane proteins, *63*
Physical stability, 116
Physicochemical complementarity, 12–14
    alpha- and beta-adrenergic receptors, *13*
    ionic and hydrophobic interactions, 13
    pharmacophore for drugs, *13*
    protein–ligand binding, 13
    regions role in binding, 13–14
    Pichia pastoris, 320
pK_a *values*
    amphoteric and polyprotic drugs, 39t
PK–PD correlation, *194*
Plasma level curves, 185, *186*
    after multiple dosing, *196*
    after oral administration, *195*
    oral formulations, *194*
    pharmacokinetic features of
        absolute bioavailability, 193
        absorption rate and extent, 186–189
        area under curve, 192–193
        half-life, 191–192
        rate of distribution, 189–190
        rate of elimination, 190–191
        route and delivery system, 193
    pharmacological features of, 195–196
Plasma protein binding, 172
Plasma renin, 268
Polyclonal antibodies, 323
Polygenic disorder, 299–300
    and monogenic disorders, *301*
Polymorphisms, 297
Polyprotic acids and bases, 39
Potentiation, 286
Presystemic metabolism, 172–173
Prodrugs, 158–159
Promethazine, 53

Proteins, 9–11
  approaches, *317*
  denaturation, *328*, 329
  drug–protein interactions, 9
  kinase receptor, 219
  levels, *318*
  regulatory protein targets, *10*, 10–11, *11*
  structure of, 9–10, 316–317
  therapeutic protein drugs, 316, *317*
Protein drugs, PEGylated, 335t
Protein-ligand interactions, 11, *11*
  binding, 13
  Protein synthesis, *336*
Proteome, 308
Proteomics, 308
Prozac® (*see* Fluoxetine)

Q
QSAR (*see* Quantitative SAR (QSAR))
Quantal dose–response curves, 254–255
  effective and toxic dose–response, *258*
  frequency of response, *255*
Quantitative SAR (QSAR), 21–22, *22*

R
Racemate, 16–17
Random screening, 3
Rapid acetylators, 303
Rational drug design, 3
Reabsorption, 142–143
  schematic diagram, *143*
Receptors
  blockade, 18, *19*
  density, 222
  downregulation, 222, 269
  dynamism, 222
  ligand-receptor interactions, 210
    allosteric modulation, 222
    ligand concentration, 222
    receptor density, 222
  noncatalytic and catalytic receptors, 210–211
  proteins, 10, 63
  selectivity, 18, *19*
  structure and classification
    cell-surface receptors, 215–219
    intracellular receptors, 219–221
  subtypes, 211–215
  upregulation, 222, 269–270
recombinant DNA (rDNA) technology, *See also*
    Genetic engineering
Reduction, 163–164
  phase I, *164*
Regulatory protein targets, *10*, 10–11, *11*
Regulatory regions, 295
Renal clearance, 146–149
  concept of, *146*
  creatinine, 147–148
  drugs, 148–149
  of inulin, 147
  p-aminohippuric acid, 148
  physicochemical properties and, 147

  rate *versus* extent, 149
Renal excretion, 144–146, 283
  rate of, 145–146
Replacement therapy, 316
Reversible enzyme inhibitors, 239
Rifampicin, 150
Ritonavir, 44
Rituximab, 326
Rofecoxib, 241

S
S-adenosylmethionine (SAM) (*see* Methylation)
Saccharomyces cerevisiae, 320
Salicylates, 151
Saliva, excretion by, 151
Salts of
  weak acids and bases, 32–33
SAR (*see* Structure-activity relationship (SAR))
Second messengers, 212
Selectivity and toxicity, 255
Semipolar solvents, 46
Shelf life, 114
Sickle cell anemia, 299
Signal transduction, 212–215
  features, 213, *214*
  representation of, *212*
  termination of, *215*
Single-nucleotide polymorphism (SNP), 298
Sinusoids, 169–171
Site-specific drug delivery, 113
Slow acetylators, 303
Slow metabolizer, 302
SNP (*see* Single-nucleotide polymorphism (SNP))
Solid state structure, 109–110
Solubility, 109
  in absorption rate, role of, 110
  principles, 42–43
    solute molecular size, 43
  product, 48–50
  solid-state structure, 43–44
    crystalline and amorphous drugs, 43–44
    polymorphs, 44
  solvent
    polarity, 44–46
    water, 46–50
Soluble proteins, 62–63
Solvent polarity, 44–46
  functional groups, order of, *45*
Spare receptors, 234–235
Specificity of actions, 209–210
Stagnant layer, 107
Stereoisomers, 14
Steric complementarity, 14–17
  chiral center, *15*, 15–16
  enantiomers and chirality, 14–15
  geometric isomers, 16, *16*
  hypothetical enantiomers, binding, *15*
  racemic mixtures, 16–17
  stereoisomers, 14
Steroid hormones, 205
  structures of, 206

Strong acids and bases, 28–29
Structure-activity relationship (SAR), 21–22
    antipsychotic chlorpromazine, *21*
    quantitative SAR, 21, 22
Sulfacetamide, 18
Sulfanilamide, 151
Sulfapyridine, 151
Sulfation, 165–166
    sulfate conjugation process, *166*
Surface tension effect, 54
Susceptibility genes, 300
Sweat, excretion by, 151
Synapse, 208
Synergistic interaction, 286
Systemic administration, 89

T
Targeted drug delivery, 113–114
Targetor, 114
Taxanes, 271
Teratogenicity, 267
Therapeutic index, 256–258
    effective and toxic dose–response, *258*
    Therapeutic proteins, 316
Therapeutic range, 196
Therapeutic ratio, 257
Therapeutic variability
    drug allergy, 272–273
    immunological variability, 271
    individualization of, 273–274
    pharmacodynamic variability, 267–271
    pharmacokinetic variability, 264–267
    types of, 263–264
Therapeutic window, 196, 264, 269
Thyroid hormones, 206
Tight junctions, *80*, 80–81
Tissue, 78–85
    endothelium
        drug transport across, 83–85
    epithelial, 78–79
        cell junctions, 79–80
        drug transport across, 81–83
        structure of, *79*
        tight junctions role, 80–81
Tofranil® (*see* Imipramine)
Tolcapone, 238
Tolerance, 269
Topotecan, 271
Total body clearance, 174
Total body water, 129
Transcription, 295
Transcytosis, 82, 97
    illustration of, *81*
Transgenic animal, development process, 321t
Transgenic plant, 322
Translation, 295
Transporters, 11, 73–74, *75*
Transport proteins, 63
Trastuzumab, 326
Tubular reabsorption, 142–143
    of drugs, 144–145

Tubular secretion, 143–144, 283
    of drugs, 145
Tyramine, 287

U
UDP glucuronosyl transferases (UGT), 165
UGT (*see* UDP glucuronosyl transferases (UGT))
Unbuffered solutions, ionization in, 37–38
Uniporters, 74
Urinary pH, 283
Urine formation, 140–144

V
van der Waals forces, 45–46, 295
Vascular endothelial growth factor (VEGF), 202
Vector groups, 12
VEGF (*see* Vascular endothelial growth factor
        (VEGF))
Vesicles, 54
Vesicular transport processes, 77
Vinca alkaloids, 271
Voltage-dependent ion channel, 217
Volume of drug distribution, 130–133
    binding and accumulation, 133
    measuring, 131–132
    protein binding and, 132–133
Vulnerable groups, 12

W
Warfarin, 150, 237
Water as solvent, 27–28, 45–46
    pH concept, 28
    pH of pharmaceutical systems, 28
Water solubility, 46–50
    drug salts, 48–50
    intrinsic aqueous solubility, 46–47
    solubility profiles, 48
    weak acids and bases, 47–48
Weak acids and bases, 29–32
    conjugate acid–base pairs, relative strengths,
        32t
    functional groups, *29*
    ionization of, 30–31
    pK_a ranges, 32t
    pK_a value, 31–32, 32t
    quaternary ammonium salts structure, *30*
    salts of, 32–33
    solubility of, 47–48
    strength of, 31
Weak electrolytes, 27
Wetting agents, 54

X
Xenobiotics, 156
    detoxification, 156
X-linked diseases, 299
X-linked hypophosphatemia, 299

Z
Zwitterionic ampholyte, *39*
Zyrtec® (*see* Cetirizine, antiallergy drug)